Advance praise for *Bread + Medicine*

"I was quite unaware of the degree of suffering, tragedy, and heroism playing out in Russia after the Great War—six million people succumbed in that 1921 famine. Were it not for six American physicians working with their Russian counterparts to feed and vaccinate, that number would have been far greater. Patenaude and Stevenson's beautifully researched tale is compelling reading."

—*Abraham Verghese, MD, author of* Cutting for Stone

"The response of Herbert Hoover's American Relief Administration to the 1921 famine in Soviet Russia is a story of generosity and tenacity. America's aid workers understood that fighting starvation required a combination of food and medical relief. This book, strikingly illustrated with photographs, posters, and documents, focuses on the unsung yet vitally important battle against the ravages of disease and malnutrition in the midst of famine."

—*Mary Cox, assistant professor of international relations, Central European University*

"A beautifully compelling and deeply inspiring story of altruism and ingenuity at its best; this tour de force account of the origins of large-scale humanitarian aid through Herbert Hoover's nongovernmental American Relief Administration, simultaneously addressing hunger and associated diseases in conflict-torn Soviet Russia, is essential reading for anyone interested in the human face of public health, medicine, and international relations."

—*Gary Darmstadt, MD, MS, associate dean for maternal and child health and professor of pediatrics at the Stanford University School of Medicine*

bread + medicine

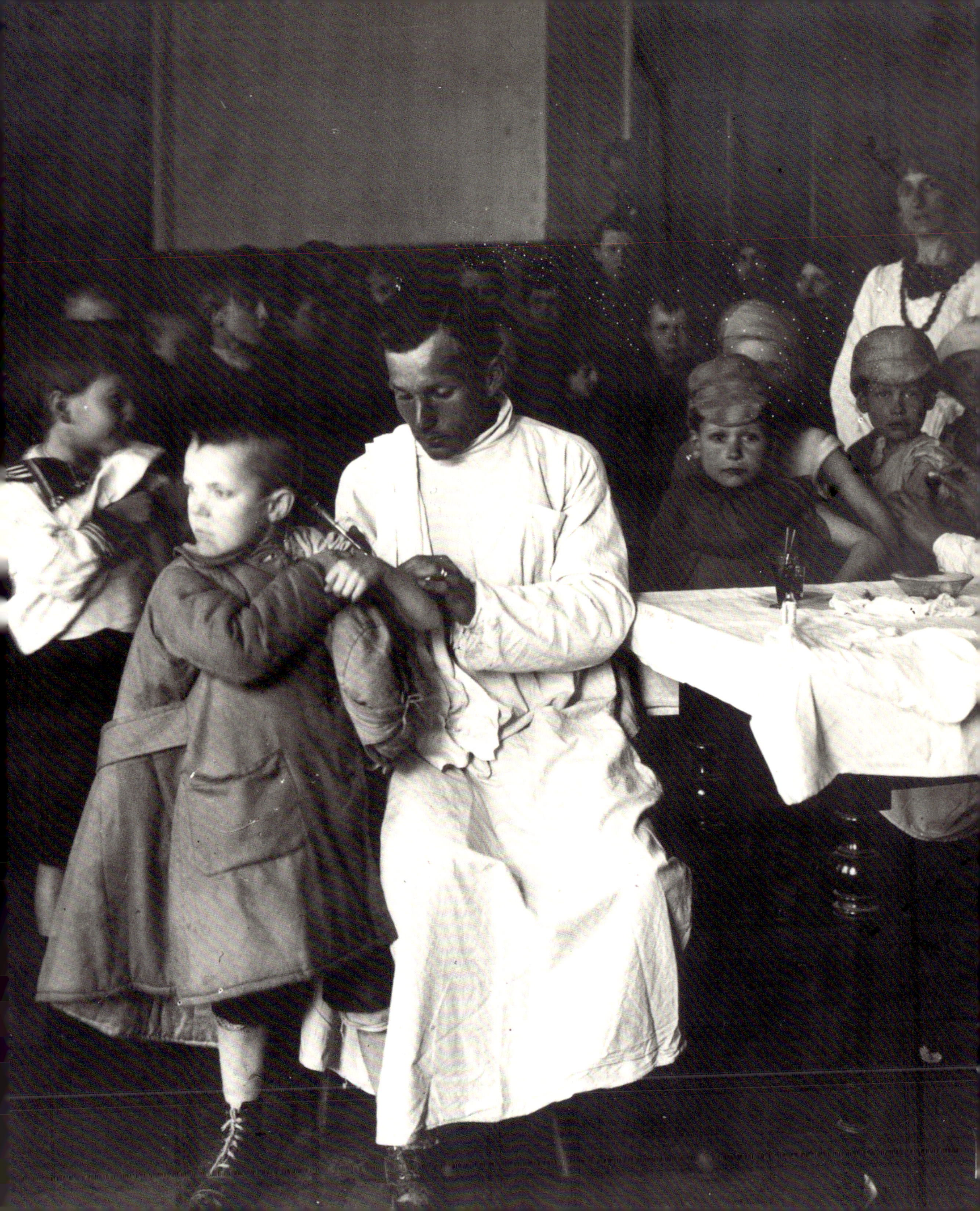

bread + medicine

American Famine Relief in Soviet Russia, 1921–1923

BERTRAND M. PATENAUDE

JOAN NABSETH STEVENSON

HOOVER INSTITUTION PRESS
Stanford University
Stanford, California

hoover.org

Hoover Institution Press Publication No. 731

Hoover Institution at Leland Stanford Junior University,
Stanford, California 94305-6003

First printing 2023
29 28 27 26 25 24 23 7 6 5 4 3 2 1

Manufactured in Canada
Printed on acid-free, archival-quality paper

Design and composition by Yvonne Tsang

Library of Congress Cataloging-in-Publication Data
Names: Patenaude, Bertrand M., 1956- author. | Stevenson, Joan Nabseth, author.
Title: Bread + medicine : American famine relief in Soviet Russia 1921-1923 / Bertrand M. Patenaude, Joan Nabseth Stevenson.
Other titles: Bread and medicine | Hoover Institution Press publication ; 731.
Description: Stanford, California : Hoover Institution Press, Stanford University, [2023] | Series: Hoover Institution Press publication ; no. 731 | Includes bibliographical references and index. | Summary: "Recounts how medical intervention, including a large-scale vaccination drive, by the American Relief Administration saved millions of lives in Soviet Russia during the famine of 1921-23"— Provided by publisher.
Identifiers: LCCN 2022059569 (print) | LCCN 2022059570 (ebook) | ISBN 9780817925758 (paperback) | ISBN 9780817925789 (PDF)
Subjects: LCSH: American Relief Administration—History—20th century. | Medical assistance, American—Russia (Federation)—History—20th century. | Vaccination—Russia (Federation)—History—20th century. | Soviet Union—History—Famine, 1921-1922.
Classification: LCC DK266.5 P24 2023 (print) | LCC DK266.5 (ebook) | DDC 614.4/70947—dc23/eng/20221214
LC record available at https://lccn.loc.gov/2022059569
LC ebook record available at https://lccn.loc.gov/2022059570

page ii: inoculation of children with the tetra vaccine at the ARA kitchen on Gagarin Street in Petrograd, spring 1922 (detail; full image shown on page 61)

page vi: ARA kitchen at the Obukhovskaya hospital in Petrograd, ca. 1922 (detail; full image shown on page 111)

page xiv: ARA pharmacy, Saratov, ca. 1922 (detail; full image shown on page 83)

“Trying to kill people may sound more
exciting than trying to keep them alive,
but don’t you ever believe it’s so.”

—*George McClintock, Samara on the Volga, 1922*

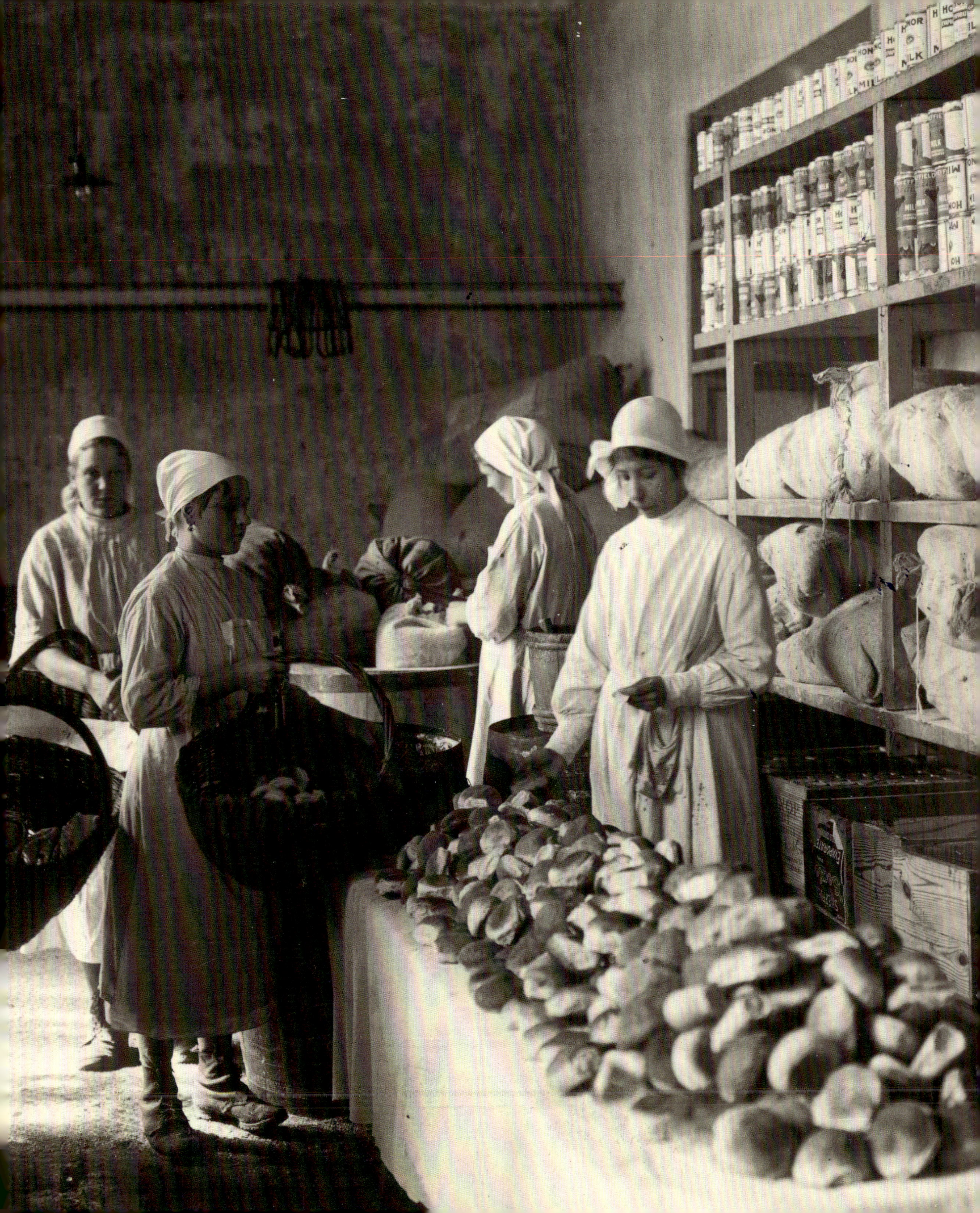
MILK

Contents

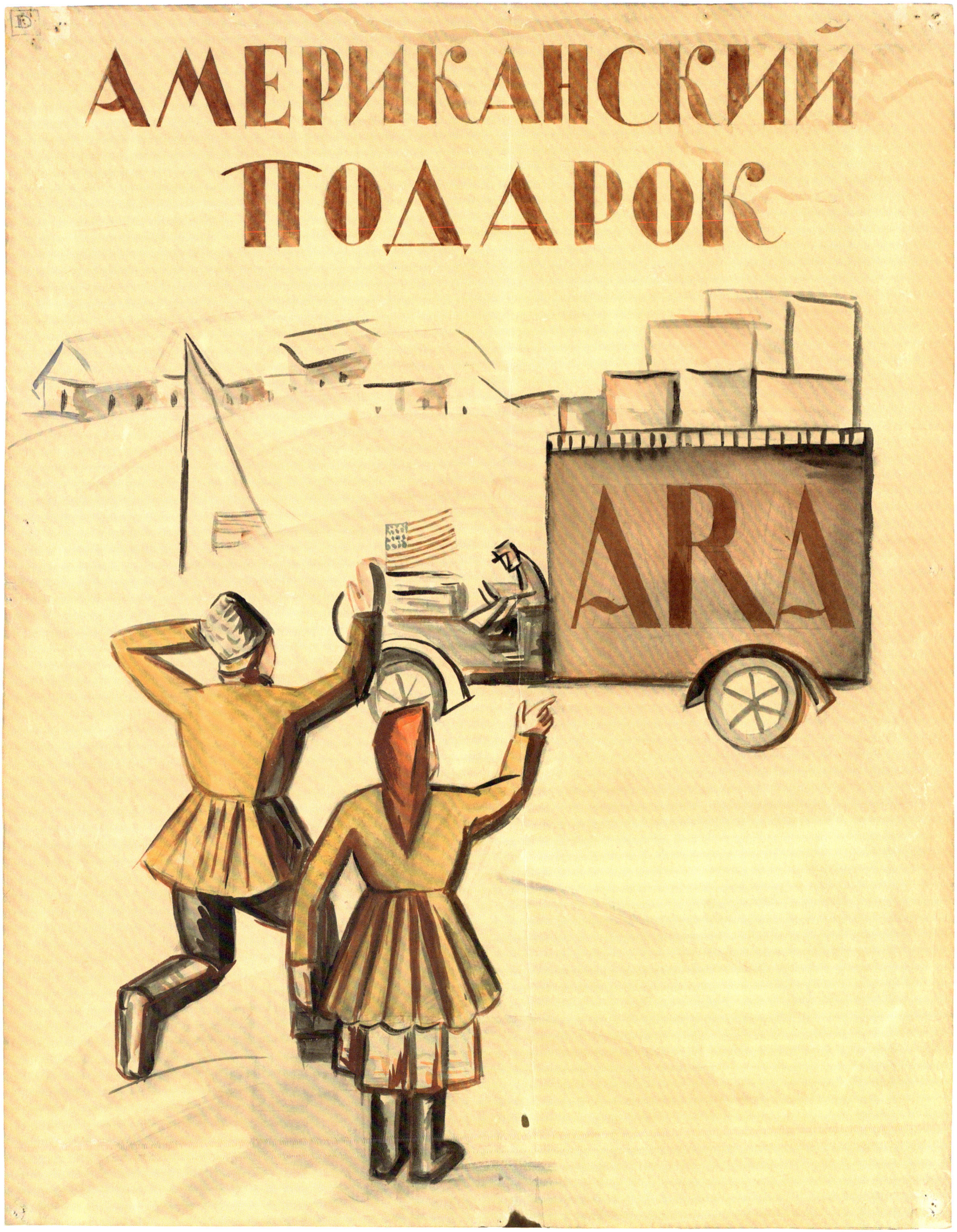
АМЕРИКАНСКИЙ
ПОДАРОК
ARA

Foreword

Bread + Medicine tells a story that will captivate infectious-disease specialists and students of humanitarian intervention. The famine that descended on Soviet Russia in 1921 and eventually claimed more than six million lives would have had far worse consequences but for the large-scale delivery of American food and medical relief, which included an aggressive campaign to combat the spread of contagious disease. Epidemic outbreaks of cholera, typhoid, and typhus threatened, fueled by an enormous wave of refugees in flight from famine. At the same time, hunger-related deficiency diseases took a steep toll, especially among children.

Beginning in the fall of 1921, American physicians—thirty altogether—raced to organize the delivery of medicines and medical supplies and equipment to meet the emergency they called a "medical famine." They were truly "doctors without borders" when it came to the feelings of solidarity they shared with the local doctors and other medical workers, who were their essential collaborators in the medical campaign. The ranks of Russian physicians had diminished as a result of wartime deaths and emigration, as well as their high mortality rates during the epidemics of the previous several years. Those who survived were overworked and underfed, yet they fought on heroically, earning the admiration of their American colleagues, who praised their fortitude and courage. An American Red Cross doctor visiting Soviet Russia in the fall of 1922 wrote: "When I see what the doctors of this country have done, are doing now and are going to try to do this winter I am proud to be a doctor." Physicians reading this narrative a century later will share that sense of pride.

The relief story offers a fascinating window into the state of medical knowledge at that time, as well as the limited tools available to medical workers to treat disease, two decades before the arrival of antibiotics. Prevention was the principal means used to combat the spread of epidemic disease, including a massive vaccination campaign in the summer of 1922 that immunized more than five million people against cholera, typhoid, paratyphoid A and B, and smallpox with vaccines supplied by the Pasteur Institute in Paris. There was of course no vaccine for typhus, which posed the major threat in the winter and spring of 1922. The Americans worked to prevent its spread within Soviet Russia and westward into Europe through a campaign of hygiene and disinfection to eradicate lice. The human body louse had been identified as the vector for epidemic typhus only a dozen years earlier, in 1909. The image of the louse struck fear in the American relief workers, who felt especially vulnerable when forced to share a railway compartment with lice-infested fellow travelers. Of the three hundred Americans who served in the two-year relief mission, only eight contracted typhus, with just one fatality.

Unidentified artist (Russian), Американский подарок [American gift], gouache and ink on paper, 1922.
Poster Collection RU/SU 1448

Reading this book, I kept thinking about the globalization of disease over the past century, which now spreads rapidly by commercial air travel rather than by rail. COVID-19 and Ebola are recent cases in point, as is monkeypox, which has been present in Africa for decades but is only now spreading globally through air travel. A story such as this one, involving a vaccination campaign and the imposition and enforcement of measures of sanitation and hygiene, is bound to remind readers of the struggle for the adoption of PPE, vaccines, and other public health measures to prevent the spread of COVID-19. Even without those vivid parallels, this history is an absolute page-turner for any infectious-disease physician, and for any reader interested in untold stories of humanitarian collaboration across borders.

Michele Barry, MD FACP FASTMH
Drs. Ben and A. Jess Shenson Professor of Medicine and Tropical Diseases
Director of the Center for Innovation in Global Health
Senior Associate Dean for Global Health
Stanford University

Director's Foreword

The Great Famine in Soviet Russia, and the American relief mission it prompted, have a special significance for the Hoover Institution Library & Archives, founded by Herbert Hoover in 1919 while he was in Paris among the peacemakers at the end of the First World War. The Soviet famine was the unfortunate occasion for the remarkable collecting achievement of Stanford professor and Hoover curator Frank Golder, who signed on with the American Relief Administration (ARA) mission and who, over the course of nearly two years, laid the foundation for Hoover's unparalleled Russia collections. Golder was born near Odessa in tsarist Russia before emigrating to Germany and then the United States. He had made research trips to Russia before and during the Revolution. In returning with the ARA in 1921, he drew on his contacts with archivists, scholars, librarians, and cultural officials to acquire an enormous quantity of documentary and other material on late Imperial Russia, the 1917 Revolution, and the nascent Soviet state for the Hoover Library, including rare books, periodicals, personal manuscripts, government documents, posters, and original artworks. Collecting documentary materials in areas of conflict in order to preserve records of enduring historical value is a mission that continues today at Hoover.

The relief mission itself bequeathed to the Hoover Institution the massive ARA collections, both for Soviet Russia and for the country missions in Central and Eastern Europe that began in 1919, when the ARA was established. To appreciate the value of these archival records, one must understand the vast scope of the record keeping undertaken by Hoover's humanitarian organizations, which prepared detailed reports on political, economic, and social conditions and forces in each country where they operated. It was the comprehensive character of these first archival collections that would influence the increasingly ambitious reach of the Hoover Institution's collecting in the years ahead. What began as a repository for documentation on the causes and course of the First World War evolved into a special-collections research center for the study of war, revolution, and peace.

So voluminous were these ARA files that Harold Fisher, head of the ARA's Historical Division, was brought from New York to Stanford in 1924 to serve as curator of the ARA archive. Fisher went on to author the first history of the ARA mission, *The Famine in Soviet Russia* (1927), and eventually became director of the Hoover Institution. Today, researchers continue to use these files to examine the causes and consequences of war, famine, and revolutionary change. An indication of the extraordinary breadth of the ARA papers is the fact that only now has the story of the ARA's tremendous medical relief program in Soviet Russia been brought to light in the exhibition *Bread + Medicine* and in this companion publication. The documentation on every aspect of the medical mission is sweeping, including an extraordinary visual record, with many hundreds of photographs revealing the extent and effects of the "medical famine" and the American effort to address the crisis, including a major vaccination campaign to combat infectious disease. It is a story that resonates a century later as we experience the impacts of the COVID-19 pandemic.

Herbert Hoover's career as humanitarian began with the wartime relief in Belgium. In September 1914, German-occupied Belgium was threatened with famine. Hoover, at the time a businessman living in London, agreed to take the helm of a neutral commission to deliver food supplies. Hoover's Commission for Relief in Belgium (CRB) secured approval from Great Britain to let food relief pass through its naval blockade, while the German government promised not to requisition the food once it arrived in Belgium. The CRB took on the responsibility of feeding the entire Belgian nation of 7.3 million, and operations were later expanded to encompass an additional two million residents in occupied northern France.

The extensive records of the CRB, which arrived on the Stanford campus in three shipments in the early 1920s, were referred to in early descriptions of the Library & Archives as the "nucleus" of the Hoover Library. Together, the CRB and ARA records were the library's founding collections. As it happens, the CRB and the ARA were also among the first-ever nongovernmental organizations, or NGOs. In fact, the CRB would serve as an inspiration and prototype for the Oxford Committee for Famine Relief—Oxfam—formed in October 1942 to address the famine in German-occupied Greece during the Second World War. Today, humanitarian relief agencies are often criticized for showing up at the scene of a crisis, exploiting the occasion for fundraising purposes, then moving on to the next disaster—the so-called "crisis caravan." Herbert Hoover's humanitarian endeavors were dedicated to finding lasting solutions. The importation of wheat seed, in addition to lifesaving food, into Soviet Russia in the spring of 1922 is a prime example. And always Hoover relief sought to inculcate a sense of self-reliance. As the head of the American medical program in Soviet Russia, Colonel Henry Beeuwkes, observed in 1922: "It is part of the gospel of the A.R.A. in Europe to teach people to help themselves and as soon as possible become independent of outside aid."

While the country that the ARA came to assist in 1921 was popularly known as "Soviet Russia," it included the nominally independent republic of Ukraine, whose people also received American food and medical relief. Readers will recognize the names of cities such as Kiev (Kyiv), Kharkov (Kharkiv), and Odessa (Odesa) from recent news coverage. A century ago, the residents of these places were contending with a catastrophic famine that resulted from the disruptions of the world war, revolution, and civil war. Today they are caught in a crisis brought on by Russia's military invasion, one that has set refugees on the move and given rise to calls for humanitarian intervention. The impact of Russia's war against Ukraine reminds us that it was humanitarianism that laid the foundation for the Hoover Institution. It should also serve as a reminder of the vital importance of *peace* in the Hoover triad of war, revolution, and peace. The search for peace, for a way to prevent a recurrence of total war and the upheaval and suffering that inevitably spring from it, was at the heart of Herbert Hoover's enterprise.

Eric Wakin

Director, Hoover Institution Library & Archives

Deputy Director, Hoover Institution

Acknowledgments

We wish to thank Eric Wakin, director of the Hoover Institution Library & Archives, for his support of the project, both the exhibition *Bread + Medicine: Saving Lives in a Time of Famine* and this companion publication. We owe a special debt of gratitude to Samira Bozorgi and her colleagues Marissa Rhee and Kiera Peacock on the Hoover exhibitions team, who have been a steady source of creative ideas and inspiration in helping us tell the story of America's medical relief campaign. At the Hoover Archives reading room, Chris Marino and David Sun generously accommodated our many requests for documents and last-minute appointments. The expert and expedited service of Hoover's preservation, description, and digitization teams has enabled us to access and present high-quality images—photographs, posters, and documents—from the American Relief Administration papers and associated collections. Thanks to our student researchers Danielle Healy, Sorcha Whitley, and Daniel Wu. At the Hoover Institution Press, Barbara Arellano, Danica Michels Hodge, Alison Law, and John O'Rourke patiently guided us along through every stage of the publication process. Thanks to our copy editor, Beverly Michaels, and our book designer, Yvonne Tsang. We are grateful for the assistance of Olga Ovcharskaia, Bess Rattray, David Stevenson, and Craig Wright.

We also wish to thank those who contributed to the preparation of the exhibition *Bread + Medicine*, guest curated by Bertrand Patenaude: Samira Bozorgi, Laurent Cruveillier, Irena Czernichowska, Douglas Emery, Simon Ertz, James Fayne, Rayan Ghazal, Kurtis Kekkonen, Jessica Lemieux, Lisa Nguyen, Talia Olshefsky, K. Sarah Ostrach, Kiera Peacock, Liz Phillips, Marissa Rhee, Mireya Salinas, Anatol Shmelev, Emma Stanford, Colin Stinson, Maryann Villavert, and Spencer Zidarich. Special thanks go to the director of the Hoover Institution, Condoleezza Rice, and to the many supporters of the Library & Archives.

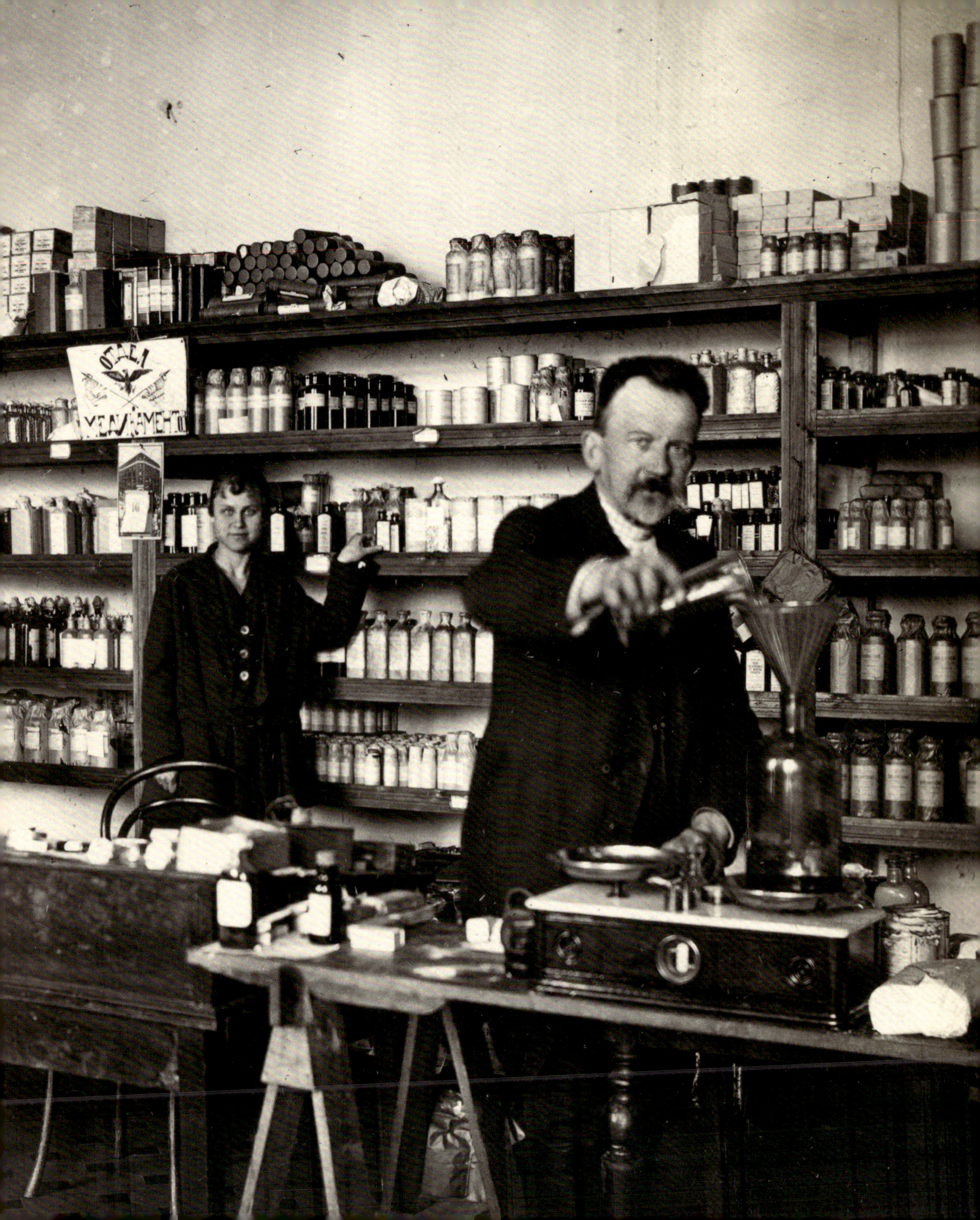
ОТДЕЛ
МЕДИКАМЕНТО

Note to the Reader

The names of places and things can change over the course of history. For this publication, the spellings and terminology in use during the early 1920s have been maintained to reflect the primary-source documents as well as the culture and context in which the material was created.

Unless otherwise noted in the caption, all photographs, posters, documents, and other visual materials shown in this publication are from the American Relief Administration (ARA) Russian operational records, Hoover Institution Library & Archives.

Many photographs in the ARA collection contain annotations, written directly on the photo, providing location information and identifying individuals pictured. These were made by staff at ARA headquarters in New York at the time the developed film arrived there, in 1922 and 1923.

bread + medicine

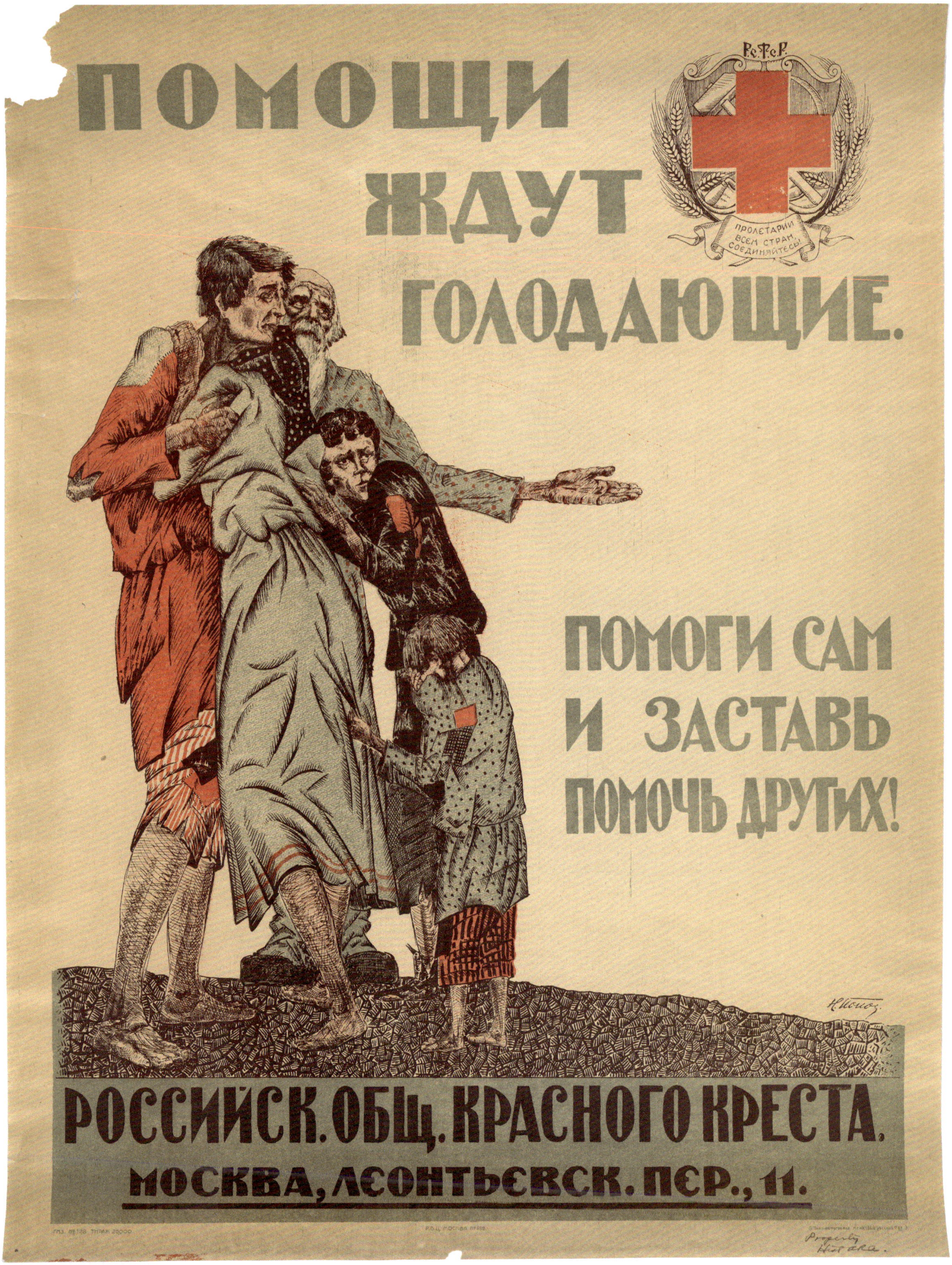

ПОМОЩИ
ЖДУТ
ГОЛОДАЮЩИЕ.
Р.С.Ф.С.Р.
ПРОЛЕТАРИИ ВСЕХ СТРАН, СОЕДИНЯЙТЕСЬ!
ПОМОГИ САМ
И ЗАСТАВЬ
ПОМОЧЬ ДРУГИХ!
РОССИЙСК. ОБЩ. КРАСНОГО КРЕСТА.
МОСКВА, ЛЕОНТЬЕВСК. ПЕР., 11.
Property
Hoover

CHAPTER 1

"Give Bread and Medicine"

"Out of the darkness came a friendly hand bringing help and human sympathy from the world unshaken by the storm."

—*Harold Fisher,* The Famine in Soviet Russia *(1927)*

In July 1921, newspaper reports told of a catastrophic famine in Soviet Russia. Russian writer Maxim Gorky issued a call "To All Honest People" for help. He announced that a crop failure caused by drought was threatening the lives of millions of Soviet citizens. He invoked the common cultural heritage of Russia and the West. "Gloomy days have come to the country of Tolstoy, Dostoevsky, Mendeleyev, Pavlov, Mussorgsky, Glinka, and other world-prized men," he wrote. In other words, forget for the moment the names of Bolshevik leaders Lenin and Trotsky: "I ask all honest European and American people for prompt aid to the Russian people. Give bread and medicine."

Gorky's appeal was read by millions in the West, but only one person was in a position to answer the call: Herbert Hoover. Hoover was chairman of the American Relief Administration (ARA), founded in 1919, and was now also serving as Secretary of Commerce in the administration of President Warren G. Harding. Hoover had achieved worldwide fame as the organizer and administrator of large-scale humanitarian relief operations, first in German-occupied Belgium during the Great War, and then as food administrator for the Allies after the armistice of November 1918. In 1919 and 1920, Hoover's ARA successfully executed a massive food relief campaign across Central and Eastern Europe, first as a US government relief agency, and then, after the signing of the Versailles treaty in June 1919, as a private relief organization. Altogether, from 1919 to 1921, this private ARA delivered food worth over $150 million (more than $2 billion in today's dollars) to children in fifteen countries in Central, Eastern, and Southeastern Europe and the Near East, functioning either independently or in conjunction with other private relief organizations.

The famine in Soviet Russia was caused by the disruptions of the First World War, the Russian Revolution of 1917 and the ensuing civil war, and also by the Soviet government's draconian economic policies, not least the forcible requisitioning of grain. Drought triggered successive crop failures in 1920 and 1921. As many as twenty-five million Soviet citizens, of an estimated total population of 138 million, were threatened with starvation and hunger-related disease, most of them living in and beyond the Volga River valley and in southern Ukraine. Unable to cope with the disaster on its own, the Soviet government was compelled to seek foreign assistance, and thus it encouraged Gorky's appeal.

Russian Red Cross poster, Помощи ждут голодающие. Помоги сам и заставь помочь других! [The starving await help. Do your part and get others to help!], 1921.
Poster Collection RU/SU 1350

Founded in 1867, when Imperial Russia ratified the Geneva Convention, the Russian Red Cross had evolved into one of the foremost charities in tsarist Russia by the time of the First World War. The Revolution of 1917 led to its unraveling as members of the original organization set up headquarters in Paris and a new Soviet-sponsored Red Cross Society was established. On October 15, 1921, the International Committee of the Red Cross in Geneva recognized the new Soviet body, the Russian Red Cross Society, as the sole entity representing Soviet Russia.

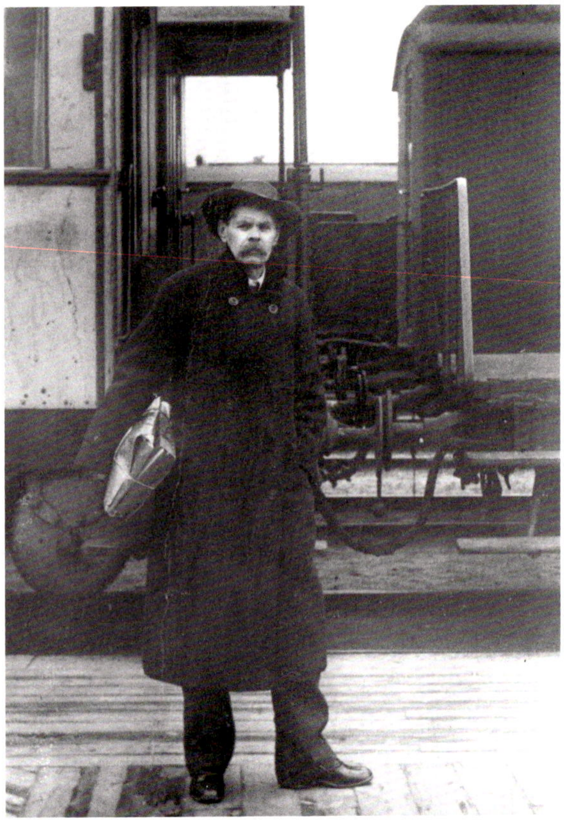

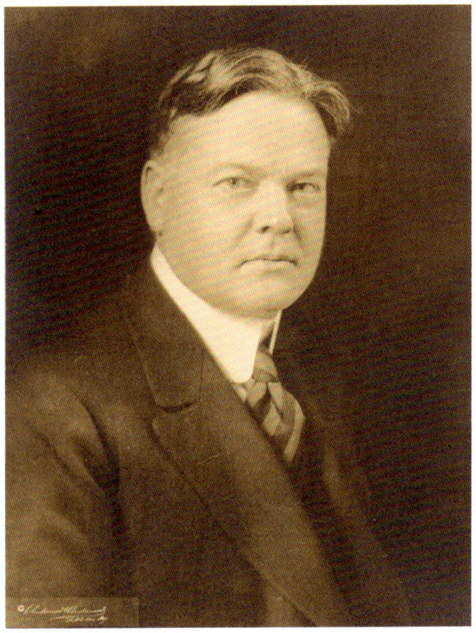

TOP: Maxim Gorky, ca. 1920.

ABOVE: Herbert Hoover, 1917.

Hoover's cabled response to Gorky led to negotiations with Soviet government representative Maxim Litvinov, Deputy People's Commissar of Foreign Affairs, in Riga, Latvia. The United States had not granted diplomatic recognition to the Soviet government, which added an air of awkwardness to the negotiations. Against the backdrop of his reputation as an implacable foe of communism, Hoover's insistence on American control of food distribution inside Soviet Russia put Soviet leader Vladimir Lenin and his Kremlin comrades on their guard. The signing of the Riga Agreement on August 20, 1921, committed Hoover's ARA to provide a daily meal to one million Soviet children. The essential terms of this contract granted the ARA control over its operations inside Russia; in return it pledged to conduct nonpartisan famine relief and not to mix in Soviet politics.

This was a precarious time for the Soviet regime. Stormy protests in the cities and antigovernment violence in the countryside in the winter of 1921 convinced Lenin and key Party leaders of the absolute necessity to pull back from the extreme economic policies known as War Communism, among whose hallmarks were the nationalization of industry and the prohibition of free trade. At the Tenth Party Congress in Moscow in March, overcoming the doubts and fears of the assembled delegates, Lenin initiated a retreat from War Communism by muscling through a resolution ending grain requisitions and allowing limited free trade. These concessions were merely the first step in a yearlong transition to a first-of-its-kind partial market economy called the New Economic Policy, popularly known by the acronym NEP. Retail trade and small-scale industry were left unfettered, while the state retained control over the economy's "commanding heights": heavy industry, the railroads, utilities, and foreign trade.

Hoover's original plan to provide a daily meal to one million Soviet children had to be revised after the American relief workers made their way to the towns and villages in the Volga region and filed reports with descriptions of the piles of tangled corpses; of hundreds of thousands of ragged and vermin-ridden refugees fleeing the famine zone in search of food; of the cries of the children, many with bellies swollen from eating grass, leaves, and bark.

This was not simply hunger, but widespread starvation. Clearly the relief efforts would have to cover adults as well as children. In December 1921, Hoover appealed to President Harding to request an appropriation from the US Congress for Russian relief. Passage of the bill on December 22 cleared the way for the allocation of $20 million for relief to Soviet Russia, primarily in the form of corn. Hoover persuaded the Soviets to spend $10 million from their gold reserve for the purchase of wheat seed. Eventually the funds used to support ARA operations in Soviet Russia totaled $60 million, worth over $1 billion today. Of this total, about $5 million was raised by several American relief organizations affiliated with the ARA in Russia, notably the American Jewish Joint Distribution Committee, the American Friends Service Committee (Quakers), and the American Mennonite Relief organization.

In the first half of 1922, the ARA undertook a massive campaign to transport corn and seed from the American Midwest to the Russian heartland. The obstacles to success were many. The key physical obstacle was the state of Russia's railroads. European Russia was scarred with "locomotive graveyards," rows of rusted and dilapidated locomotives that had gone unused for years, their tenders missing, piston rods removed, and boilers open, "resting there soundlessly, like

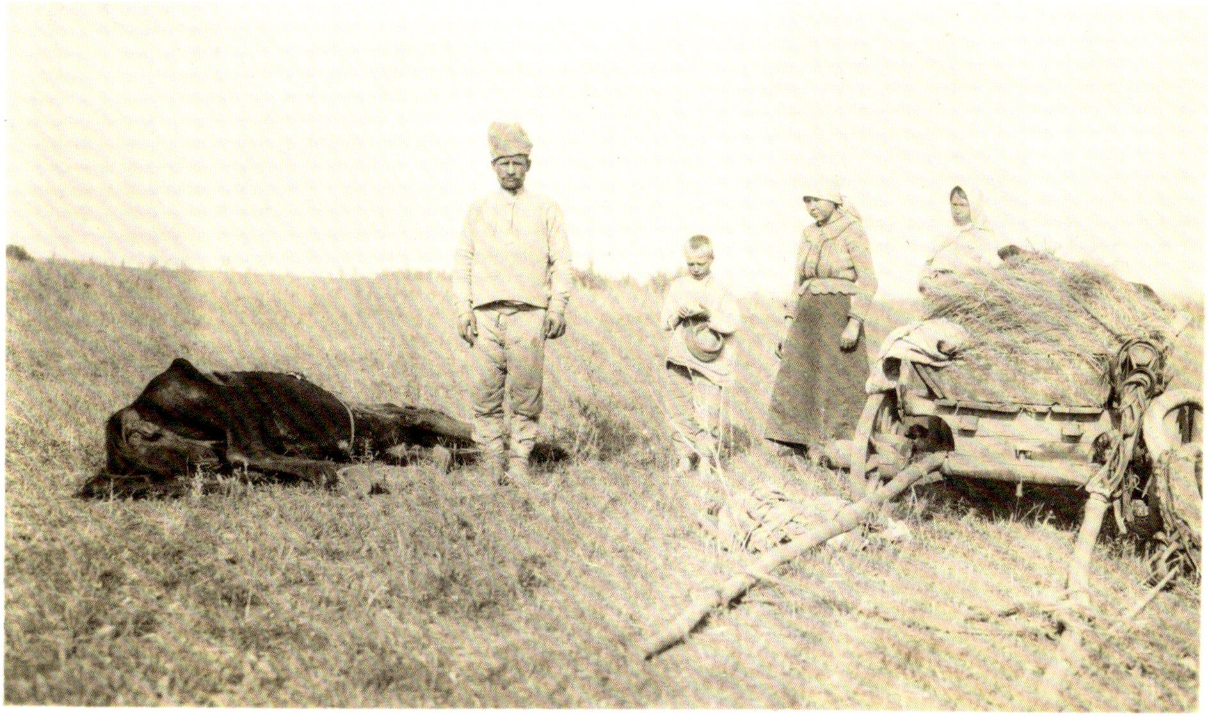

sleeping monsters," in the words of American journalist Edwin Hullinger. The central drama of the relief story is how the ARA—against all odds and after a near-disastrous logjam of corn trains west of the Volga—delivered its lifesaving corn and wheat seed to the villages in the nick of time, breaking the back of the famine and securing the harvest of 1922.

The famine of 1921 was triggered by a drought and a failed harvest in 1920, but major contributing causes were the disruptions of the Great War, the Russian Revolution of 1917, and the ensuing civil war; and also the Soviet government's forcible requisitioning of grain from the peasantry. The lack of fodder took a severe toll on livestock. The photograph shows a peasant family whose horse has just succumbed to malnourishment. American Relief Administration European operational records

By summer 1922, the ARA was providing a daily meal to some 10.5 million Soviet citizens. Thousands of ARA kitchens in cities, towns, and villages served children a daily meal consisting of white bread, corn grits—*kasha* in Russian—rice, lard, milk, cocoa, and sugar. Adults received daily rations of corn grits. ARA food turned the tide of refugees who had set off in search of food and were spreading contagious disease. Beyond saving lives, the ARA played an important role in the reconstruction of the Soviet economy, most crucially in the revival of the railroads, which might have shut down entirely had not American corn shipments kept them running through the winter of 1921–1922 and forced them to ramp up operations for the spring corn campaign.

The ARA—locals pronounced the initials as one word, "Ahrah"—became hugely popular in Soviet Russia. The Americans were regarded with wonder for the energy, speed, and efficiency of their organization, for the "rhythm" and "tempo" of their methods. There is considerable evidence that for a population numbed by war, hunger, and politics, the American presence was an object of intense interest. This enthusiasm for the ARA grew out of the tradition, reaching back into the previous century, of Russian fascination with *Amerika*. The mission would stay on in Soviet Russia for a second year, into summer 1923, on a much-reduced scale. In all, some three hundred Americans served with the ARA in Soviet Russia—never more than two hundred at one time—administering American relief through a staff of over 120,000 Soviet citizens.

+ + +

Food might save hundreds of thousands from starvation, but a greater number would be carried off by hunger-related disease. Since the Revolution of 1917, Soviet Russia had seen major outbreaks of typhus and cholera resulting from the displacement caused by the war. Now the famine set off a new wave of disease, and a rising tide of refugees in flight from famine fueled its spread. Not only were millions vulnerable to contagious disease, but the Russian medical establishment was severely underequipped to deal with the emergency, to such an extent that the ARA referred to the condition as a "medical famine." Not for nothing did Gorky's appeal end with a plea for "bread and medicine."

In tsarist times, Russia had acquired most of its medicines and medical equipment from abroad. The Great War cut off this supply at the same time that the ravages of war sharply increased the demand. With the Revolution of 1917 came a breakdown in basic sanitation in the cities and the attendant appearance of epidemic diseases. The carnage of the Russian Civil War (1918–1920) severely depleted both the number of medical personnel and the country's unreplenished supplies.

Soviet Russia's cities had seen outbreaks of typhus, relapsing fever, cholera, smallpox, and typhoid during the civil war years, when the movements of the Red and White armies ebbed and flowed. These had largely subsided by 1920. Typhoid fever and dysentery, the latter frequently resulting from the consumption of food substitutes, were still widespread, as was relapsing fever, while cholera had almost completely disappeared by the time the ARA came on the scene. Tuberculosis, meanwhile, continued to wage the war of attrition it had begun in 1914.

American relief transport column on the frozen Volga River at Tsaritsyn, March 1922.

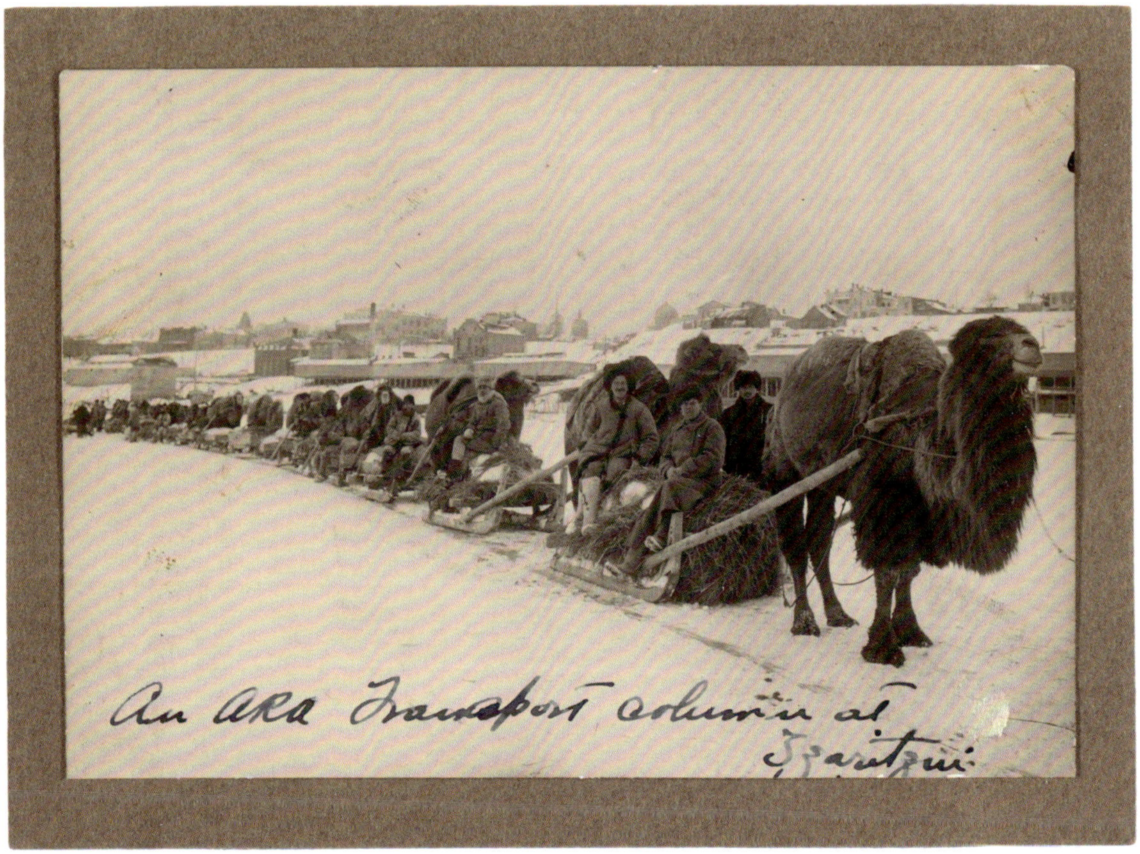

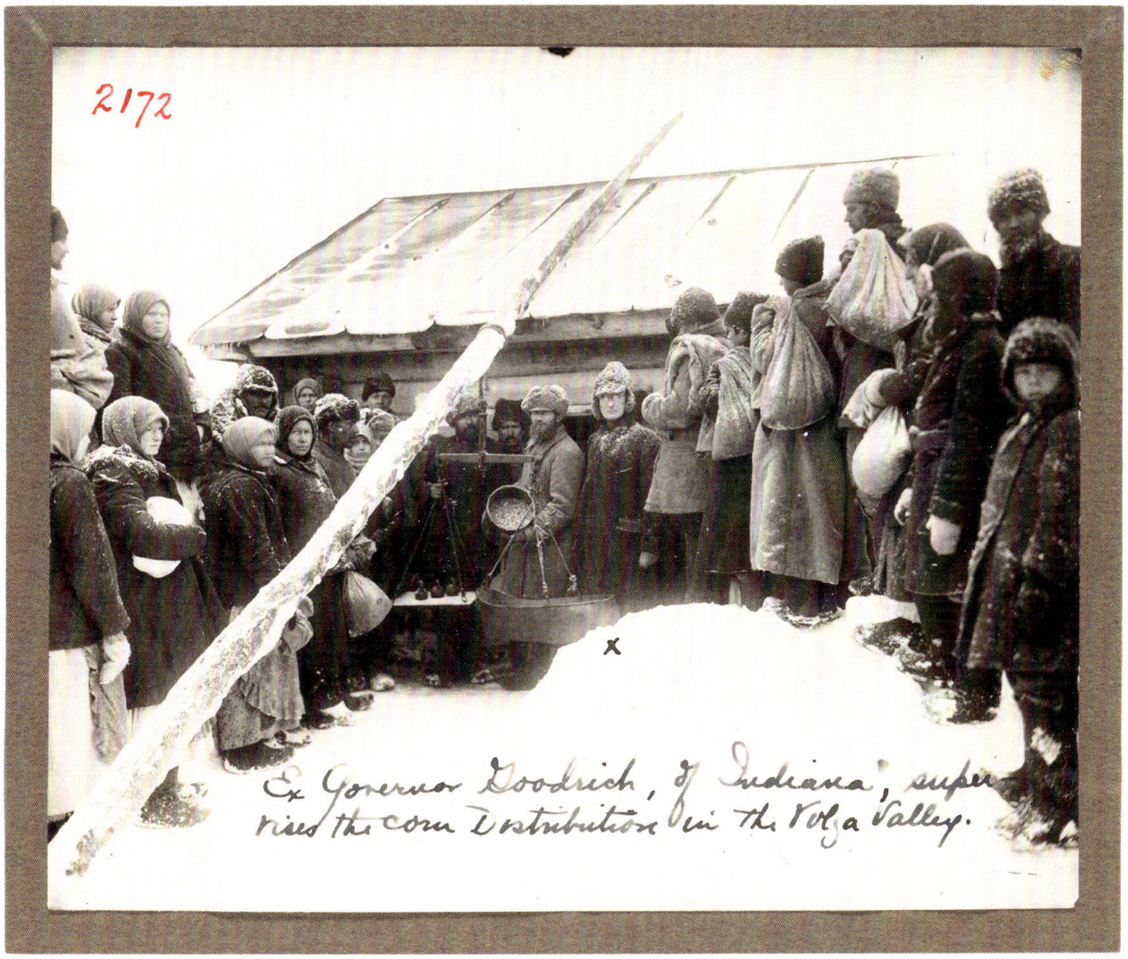
2172
Ex Governor Goodrich, of Indiana, supervises the corn Distribution in the Volga Valley.

ARA special investigator James P. Goodrich, former governor of Indiana, at center, in peaked hat and glasses, distributing corn in a village near Samara, March 27, 1922.

Malaria was widespread, and numerous cases were chronic because there was no quinine to treat it. There was also a high rate of the deficiency diseases, especially among children, including rickets, scurvy, and hunger edema. The famine portended a second, much deadlier wave of pestilence. Cholera posed the most immediate threat, but there was far greater concern about an inevitable and looming epidemic of typhus.

In order to meet this danger, the ARA mounted a large-scale medical relief effort. The ARA had not conducted a medical program in any of its previous missions, but Russian conditions demanded it. This task would normally have fallen to the American Red Cross, which had operated throughout wartime and postwar Europe, but that organization had earned the suspicion of the Soviet government in recent years by providing assistance to civilians behind the lines of the White armies in Russia's north and south and in Siberia during the civil war. The Soviet government eyed the Red Cross warily, perceiving it as an arm of the US government. The ARA, despite Hoover's avowed anti-Bolshevism, was viewed more positively, if also with suspicion.

The foundation of the ARA's medical program was an agreement made with the American Red Cross on September 2, 1921, by which the latter undertook to furnish the Russian unit with supplies and funds totaling $3 million, a sum later increased to $3.8 million. In January 1922, the ARA secured an additional $4 million worth of US Army surplus medical stocks. The Red Cross also endorsed the ARA's selection of a chief medical officer, Colonel Henry Beeuwkes (pronounced "bee-YOO-kees"), of the US Army Medical Corps. Beeuwkes's staff eventually

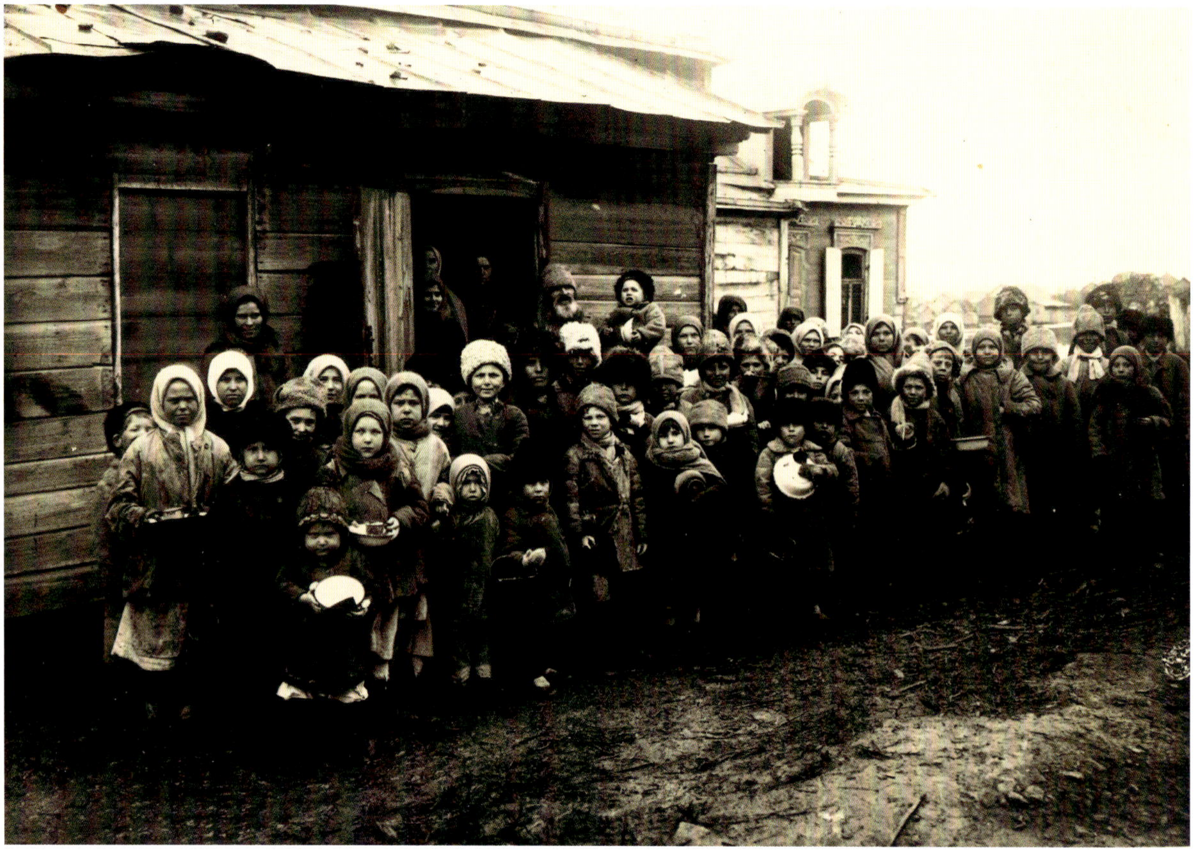

ABOVE: An ARA village kitchen in Tsaritsyn, late winter 1922.

FACING: Unidentified artist (Russian), Дар американского народа, A.R.A. [Gift of the American people, A.R.A.], 1922. Poster Collection RU/SU 502

drew on the services of thirty American doctors supported by a staff of fifteen clerks and two stenographers. The maximum number of American medical personnel on duty at any one time was forty, reached during the month of July 1922.

The ARA Medical Division would work to improve basic sanitary conditions in cities, towns, and villages through major reconstruction of dilapidated sanitation systems; would launch cleanup campaigns to rid streets, institutions, and homes of a nearly four-year accumulation of filth; and would provide chlorinators and chloride of lime to secure safe drinking water supplies. The Medical Division would combat infectious diseases with the drugs Neosalvarsan and quinine, and it would work to prevent disease through a massive vaccination campaign against five communicable diseases. All the while, American physicians would inspect hospitals and children's homes and stock them with badly needed medicines, surgical equipment, and basic supplies such as soap. To further ensure that Soviet Russia's physicians could once again practice the art of healing, the ARA supported them with lifesaving food and clothing packages and with the medical literature they had been deprived of since 1914, when the war cut off contact with the outside world. All these efforts were designed to address the many dimensions of the "medical famine" that had overtaken Soviet Russia and threatened to compound the existing famine with concurrent deadly disease.

In the end an estimated six million people perished in the famine, but millions survived thanks to American famine relief. The lifesaving role of American food has dominated accounts of the relief campaign, overshadowing the achievements of the vast American medical relief program. Yet most famine victims succumb not to starvation but to famine-related disease. The ARA's medical relief program proved to be essential to the overall success of the mission. *Bread + Medicine* tells that story.

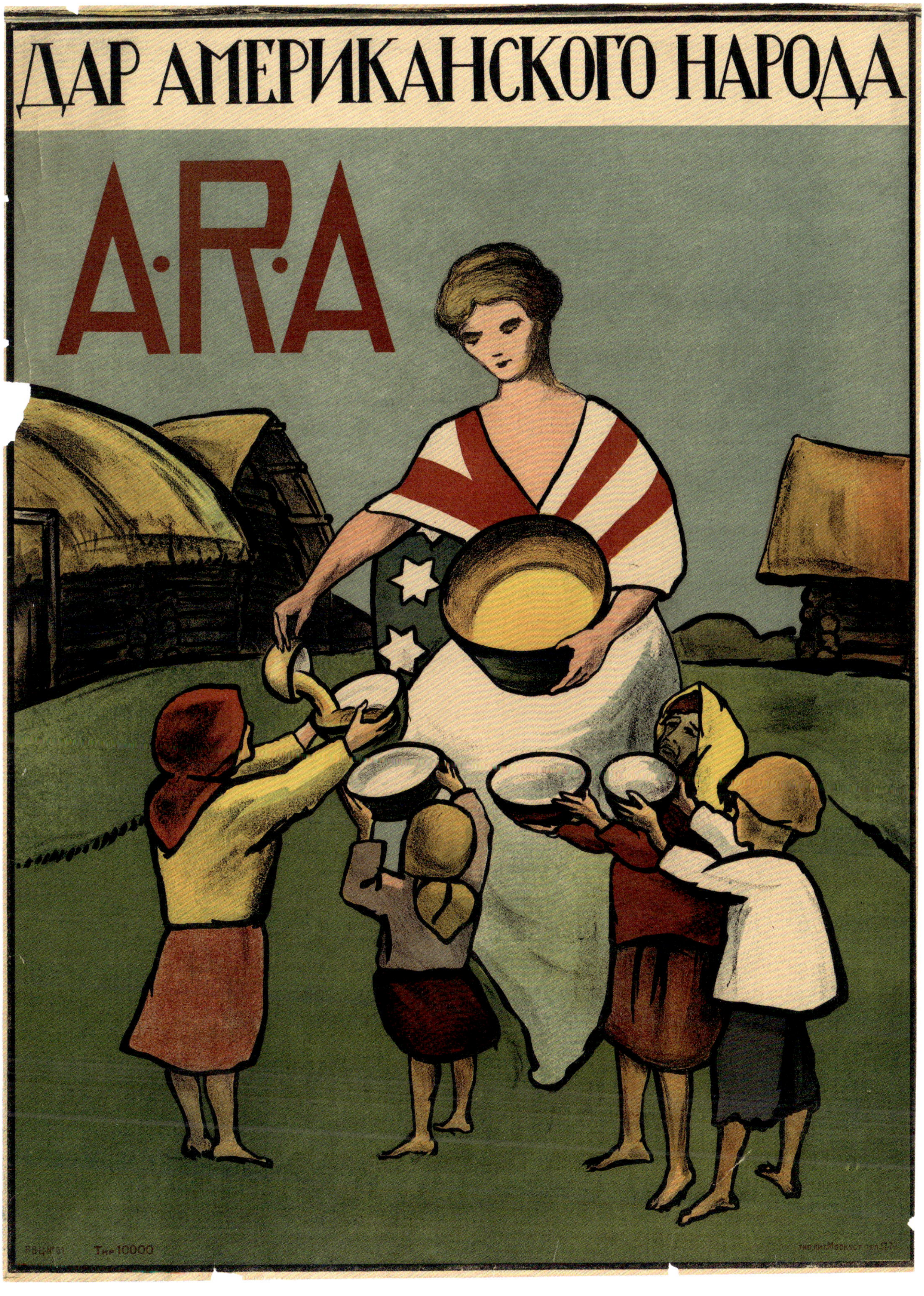
ДАР АМЕРИКАНСКОГО НАРОДА
A·R·A
Тир 10000

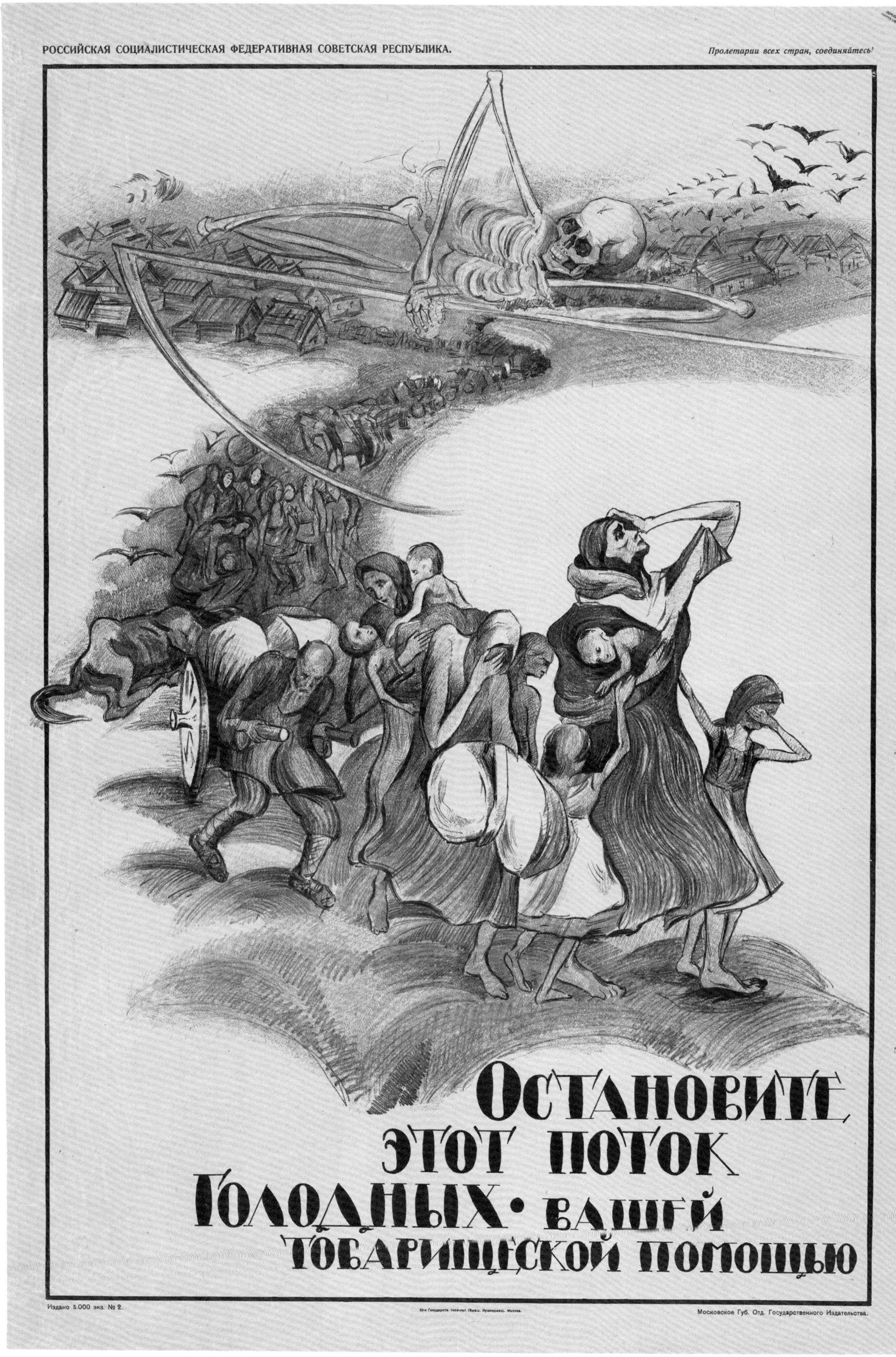
РОССИЙСКАЯ СОЦИАЛИСТИЧЕСКАЯ ФЕДЕРАТИВНАЯ СОВЕТСКАЯ РЕСПУБЛИКА.
Пролетарии всех стран, соединяйтесь!
Остановите этот поток голодных • вашей товарищеской помощью
Издано 5.000 экз. № 2.
10-я Государств. типо-лит. (бывш. Кушнерева). Москва.
Московское Губ. Отд. Государственного Издательства.

CHAPTER 2

Medical Famine

> "There are twenty-six hospitals in Samara, every one of which I have personally inspected. The name 'hospital' in the case of two thirds of them is a misnomer. The local population and peasants call them 'houses of death.'"
>
> *—Dr. Walter Davenport, January 3, 1922*

One week after the signing of the Riga Agreement, the ARA advance party of seven Americans arrived in Moscow from Riga on August 27. After having a look around, Will Shafroth, a veteran of ARA relief missions in Central Europe, wrote his mother that Moscow was "the most depressing city in the world today." It appeared to him that the regular residents had abandoned the metropolis and their places had been taken by peasants from the surrounding countryside, "with no notion of cleanliness or sanitation." The city, he wrote, "seems to have started back on the road to the civilization of the middle ages."

Generally, the newly arrived Americans expressed a sense of relief as they looked around. They had expected hunger to be much worse. The men of the ARA, in their encounters with hardship across Central Europe, had found conditions worst in the urban centers, not least in the capital cities, where bread was scarcest, whereas the countryside was, generally speaking, not nearly as bad off. Thus the Russian situation required of these relief workers some mental adjustments, beginning with the fact that the crisis at hand was a full-blown famine, striking directly at the actual producers of food. Moscow itself was hardly affected, since the actual scene of the catastrophe was several hundred miles east of the capital. Once they arrived on that scene, they would discover that it was those who worked the land, the peasants themselves, who were starving in large numbers.

During the years of war, revolution, and civil war, the urban population dropped sharply, as people moved to the countryside in search of food or in order to escape the notice of the Soviet authorities. The number of Moscow's residents had fallen by nearly half since 1914, while Petrograd's declined by more than two-thirds. Until 1918, Petrograd—the former and future St. Petersburg—was the Russian capital. ARA representative Carlton Bowden, a former Rhodes Scholar who served with the wartime Commission for Relief in Belgium and with the ARA in Hungary, arrived there in the first days of September. "Compared to Russia, the other countries in which we have worked are paradises of plenty," he wrote to ARA London headquarters on September 18.

> Hungary seems like a land flowing with milk and honey. There is absolutely nothing here. More than half the children in Petrograd are without shoes of any sort, and with no clothing to speak of. It will be impossible for them to

Unidentified artist (Russian), Остановите этот поток Голодных вашей товарищеской помощью [Stop this flow of the starving by your comradely help], 1921.
Poster Collection RU/SU 575

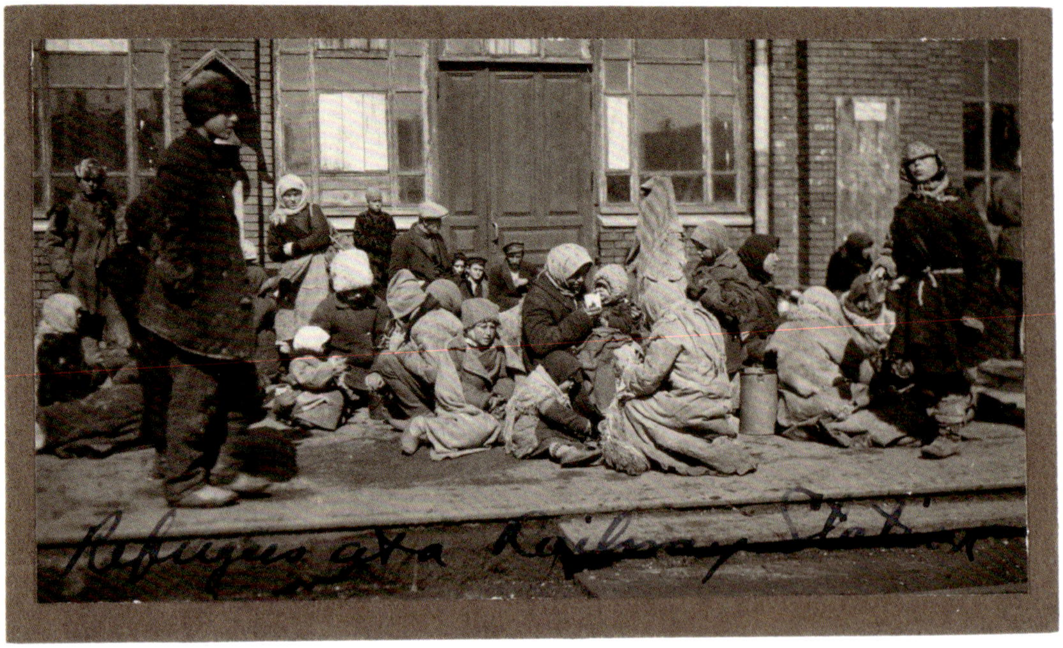

Refugees at a railway station in the Volga region, autumn 1921.

> attend school, and in many cases they will not be able to come to our kitchens. Many hospitals will be closed on account of the lack of fuel. I generally expect the worst wherever I go, but this place is in a far more desperate plight than I had ever imagined, and I am told that the situation here is excellent compared to other parts of Russia. We have certainly come to the right place.

Five days after the ARA advance party reached Moscow, a team of three relief workers was dispatched to the Volga: Shafroth, veteran relief worker John Gregg, and Frank Golder, a Stanford history professor and curator at the new Hoover War Library at Stanford, who served as guide and translator. Their first destination was the city of Kazan, on the northern Volga, about 650 miles directly due east of Moscow.

The American investigators got their first look at actual famine conditions upon arrival at the Kazan railway station, which was overflowing with refugees, most lying on the floor and seemingly incapable of getting up. Near the station, the trio came upon an encampment of refugees—about a thousand strong, in Shafroth's estimation.

> They were the most pitiable sight I have ever seen. Little ragged, white faced, wizened up children, old from the look of suffering on their pinched faces, without hope and without spirit, and with barely enough patched together tatters of clothing to cover their emaciated arms and toothpick legs. They were clustered together like sheep and among them were mothers with babes in their arms. One of these we stopped to talk to, and she showed us the little bit of humanity wrapped up in her old shawl. She knew that it was going to die. Her lips began to quiver in spite of her efforts to control herself, and as she showed us all she had to give it to eat—a bit of black bread, so hard and so earthy and so full of grass and straw that it seemed impossible anyone could use it for human food—the tears began to run down her cheeks. It was heartrending. And there are thousands like her in the famine belt.

The men inspected the city's hospitals and children's homes. Of the latter the most revolting were the emergency institutions known as "collectors" or "receiving homes" (*priyëmniki* in Russian), where refugee children, orphaned or abandoned by their parents, were taken in. Here Shafroth and Gregg witnessed scenes of horror unlike any they had encountered in Central Europe. Shafroth tells of "emaciated little skeletons, whose gaunt faces and toothpick legs, around which their rags were fluttering, testified to the truth of the report that they were dying off daily by the dozen."

Many of the people in their midst were suffering from edema, the distended stomach caused by a protein deficiency from eating grass and weeds and various other food substitutes. What passed as food typically resembled black or green bread and usually contained only the slightest bit of flour, if any, the rest being grass or some similar ingredient. During the winter, the menu came to include such indelicacies as straw from the roofs of peasant huts ground into powder and baked, wood ground into sawdust, cattle dung, and bones from decaying carcasses. Starving horses would turn down such offerings, as would other domestic animals, even the few remaining dogs and cats. A very popular source of sustenance was a weed called *lebeda*, which grows among rye and resembles oats. Unlike either cereal, however, it might produce the swollen "hunger belly," the swelling sometimes affecting the legs. Children were especially vulnerable. Substances that could sustain adults could kill their young offspring.

Three days of taking in such horrors left their mark on the investigators. Gregg was in no doubt: "The need for relief in this country is beyond anything I have ever seen." His first telegram to Moscow headquarters, sent from Kazan on September 5, urged the shipment of food and the emergency recruitment of ARA veterans in Europe, whose services were desperately needed on the Volga. He emphasized the urgency of the situation: "Speed is of utmost repeat utmost importance as without exaggeration children dying actual starvation every day."

The party continued southward to Simbirsk and found conditions if anything even worse. Shafroth's trip report contains some gruesome details.

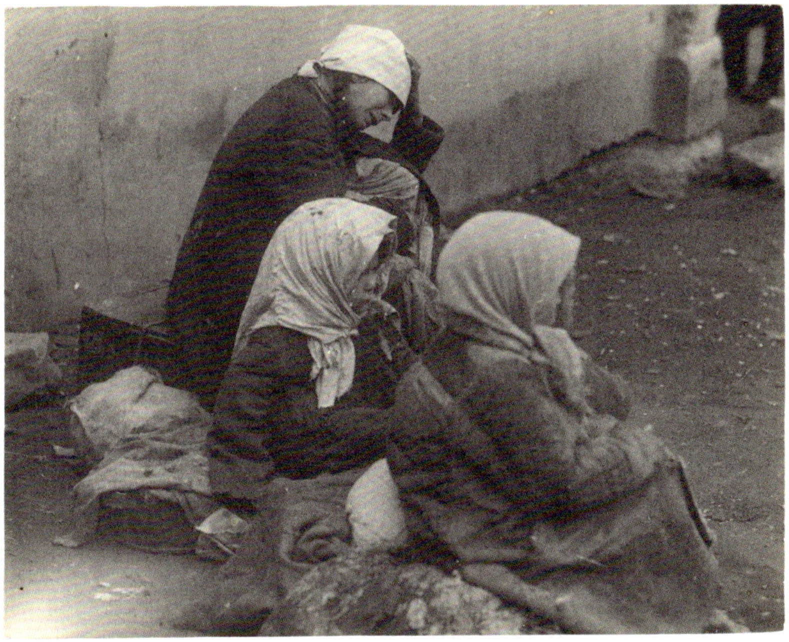

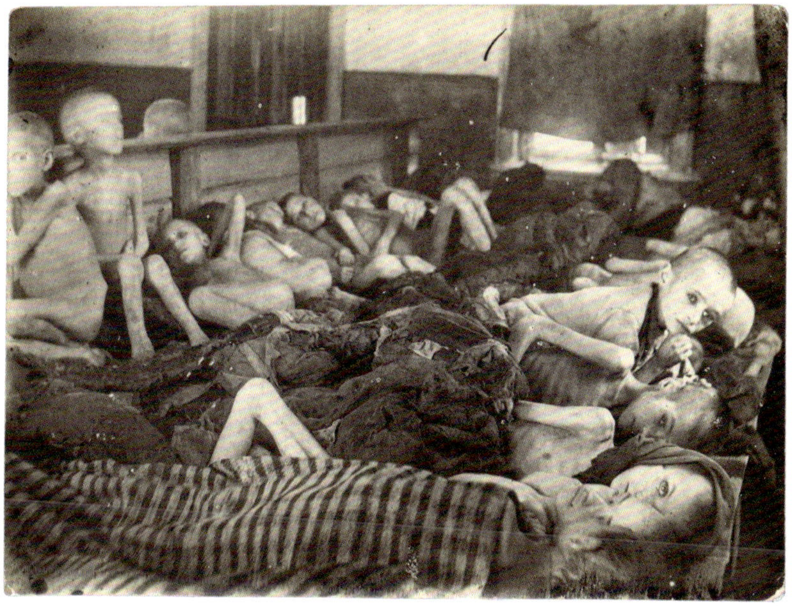

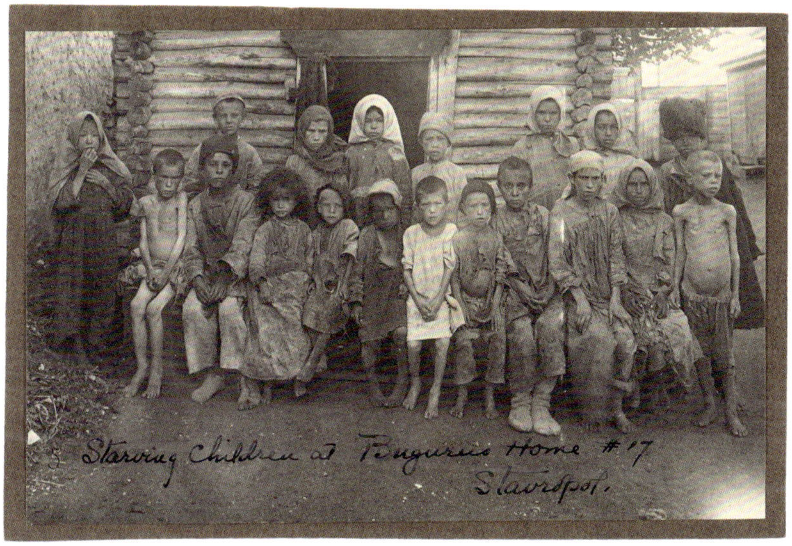

TOP: Refugees, ca. 1922. Frederick Dorsey Stephens papers

MIDDLE: A home for orphaned and abandoned children in Samara, autumn 1921. Charles L. Hall papers

BOTTOM: Lost or abandoned Muslim Tatar children outside Home No. 17, in Buguruslan, district of Stavropol, Samara province, autumn 1921.

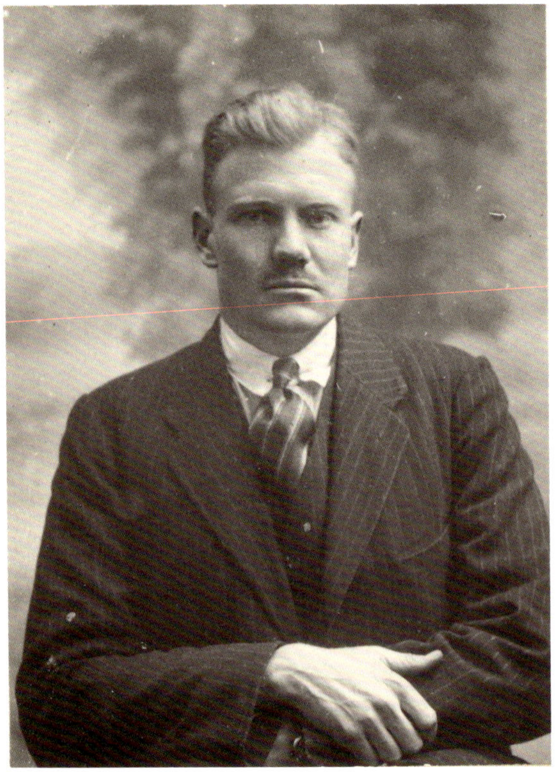

We asked to see how the people lived and were taken into a small one-room cabin. On one side of the room was the usual Russian stove, made of brick and whitewashed, with a flue extending up to the ceiling. On one side of the room was a sort of platform which served as a bed. On it were standing three children, so thin and white and emaciated looking that one almost wondered how they could stand. They had the swollen bellies of grass eaters, and then the peasant woman showed us the "flour" from which she made her bread, it was green. Those children were dying of starvation. They would hold out ten days, two weeks, maybe longer. But if food with some nourishment in it did not come soon, they would all die. As their mother looked at us we could see that she knew it. She dropped to her knees and began to pray to us, sobbing. We turned away, sick of heart. Thousands of little children dying like that! It was unthinkable.

Worse was yet to come, in Samara. Samara being a railroad junction on the Trans-Siberian, the train stations were teeming with refugees. Some were headed toward Moscow, many more toward Siberia—with little sense of the actual distance involved—and of course there was the usual quota destined for Ukraine, the proverbial breadbasket of Russia. It was a scene, like so many others, of misery, suffering, and filth but on a scale and of a severity surpassing anything the investigators had witnessed thus far. F. A. Mackenzie of the *Chicago Daily News*, who came to this godforsaken spot shortly afterward, described what he saw:

> Here were lads, gaunt and tall, thin beyond any conception a Westerner can have of thinness, covered with rags and dirt. Here were old women, some of them sitting half-conscious on the ground, dazed by their hunger, their

ABOVE: Will Shafroth, ca. 1921.

BELOW RIGHT: Frank Golder's ARA passport, issued September 17, 1921. Frank A. Golder papers

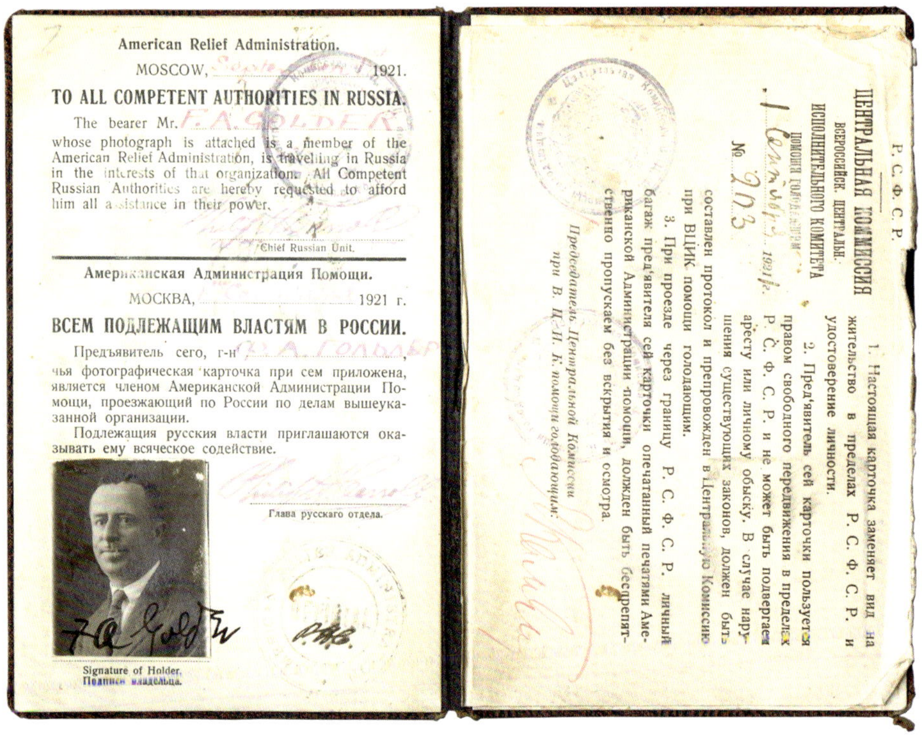

American Relief Administration.

MOSCOW, ... 1921.

TO ALL COMPETENT AUTHORITIES IN RUSSIA.

The bearer Mr. F. A. GOLDER whose photograph is attached is a member of the American Relief Administration, is traveling in Russia in the interests of that organization. All Competent Russian Authorities are hereby requested to afford him all assistance in their power.

Chief Russian Unit.

Американская Администрация Помощи.

МОСКВА, ... 1921 г.

ВСЕМ ПОДЛЕЖАЩИМ ВЛАСТЯМ В РОССИИ.

Предъявитель сего, г-нъ Ф. А. ГОЛЬДЕР, чья фотографическая карточка при сем приложена, является членом Американской Администрации Помощи, проезжающий по России по делам вышеуказанной организации.

Подлежащия русския власти приглашаются оказывать ему всяческое содействие.

Глава русскаго отдела.

Signature of Holder.
Подпись владельца.

Р. С. Ф. С. Р.

ЦЕНТРАЛЬНАЯ КОМИССИЯ
ВСЕРОССИЙСК. ЦЕНТРАЛЬН.
ИСПОЛНИТЕЛЬНОГО КОМИТЕТА
ПОМОЩИ ГОЛОДАЮЩИМ

1 Сентября 1921 г.

№ 203

1. Настоящая карточка заменяет вид на жительство в пределах Р. С. Ф. С. Р. и удостоверение личности.

2. Пред'явитель сей карточки пользуется правом свободного передвижения в пределах Р. С. Ф. С. Р. и не может быть подвергаем аресту или личному обыску. В случае нарушения существующих законов, должен быть составлен протокол и препровожден в Центральную Комиссию при ВЦИК помощи голодающим.

3. При проезде через границу Р. С. Ф. С. Р. личный багаж пред'явителя сей карточки опечатанный печатями Американской Администрации помощи, должен быть беспрепятственно пропускаем без вскрытия и осмотра.

Председатель Центральной Комиссии при В. Ц. И. К. помощи голодающим:

> misery and their misfortune. The little children played feebly around. Some had lost their parents. Other women tried to mother them a bit as best they could. Here were pallid mothers seeking to feed dying babies from their milkless breasts. Were a new Dante to come among us, he could write a new Inferno after visiting one of these railway stations.

Just as the plight of the refugees was more extreme in Samara, so were conditions in the children's receiving stations. Shafroth and his colleagues visited six of these "hell-holes," one of which he described as "a nightmare of filth, lack of equipment, unbelievable overcrowding and criminal lack of the most elementary sanitary measures." Eight months later, Shafroth departed Russia but could not leave these images behind: "I shall never forget the sights I saw in September, in Samara."

+ + +

Word arrived from Moscow that Shafroth was to remain in Samara and begin to set up feeding operations there and await the first shipment of American food. ARA food trains soon began arriving in Kazan, Samara, Simbirsk, and, by mid-October, Saratov, followed at the end of the month by Tsaritsyn, situated on the lower Volga, where the river turns left toward the Caspian. These were the Volga "districts," as the ARA called its administrative-territorial units. They were roughly coterminous with the corresponding Russian provinces—*gubernii*—which were named after their capital cities. The ARA adjusted boundaries here and there, where practical considerations such as the location of a warehouse or a railroad line argued in favor of the disposition of one or another provincial region to a contiguous district.

Alone the five Volga districts would have constituted a sizable mission, yet as American investigations had confirmed, the ubiquitous expression "the Volga famine" understated the scale of Soviet Russia's crisis. By late October, the ARA had established two sprawling districts to the east. One was centered at Ufa, on the western slopes of the Ural Mountains, and included most of the Bashkir Autonomous Republic. Feeding children at Ufa began on November 16, with food supplies for fifty thousand. The other trans-Volga district was Orenburg, capital of the Kirghiz Autonomous Republic, situated at the southeastern edge of European Russia, where the southern ranges of the Ural Mountains descend into the scrub and brush of the steppe, back then Russia's Badlands.

Both district capitals were nearly a thousand miles removed from Moscow. For the relief workers in all the districts, the problem of distance was compounded by the sparseness and wretched state of Russia's transportation and communication system. The ruinous condition of Russia's railroads was graphically conveyed in an October 20 telegram sent to Hoover by the head of the ARA mission, Colonel William Haskell: "Railroads hanging together, roadbeds unrepaired, derailed cars ditched. Thousands [of] cars deteriorating on sidings where rails and ties had been removed from under them."

A further complication in the early going was the slow and unreliable telegraph service. In autumn 1921, it generally took five days for a telegram from Moscow to reach Kazan, Simbirsk, or Samara; to Tsaritsyn it took fifteen days; to Orenburg

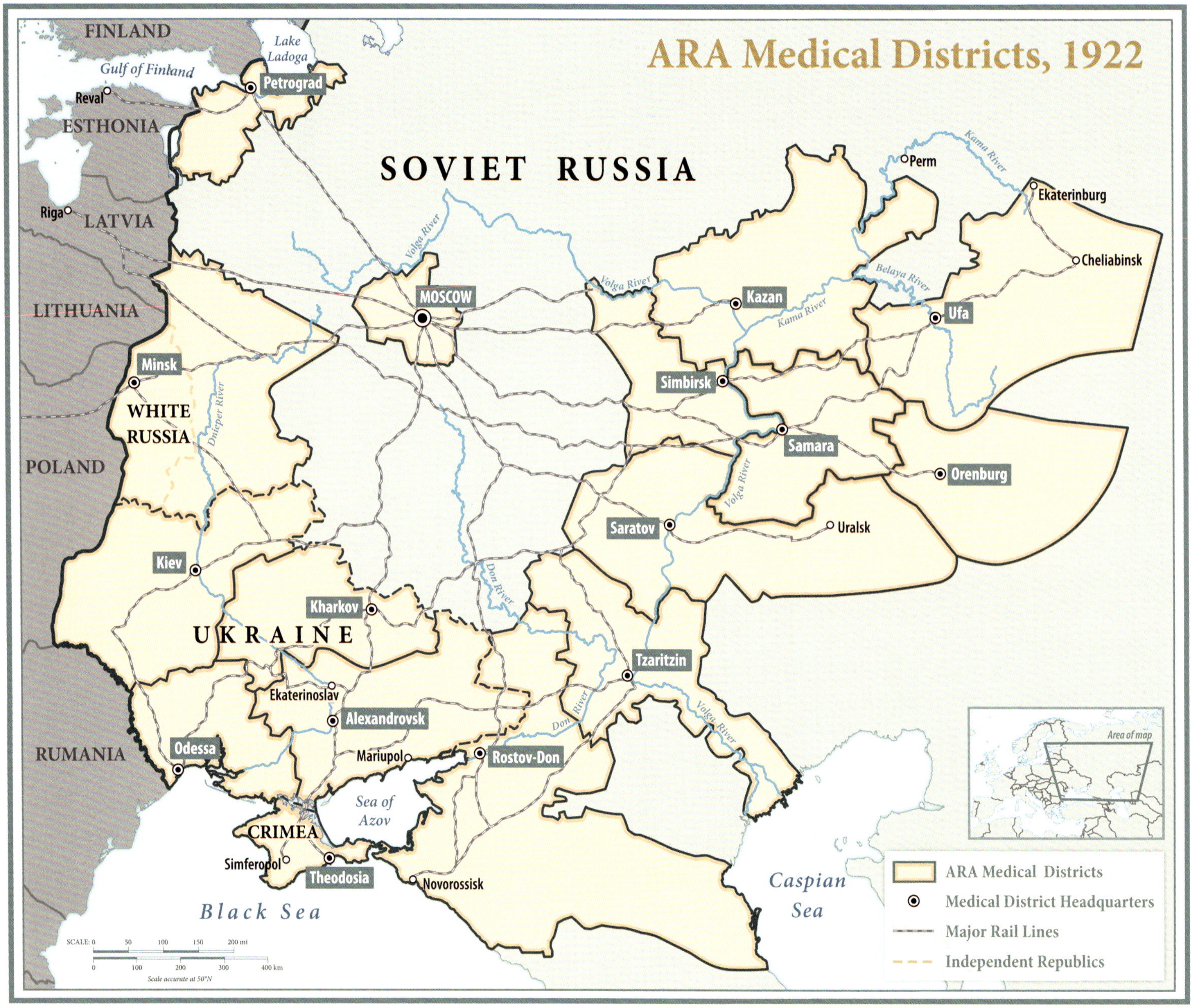

Map showing areas of operation of the ARA Medical Division as of spring 1922.

fourteen. International communication was initially slow as well: a wire from Moscow to London took six or seven days. Only by summer 1922 did this become a twenty-four-hour service.

All of that—the expansion of the mission, the establishment and staffing of ARA districts—was still to come. For now, at the moment when Gregg's September 5 telegram reached Moscow headquarters, Colonel Beeuwkes, chief of the ARA Medical Division, was aboard a ship making his way across the Atlantic.

+ + +

Colonels Haskell and Beeuwkes, as part of a company of twenty-one men, arrived in Moscow on September 21. Haskell, director of the mission, qualified for the Russia assignment by following a path markedly different from the ARA veterans. A graduate of West Point, class of 1901, he was a career soldier with a distinguished record of service. In the Great War he was a line officer in the St. Mihiel

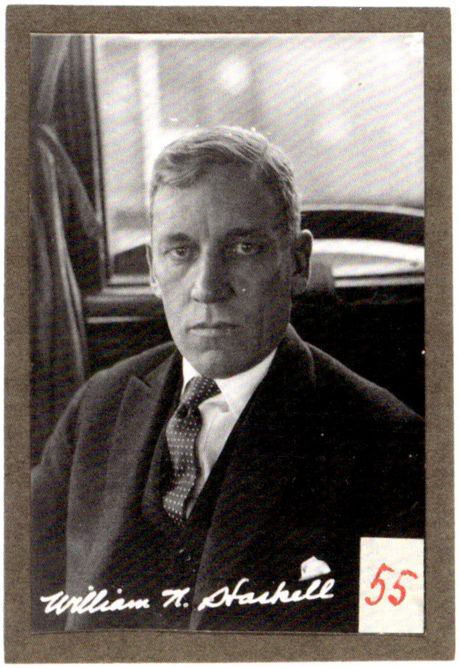

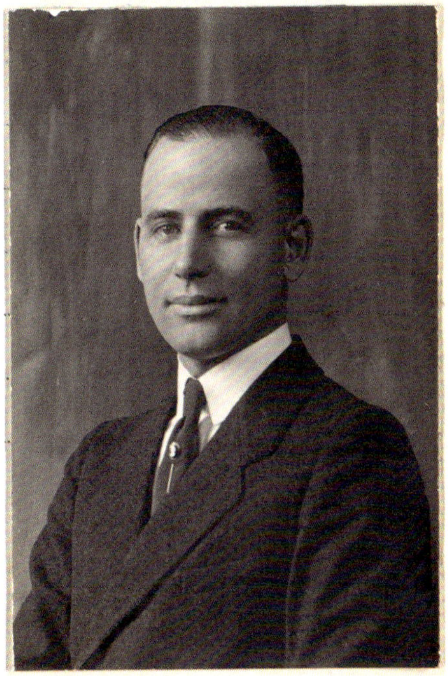
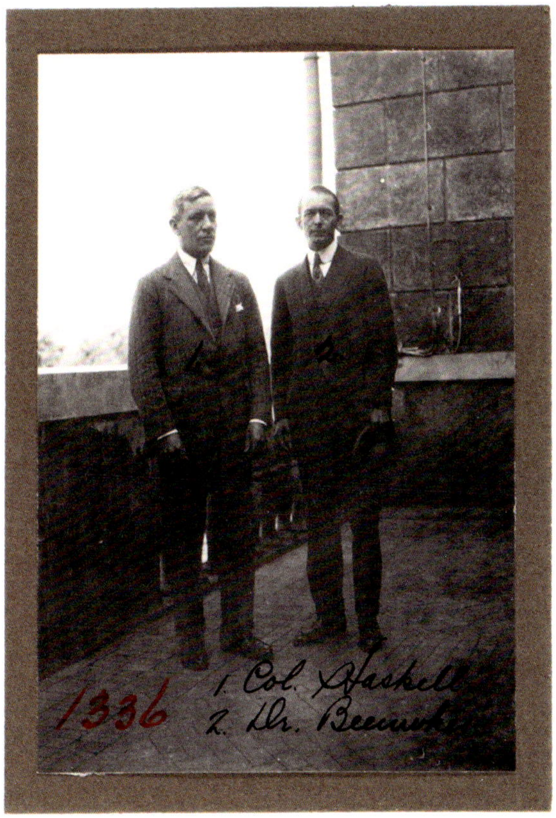

FROM LEFT: Colonel William N. Haskell, director of the ARA's Soviet Russia mission, Moscow, 1922; Dr. Walter Davenport, ca. 1921; Colonel William Haskell (left) and Colonel Henry Beeuwkes, Moscow, 1922.

offensive, before becoming deputy chief of staff and chief of operations of the Second US Army Corps on the British front.

As a relief worker, too, he had, as they used to say, large experience. After the signing of the armistice, Hoover made him chief of the American relief mission to Romania, an operation of the US Food Administration, and subsequently, in August 1919, he was selected by the Allied Supreme Council to be High Commissioner to Armenia, where he also served as director general of all American and European relief agencies in Transcaucasia. These included the Near East Relief and the American Red Cross.

Newly independent Armenia, in the wake of the 1915 genocide under the Ottoman Empire, struggled to cope with a flood of returning refugees, food shortages, contagious disease, and a looming invasion by the Red Army. The purpose of the Haskell mission had been to help stabilize the country. The mission had included a medical department headed by Major Walter P. Davenport of the US Army Medical Corps. Davenport, born in 1887, was from Appleton, Minnesota, and had received his MD from the University of Illinois. Davenport and his staff of twenty Army officers and seventy-five civilians, along with a local Armenian staff, organized hospital services for several thousand people, worked to improve health care facilities and sanitary conditions, and conducted an inoculation drive against typhoid and smallpox. They worked with an undernourished and destitute population vulnerable to cholera, typhus, relapsing fever, and dysentery, as well as rising cases of malaria and tuberculosis.

It is a testimony to the impression made on the American public by the Armenian genocide and the plight of its survivors that a second American mission was sent to Armenia at the same time, this one a military mission. Its chief was Major General James G. Harbord, who had served as the chief of staff to General John J. Pershing, the commander of the American Expeditionary Force during the First World War. Harbord's charge was to assess the military situation in the region and advise President Woodrow Wilson on US policy toward Armenia and its neighbors. The Harbord mission, too, had a chief medical officer, and that was Beeuwkes. Beeuwkes was born in Illinois in 1881. He earned his MD from

Johns Hopkins in 1906. His career in military service began in 1909, when he became a student at the Army Medical School. He served in France from 1917 to 1919 as Chief Medical Executive of the American Expeditionary Force, during which time he was the personal physician of General Pershing, commander of the AEF.

With their shared experience in Armenia, it seems only natural that Haskell, Beeuwkes, and Davenport were brought together by the ARA to fill vital roles in the Soviet Russia mission. Conditions in Armenia were not nearly as dire as those they would encounter in Soviet Russia, but Armenia provided lessons in how to conduct relief operations in a failing state and how to combat contagious disease among a hungry people. Beeuwkes took on Davenport as assistant director of the ARA Medical Division, and Davenport arrived in Moscow together with Haskell's party on September 21.

+ + +

During their initial weeks in Moscow, Beeuwkes and Davenport were busy establishing the Medical Division, hiring local staff and securing warehouse space for the anticipated deluge of medical supplies. At the beginning of November, as Red Cross supplies began to arrive in Moscow, Davenport was dispatched to the Volga to assess conditions for medical relief, preceded by a shipment of essential supplies. He arrived in Samara on November 8, welcomed there by ARA district supervisor Will Shafroth. His letters to Moscow from the famine zone provided Beeuwkes with the expert eyewitness testimony he would need to plan the ARA medical program.

Davenport's inspection of the city's hospitals told him everything he needed to know about the woeful lack of medical and basic supplies—blankets, clothing for patients, essential medicines and disinfectants—as well as fuel and food. In the hospitals, "there has been no replenishment of equipment nor repairs for the past six years," he reported to Beeuwkes.

> Only one third of the sick are housed in institutions that could by any stretch of [the] imagination be called hospitals—the other two thirds, while they have shelter and a few rags to cover them with, are without many of even the necessities, let alone the modern conveniences we associate with the word "hospital." Without fuel, sufficient food, adequate clothing, sufficient medicines, water, bathing and toilet facilities, let alone some of the refinements as delousing, disinfecting and ventilating and laundry facilities, they are called very properly "houses of death."

Davenport was struck by the paucity of doctors and of health workers generally. Some had fled the country. Others perished, weakened by hunger, disease, and demoralization. "Fully 50% of the doctors in the [province] have died during the epidemics of the past three years—the same can be said of the other trained medical personnel, feldshers, nurses and hospital attendants. As a result of this scarcity of personnel, all the doctors have been 'mobilized' and occupy various government positions—all medical facilities, including hospitals, ambulatories, dispensaries, etc. are operated by the Government." In each province—*gubernia* in Russian—all health measures and initiatives were under the purview of the

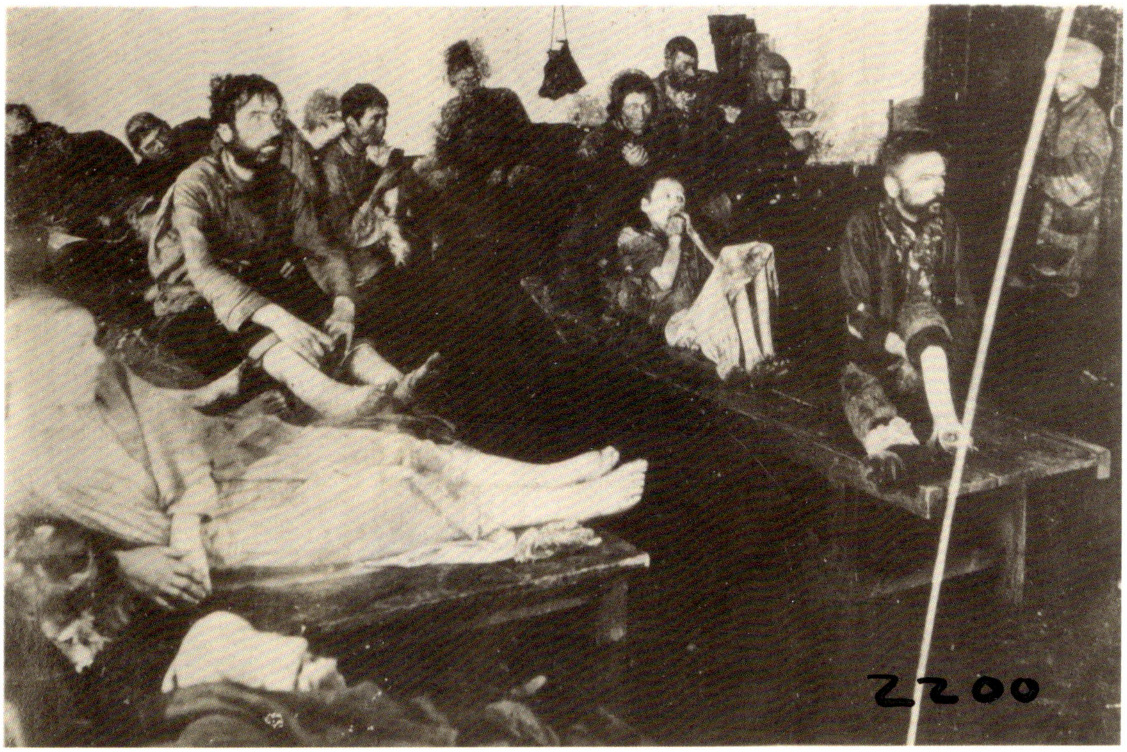

Hospital near Chelyabinsk, in the Ufa district, autumn 1921. Frank A. Golder papers

gubzdrav, the provincial public health department, the local branch of the People's Commissariat of Health in Moscow.

In his conversations with Samara's doctors, Davenport learned the rise-and-fall story of Russian medicine during the previous half-century: in the last decades of tsarist Russia, a body called the *zemstvo* emerged as "a most efficient organization and was directly responsible for the peasant, even in the remote villages, receiving to a greater or less degree scientific medical treatment when he was ill and the advantages of their well-equipped combative sanitary organization in time of epidemics." Over time, "modern hospitals and laboratories were developed in the larger towns in the [counties], with dispensaries and smaller hospitals in the smaller towns and villages," until by 1914, "the 'Zemstvo' had operating throughout the length and breadth of Russia 3,000 hospitals in two thousand seven hundred towns and villages with a bed capacity of over 50,000, these hospitals employing the whole time over 4,000 doctors." As Davenport reported to Beeuwkes, "whatever faith the peasant had at this time in scientific medicine, both preventative and therapeutic, and it was considerable, is directly due to the work of this body." That faith, he was told, had since evaporated.

The zemstvos collapsed after the Bolsheviks took power in 1917. The gubzdrav was intended to be a replacement, but had neither the resources nor the institutional reach or expertise to get the job done. In Samara, Davenport found the gubzdrav to be "an excellent organization on paper," but "it has not the means, either financially or in supplies, both medicines and food, to even attempt to carry out in the gubernia over 5% of an adequate medical program justified by present existing conditions. Only 1% of a very moderate requisition for medical supplies was sent [to] them by the Central Government this year for the whole Samara gubernia with over 11,000 hospital beds; only 300 arshines (225 yds) of surgical gauze was sent to supply the medical needs of 3,000,000 people."

Most members of the new medical establishment were clearly out of their depth. The relief workers recorded several cases in which physicians with long

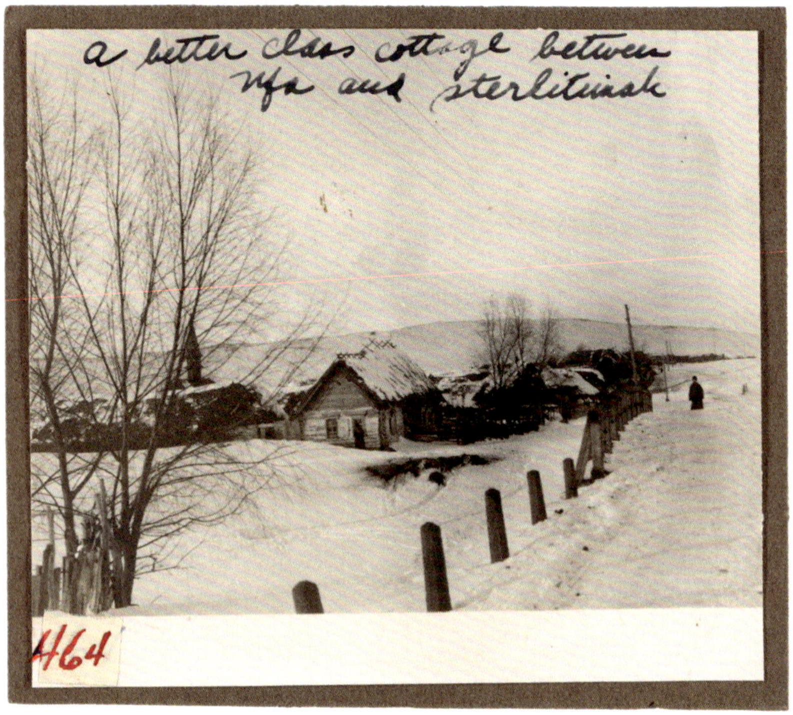

Scene along the road between Ufa and Sterlitamak in the Urals, winter 1922.

and distinguished careers as directors of hospitals and local health departments had been, after the revolution, replaced by veterinarians holding the proper Communist credentials. Davenport wrote to Beeuwkes: "In the Samara gubernia a feldsher (male nurse) heads the 'Gubzdrav,' in the Ufa gubernia a veterinary feldsher occupies the same position—in neither of these gubernias would any of the few remaining competent medical men accept these positions—principally for the reason that the holder of this office must of necessity belong to the Communist Party and also the fact that with nothing to work with the doctor in charge would lose any reputation he might previously have made." Davenport conveyed his sense of exasperation with this state of affairs in telling Beeuwkes: "the biggest thing you can do for us here is to get the central govt [in] Moscow to send down a real man to handle the health dept. which is absolutely not functioning."

In the meantime, there were steps the ARA could take to improve the situation, as Davenport illustrated in a letter from Samara.

> The 224th Evacuationary Hospital, a very needy institution and doing good work in caring for refugees with about 300 patients, was about ready to close operations on account of lack of food, clothing, medicines and fuel. We agreed to do supplementary feeding and supply hospital clothing and medicine provided the Gubzdrav would supply fuel. The Gubzdrav did manage to get a couple of loads of wood to them, then the supply ceased but, rather than quit after what we had done for them, they consented to tear up the wooden walks for fuel—the last time I was out there they were tearing down one of the wood barracks for epidemic diseases for the same purpose. If the barracks hold out, this institution should get through the winter nicely.

It was the kind of improvised arrangement most ARA doctors would make with the local authorities in the months that followed in order to prevent hospitals and medical laboratories from going under.

+ + +

Having spent more than two weeks in Samara, Davenport traveled east to Ufa, in the Ural Mountains, arriving there November 29, just in time to help attend to Colonel Walter Bell, the district supervisor, who had arrived back at Ufa headquarters from an inspection trip delirious with fever.

> Col. Bell had been ill five days—there was not much question about the diagnosis and on the day after he arrived the typical exanthematic typhus rash put in its appearance. The Colonel had been up all this period and had just taken to his bed the day we arrived.—he was in delirium and had a temperature of 104F.—it is now the 17th day of his illness and we think he

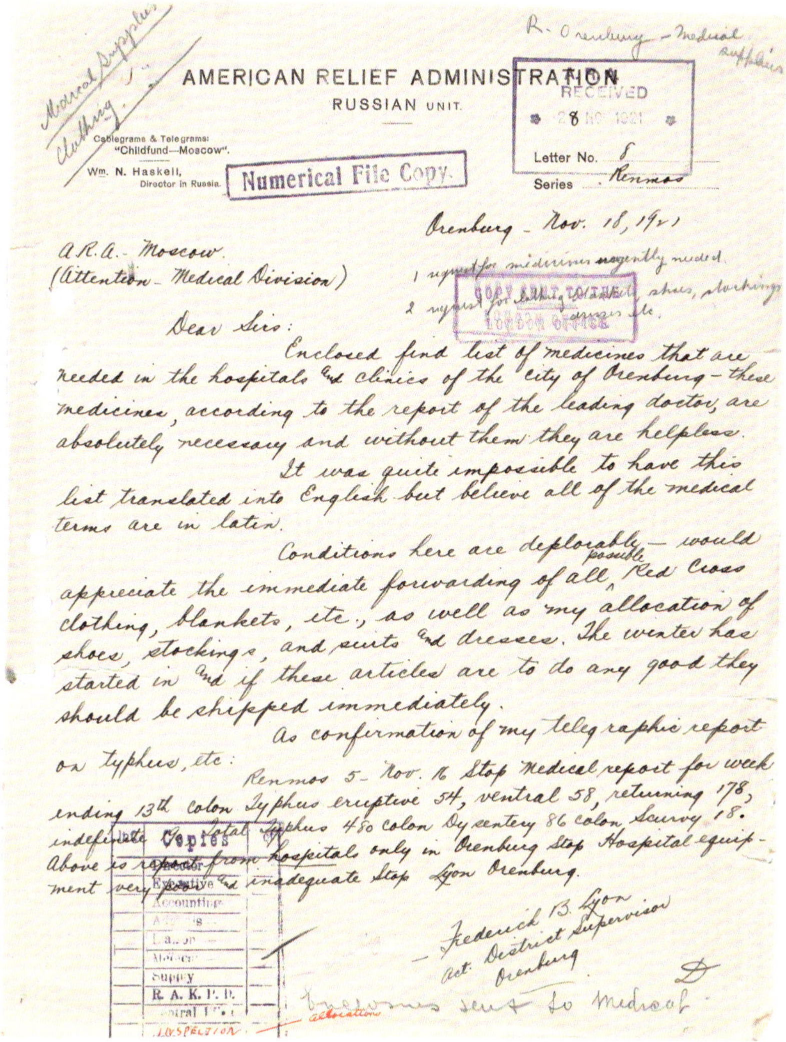

AMERICAN RELIEF ADMINISTRATION
RUSSIAN UNIT.

Cablegrams & Telegrams: "Childfund—Moscow".
Wm. N. Haskell, Director in Russia.

Numerical File Copy.

RECEIVED 28 NOV 1921

Letter No. 8
Series Renmos

Orenburg – Nov. 18, 1921

A.R.A. – Moscow.
(Attention – Medical Division)

Dear Sirs:

Enclosed find list of medicines that are needed in the hospitals and clinics of the city of Orenburg – these medicines, according to the report of the leading doctor, are absolutely necessary and without them they are helpless.

It was quite impossible to have this list translated into English but believe all of the medical terms are in latin.

Conditions here are deplorable – would appreciate the immediate forwarding of all possible Red Cross clothing, blankets, etc., as well as my allocation of shoes, stockings, and suits and dresses. The winter has started in and if these articles are to do any good they should be shipped immediately.

As confirmation of my telegraphic report on typhus, etc.:

Renmos 5 – Nov. 16 Stop Medical report for week ending 13th colon Typhus eruptive 54, ventral 58, returning 178, [illegible] Total Typhus 480 colon Dysentery 86 colon Scurvy 18. Above is report from hospitals only in Orenburg Stop Hospital equipment very poor and inadequate Stop Lyon Orenburg.

– Frederick B. Lyon
Act. District Supervisor
Orenburg

[illegible] sent to Medical

has safely passed the crisis, of course as to complications no one knows what can happen at the time of writing this though he is extremely weak and has a rather severe bronchitis—the local medical talent have been very decent and we lacked for nothing essential in the treatment.

During the Armenia mission in winter 1920, an anticipated epidemic outbreak of typhus had failed to materialize. Now, in Soviet Russia, the threat seemed ominous. The statistics in both Ufa and Samara were troubling, Davenport told Beeuwkes: "Very frankly I am very much depressed on the typhus situation—it is everywhere—one of the doctors treating Col Bell now has it, the Chief of the Ufa Office force, Mr Russ, a very fine gentleman, is also down with it, as are also two more of the [Ufa] office force—I merely mention this to show you how prevalent it is everywhere—and I think on the whole it is even worse in Samara." Davenport estimated that of the one hundred institutions he had inspected in his travels—hospitals, ambulatories, and children's homes—sixty of them harbored typhus cases.

This is the reporting of a seasoned physician with experience in medical relief. The outlook was worrying, but Davenport maintained a positive attitude. "While at times I am depressed and discouraged," he wrote from Ufa on December 8, "I feel that we are doing a good work, probably making a few mistakes, but nevertheless getting on. The doctors as they do the world over show a mighty fine spirit here and I feel that when we win their approval as I believe we have in both Samara and Ufa we are getting somewhere."

Back in Moscow, Beeuwkes was receiving less levelheaded reports from relief workers arriving in the districts, among them Frederick B. "Freddie" Lyon in Orenburg. He had traveled from Moscow to Samara with Davenport before continuing on to Orenburg. Lyon, a twenty-four-year-old University of Michigan graduate from Cleveland, signed on with the ARA from the Graves Registration Service, generally considered the source of the lowest-caliber ARA recruits. He had absolutely no background in food relief, and his charge was merely to get operations in Orenburg up and running until an experienced hand could take over. His initial reports give the impression of a young man overwhelmed and overwrought by the situation he had found. On November 10, 1921, he had inspected a children's home and was clearly shaken by the experience.

> I was taken thru a children's institution, or orphanage, this morning where there are housed 1000 threadbare, scrawny, scraggly children, ranging in age from three to twelve years. These orphans are lying on the bare-wood floor with no blankets, and are huddled together in an endeavor to keep warm. Some of them have dirty scurvy garments which are fairly alive with fleas and vermin. They are packed into a small building of not over twenty rooms and I was told that the death rate here was between forty and fifty a

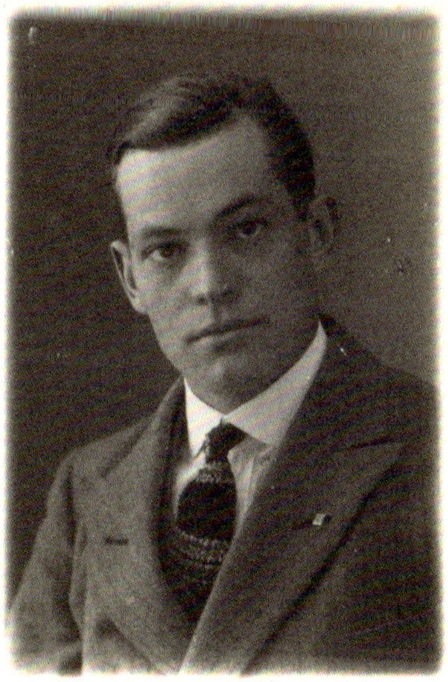

TOP: Letter from Frederick B. Lyon, acting ARA district supervisor in Orenburg, to the ARA Medical Division in Moscow, November 18, 1921.

ABOVE: Frederick B. Lyon, ca. 1921.

day. Such a demoralizing, depressing, and sickening sight I have never seen and hope never to see again. There are not words in my meager vocabulary to cover a word picture of this horrible spectacle. . . . The doctors have absolutely nothing to work with, and in my mind the situation is hopeless.

He echoed other arriving Americans in urging rush shipments of supplies. "I shall start feeding immediately upon the arrival of the food train and that will alleviate some of the suffering. The arrival of clothing, blankets, soap, etc. would be a 'Godsend.' "

At least Lyon could anticipate the arrival of a food train. Davenport's letters to Beeuwkes are punctuated by remarks about the crying need for food in the context of medical relief. "In my inspection of the hospitals nobody asks for medicine and clothing—they all clamor for food" (November 16, 1921). "The thing the officials, doctors, nurses and children cry for is not medicine and clothing, but food" (December 8, 1921). "The hospitals are very inadequately supplied with food, and in making an inspection of an institution the request is always first for food 'Americanski producti,' secondly, for clothing and last of all for medicine. . . . Quinine and aspirin can do a patient no good when he is dying of hunger" (January 3, 1922).

In Samara, he discussed with district supervisor Shafroth the possibilities for feeding in the hospitals, even though food supplies were intended for children. Once he arrived back in Moscow in early January he learned about the US congressional appropriation of $20 million for the feeding of adults. He was delighted to share this information with the newly arrived district physician in Samara, Frederick Foucar: "It's possible now that we'll be able to do a lot more with adult feeding than we had planned." Shafroth, meanwhile, had just completed an inspection tour of the lower reaches of the Samara district, where he had observed a group of peasants hollowing out a large burial pit in anticipation of future corpses. Black clouds were gathering, he later recalled, "And then into the pervading gloom of this situation, like a shaft of light came the Christmas message from Mr. Hoover." The news spread quickly into Samara's villages that the Americans were promising to supply corn to adults. "Altho it was known that this food could not reach the Volga before March, the announcement put heart into the peasants who had already learned to trust our word."

+ + +

Davenport was hoping to become a "travelling man," a roving physician setting up operations in other districts in the famine zone. He would end up spending a considerable amount of time on the road, but at that moment Beeuwkes badly needed his services at Moscow headquarters. American doctors began to arrive in Moscow and be assigned to the districts. In November, the medical program began in Kazan, Samara, Moscow, and Petrograd. In December, operations spread to Simbirsk, Saratov, Tsaritsyn, and Orenburg, and in January 1922 to the Ufa district. It was in January that word arrived of the congressional appropriation of $4,000,000 for the purchase of surplus US Army medical stocks. As Beeuwkes noted in an interview in March 1922, "Medical starvation exists throughout Russia and is not confined to the Volga famine area." By spring 1922, the medical program was expanded into Ukraine and Belorussia (today Belarus) and the provinces in western Russia. Eventually operations were organized into sixteen separate medical relief districts, including the districts of Kiev, Kharkov, Odessa and Alexandrovsk for Ukraine, the district of Minsk for White Russia, Theodosia for the Crimea, and Rostov for southeastern Russia, extending south into the Caucasus region. The central provinces of Russia proper not located in the famine zone would later be reached by the ARA Sanitary Trains.

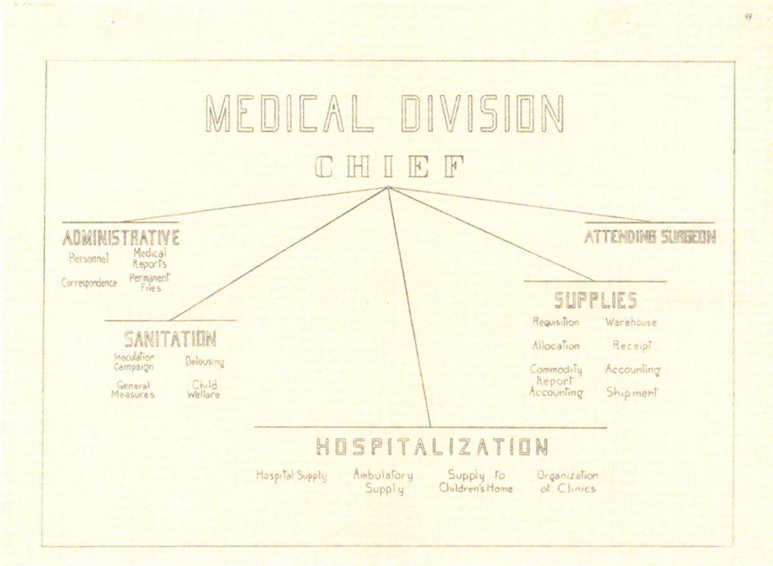

Assigned to each district was an American physician. They were recruited from the American Red Cross, the US Army, and civilian American medical facilities. Their chief responsibility was to supervise the distribution of the many varieties of medical supplies imported into Soviet Russia by the ARA. In other words, the district physicians were intended to be inspectors and controllers and not to practice medicine unless an ailing relief worker required their professional attention. The job entailed frequent inspections to determine institutional needs and to ensure proper use of supplies upon delivery, and also involved a considerable amount of paperwork, mostly in the form of monthly medical reports sent to Moscow. It was an ARA practice that nothing could simply be given away, that absolutely everything had to be accounted for.

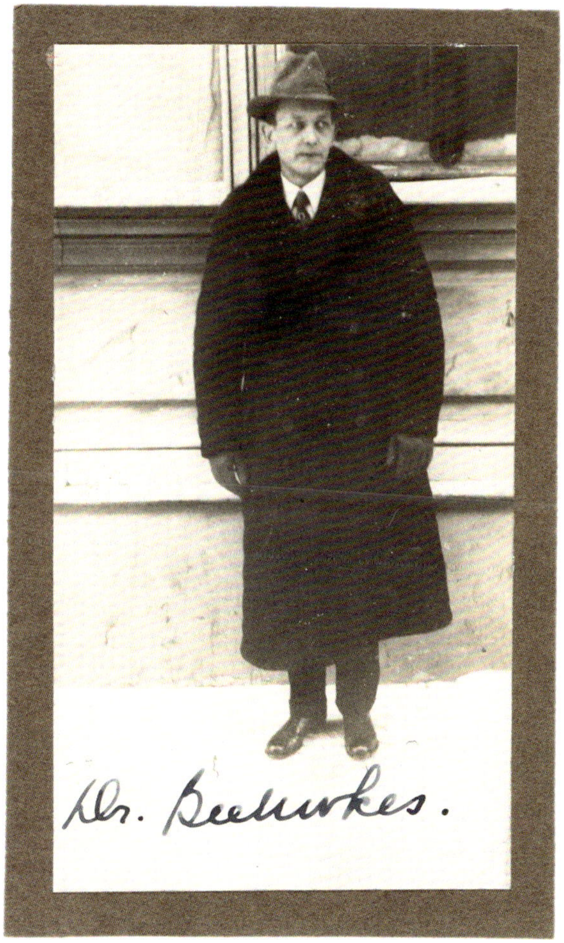

In the initial weeks of the medical program, supplies were slow in arriving in the districts, prompting importuning and complaining from the ARA physicians. The reason for this dearth was the delayed arrival of the Red Cross supplies. "The great bulk of American Red Cross supplies were purchased in America according to our requisitions, being shipped either direct to Riga or Petrograd from the United States, or forwarded to these ports after transshipment at Hamburg," Beeuwkes wrote.

> We had been informed by Red Cross officials that we might expect supplies within a month or six weeks after the receipt of requisitions. That estimate was entirely too optimistic; the first requisition was submitted on September 3, 1921, before we left America, and the corresponding shipments were not complete in Moscow until January 10, 1922, while the average time required was between three and four months with a maximum of six months. This adverse time element was due to delays in purchasing and shipping supplies in the United States and also due to the severity of the winter of 1921 [in Europe], and the blocking of northern seas by ice, making shipping very difficult for a considerable period.

But Beeuwkes had done some contingency planning. When Haskell's party arrived in England, he went directly to Paris, on September 10, where the Red Cross had identified surplus stocks totaling $600,000, which could be sent to Soviet Russia by train. "Though these stocks were not well rounded," Beeuwkes observed, "they included quantities of essential drugs, disinfectants, surgical dressings and hospital clothing, and as they arrived in Russia very promptly by overland shipments, we were able to begin work without material delay."

TOP: ARA Medical Division district organizational chart, 1922.

ABOVE: Dr. Henry Beeuwkes, Moscow, winter 1922.

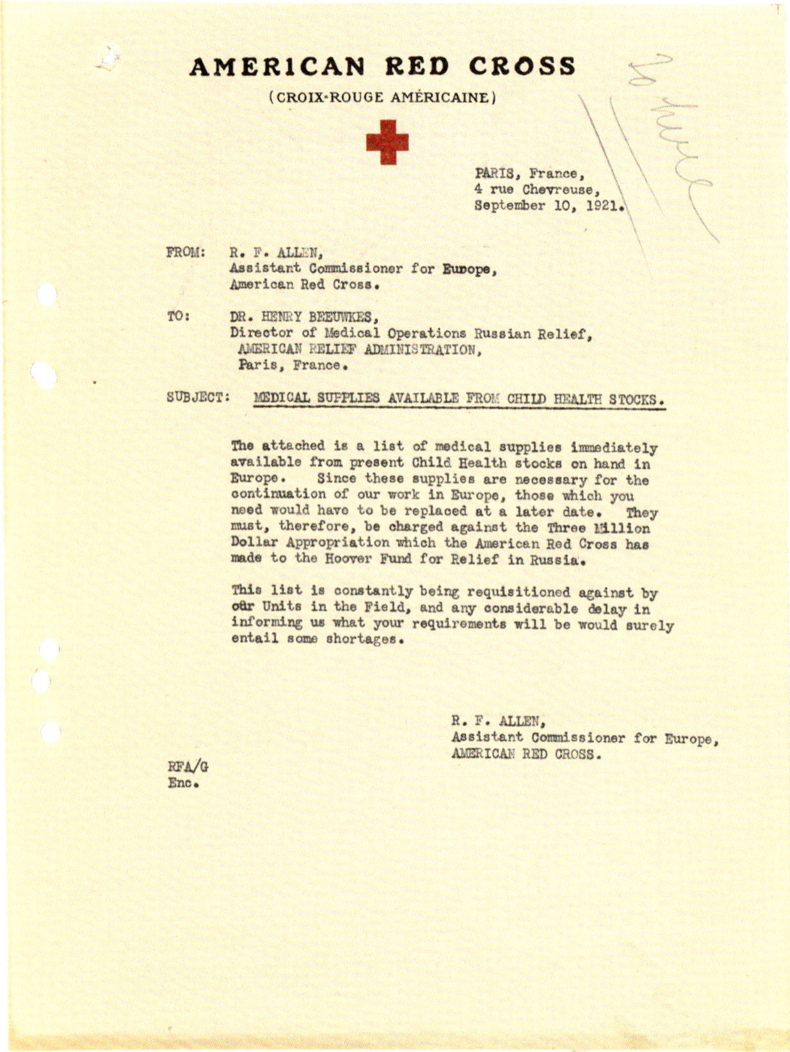

AMERICAN RED CROSS

(CROIX-ROUGE AMÉRICAINE)

PARIS, France,
4 rue Chevreuse,
September 10, 1921.

FROM: R. F. ALLEN,
Assistant Commissioner for Europe,
American Red Cross.

TO: DR. HENRY BEEUWKES,
Director of Medical Operations Russian Relief,
AMERICAN RELIEF ADMINISTRATION,
Paris, France.

SUBJECT: MEDICAL SUPPLIES AVAILABLE FROM CHILD HEALTH STOCKS.

The attached is a list of medical supplies immediately available from present Child Health stocks on hand in Europe. Since these supplies are necessary for the continuation of our work in Europe, those which you need would have to be replaced at a later date. They must, therefore, be charged against the Three Million Dollar Appropriation which the American Red Cross has made to the Hoover Fund for Relief in Russia.

This list is constantly being requisitioned against by our Units in the Field, and any considerable delay in informing us what your requirements will be would surely entail some shortages.

R. F. ALLEN,
Assistant Commissioner for Europe,
AMERICAN RED CROSS.

RFA/G
Enc.

Letter from R. F. Allen, American Red Cross office in Paris, to Dr. Henry Beeuwkes, September 10, 1921.

The American doctors in the field were unaware of the reasons for all the delays, and some assumed their requests had been forgotten or were being ignored. An intemperate blast to this effect from Dr. Foucar in Samara elicited a firm but friendly response from Beeuwkes, who informed Foucar, in a letter dated January 25, that Moscow was doing the best it could under the circumstances. "You know it is almost inconceivable that we are now distributing to the districts what we ordered September 3rd before leaving New York," he explained. "We fully expected that Requisition No. 1 would reach us in approximately six weeks, and yet it required about three and a half months time." What is more, transport from Moscow to the districts was often held up without headquarters being aware. "As an example: a carload of compresses, etc. which was turned over to the Supply Department on December 21st was not sent out to you until January 9th, together with two other loads. I fully thought you had received that long before it even left Moscow."

And there were more delays en route. In Orenburg, where weeks earlier Lyon had felt the situation to be "hopeless," Dr. A. B. Musa wrote to Beeuwkes on January 5, 1922: "Arriving at Orenburg 29 December 1921, I find that the cars containing the medical supplies are still buried in the snow within sixty miles of this city. We are told that fifteen hundred men are working to clear away the snow and that the cars will probably reach here within a week." Much greater logistical challenges lay ahead, especially once the American corn and wheat seed began to arrive in the Soviet ports.

\+ + +

At ARA headquarters in Moscow, Beeuwkes was absorbing all the information from the district and outlining a plan of action for the medical campaign. He later wrote:

> Our early medical surveys revealed a poverty stricken people existing on scanty rations, living under the most unhygienic conditions, more or less riddled by constitutional disease; great epidemics of typhus, relapsing and typhoid fevers sweeping the country; cholera quiescent but threatening in the spring; twenty-four millions facing starvation; a great uncontrolled refugee mass carrying disease; and a medical famine existing throughout the whole of Russia: patients without clothing; beds with few blankets and no sheets; operating rooms with scanty dressings; pharmacies without essential medicines; kitchens with little food.

With Davenport's assistance, Beeuwkes formulated a plan of operations for the district physicians. *Prevention* of disease would be a central component: cleanup campaigns of the hospitals and children's homes, streets, railway stations, and all

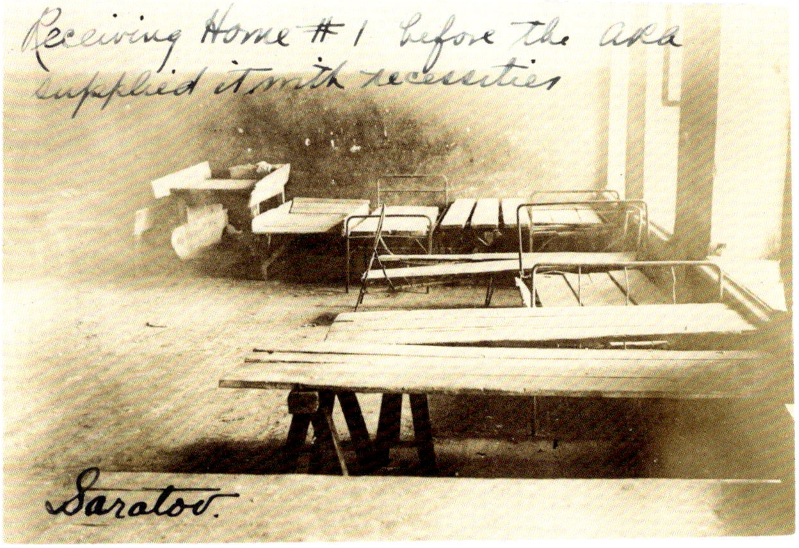
Receiving Home #1 before the ARA supplied it with necessities
Saratov.

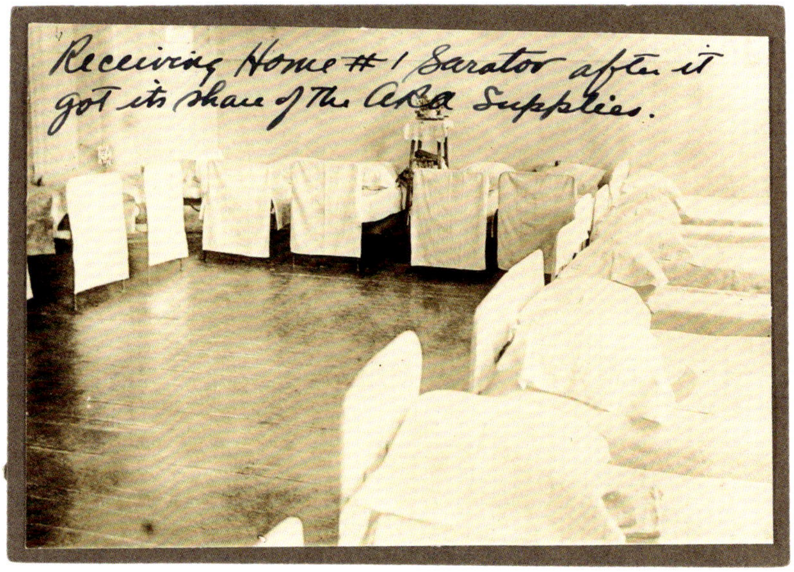
Receiving Home #1 Saratov after it got its share of the ARA Supplies.

Children's Receiving Home No. 1, Saratov, before and after being supplied by the ARA, fall 1921 and likely spring 1922.

other public places, especially where refugees gathered; bathing campaigns with ARA-supplied soap; disinfecting campaigns of clothing and interior spaces using sulphur; repair of water systems and the use of chloride of lime to purify water; and a vaccination campaign against typhoid, paratyphoid A and B, and cholera, with an additional vaccine against smallpox. These actions would help to contain and mitigate the spread of the epidemics of disease.

Beeuwkes also planned for the *treatment* of disease by sending massive quantities of essential medicines and all manner of hospital supplies to the American physicians in the outlying districts, and they, in turn, supplied hospitals, children's homes, refugee centers, ambulatories, and dispensaries with much-needed tools for disease treatment. Fully equipped and staffed hospitals would once again be able to house and care for patients who needed to isolate. Laboratories in major cities would receive supplies to make diagnostic medical tests and would increase staffing in order to begin producing a bivalent vaccine against typhoid and cholera.

Even the most modern preventive and therapeutic measures would amount to little, Beeuwkes reasoned, without the knowledge and expertise of Russian physicians and medical staff to employ them wisely and effectively. To fortify and sustain this essential workforce, Beeuwkes arranged for essential food and clothing packages to be sent out to the districts for distribution among those health care workers associated with the ARA medical campaign. As the American corn began to arrive, the Medical Division was able to support local medical personnel and hospital patients with rations of corn grits. Once fortified, Russian physicians, feldshers, nurses, midwives, pharmacists, medical students, and laboratory scientists would regain the physical and mental stamina necessary to serve the health needs of the Soviet people. The ultimate goal of the medical program, as of all Hoover relief campaigns, was self-reliance. As Beeuwkes reflected in a March 1922 press interview: "It is part of the gospel of the A.R.A. in Europe to teach people to help themselves and as soon as possible become independent of outside aid."

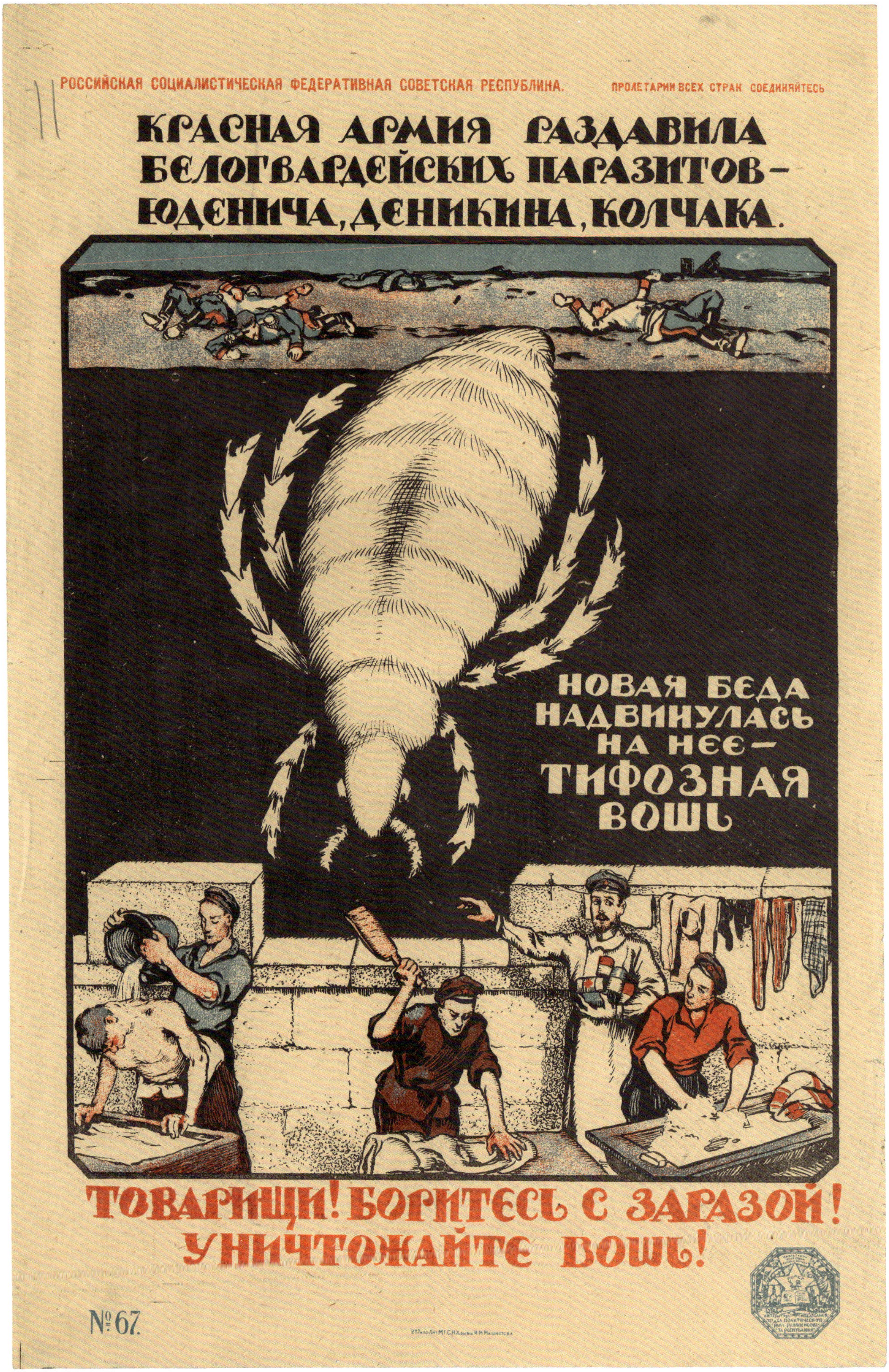
РОССИЙСКАЯ СОЦИАЛИСТИЧЕСКАЯ ФЕДЕРАТИВНАЯ СОВЕТСКАЯ РЕСПУБЛИКА.
ПРОЛЕТАРИИ ВСЕХ СТРАН СОЕДИНЯЙТЕСЬ
КРАСНАЯ АРМИЯ РАЗДАВИЛА БЕЛОГВАРДЕЙСКИХ ПАРАЗИТОВ – ЮДЕНИЧА, ДЕНИКИНА, КОЛЧАКА.
НОВАЯ БЕДА НАДВИНУЛАСЬ НА НЕЕ – ТИФОЗНАЯ ВОШЬ
ТОВАРИЩИ! БОРИТЕСЬ С ЗАРАЗОЙ! УНИЧТОЖАЙТЕ ВОШЬ!
№ 67.

CHAPTER 3

The Terror of Typhus

> "Either socialism will defeat the louse, or the louse will defeat socialism."
>
> —*Vladimir Lenin, Moscow, December 1919*

In December 1919 the Soviet regime had survived the worst onslaughts of the White armies in the Russian Civil War. Yet it found itself contending with another existential threat in the form of epidemic typhus. Between 1918 and 1922 there were as many as twenty-five million cases of typhus in Soviet Russia, causing two to three million deaths. At the moment Lenin was warning of the threat posed by lice, the Soviet government found it could barely cope with the situation.

The epidemic in Russia developed over many years and in several surges. From the late nineteenth century up to 1917, there was an estimated average of ninety thousand typhus cases a year but there were no nationwide epidemics, primarily because people remained in their relatively isolated villages. With little need for widespread travel, disease was not disseminated geographically. In 1918, at the end of the Great War, the roughly fifteen million men who made up the Imperial Russian Army began to return home, precipitating a disruption of the social order that would lead to a massive epidemic of typhus fever or spotted typhus.

There were three louse-borne diseases prevalent in the second decade of the twentieth century: trench fever hit the armies fighting on the Western Front hardest during the world war; troops on the Eastern Front were spared from trench fever but instead had to combat both typhus fever—also known as epidemic typhus, typhus exanthematicus, and spotted typhus—and relapsing fever, also called typhus recurrens. These latter two louse-borne diseases ravaged the soldiers alongside the influenza pandemic of 1918–1919. When wounded and sick Russian soldiers were evacuated from the front, protocol required that they first be examined for infectious disease and, if necessary, isolated at a local hospital. In the chaos of the evacuation and the urgency of wound treatment, many soldiers ill with typhus and relapsing fever nevertheless boarded trains and headed to medical facilities in the Russian interior, carrying infected lice with them.

Wounded soldiers may have launched the exposure of Russian civilians to typhus and relapsing fever, but the first large surge of disease occurred after the Bolshevik overthrow of the Provisional Government in November 1917, as upwards of fourteen million soldiers "self-demobilized" and flooded railway stations, overwhelmed the trains, and ultimately left thousands of people stranded at the stations. This influx of soldiers constituted the first surge of typhus into civilian Russia.

Unidentified artist (Russian), Красная Армия раздавила белогвардейских паразитов . . . Новая беда надвинулась на нее—тифозная вошь. Товарищи! Боритес с заразой! Уничтожайте вошь! [The Red Army crushed the White Guard parasites. . . . A new disaster looms over it—the typhus louse. Comrades! Fight the infection! Destroy the louse!], ca. 1921.
Poster Collection RU/SU 11

Another surge followed late in 1917 and into 1918, as nearly six million wartime refugees made their way from exile in eastern Russia back to their homes in the provinces abutting the western Russian border. At the same time, heading in the opposite direction were some four million repatriated Russian prisoners of war, which constituted a third wave. Often they crossed paths with their counterparts—and with members of a fourth wave: about 2.5 million German and Austrian prisoners of war, together with refugees traveling west toward Poland, less than half of them Poles.

By 1918, a frightening trio of conditions had come together in Russia to incite a deadly epidemic of typhus: an infected louse as the agent or vector of transmission; an exhausted civilian population with little or no health care because the medical systems and institutions had been devastated; and the crowded trains that crisscrossed Russia, transporting decommissioned troops, prisoners of war, and civilian refugees—"pools of human misery," in Harold Fisher's words—many of whom carried typhus over the vast expanse of Soviet Russia.

Typhus spread throughout Soviet Russia during 1919–1920 at a time when systems of basic medical care and sanitation were being dismantled or destroyed in the ebb and flow of the civil war. The rudimentary Soviet replacement, the People's Commissariat of Health, had yet to establish itself, and the most basic sanitary supplies—soap, disinfectants, fuel to run water pumps, even water—were scarce or absent altogether. Like all diseases, typhus took advantage of people with already weakened immune systems, the victims of the debilitating effects of the influenza pandemic, endemic tuberculosis, and sporadic outbreaks of seasonal cholera. The onset of famine in the summer of 1921 promised to catalyze the spread of the disease in the coming winter.

Without any curative treatment for typhus beyond rest and care of symptoms, prevention—through isolation, personal hygiene, and, on a larger scale, the use of sanitizing and disinfecting equipment—was the principal tool to combat the spread of lice infected with typhus. Military disinfecting stations had been successfully deployed throughout Europe during the world war, and in many countries they were repurposed at war's end for use in the civilian population. But Russia experienced successive revolutions in 1917 followed by a barbarous civil war, which deprived the country of the opportunity to recover and rebuild, and further disrupted the social order and eroded modern public utilities such as sanitation and water supply systems. Without these basic preventive measures, susceptibility to typhus in the civilian population rose exponentially. The prewar average annual number of cases—90,000—grew to about 142,000 in 1918 and close to five million in the years 1919–1920.

By November 1919, an alarmed Soviet government had implemented a major anti-typhus campaign, erecting nearly three hundred disinfection stations along the congested railways and waterways. At one point, disinfecting teams ministered to forty to fifty thousand passengers daily in Moscow train stations. Stories were told of military disinfection stations where, at the end of the day, the floor was carpeted in a two-inch layer of dead lice.

The government stepped up its propaganda campaign. Posters, pamphlets, and public lectures urged the public to practice cleanliness and hygiene. For illiterate peasants, graphic pictures were used to get the point across. The Sanitary Equipment Section of the People's Commissariat of Health (Narkomzdrav) ordered the production of more medical supplies and equipment. The edict met with shrugs and disbelief on the part of those tasked with acting on the order. They pointed to a lack of fuel and electricity, insufficient food rations, and the threat of conscription into the Red Army as ample reason for not fulfilling the government's request. Notwithstanding the government's efforts, 1920 witnessed a new wave of typhus throughout the country, the greatest surge yet, which peaked in February and only ended in June. Official data submitted to the League of Nations cited 3,962,201 cases in Russia in 1920.

CORDON SANITAIRE

Epidemic typhus initially appeared in wartime Poland in 1916 and persisted for four years afterward, largely due to reinfections caused by the reentry of waves of refugees displaced by war and POWs returning to Germany and Austria from Russia. Nearly twenty thousand Poles died of typhus in 1919. In response to the ongoing threat, the Supreme War Council, which included the heads of state of Great Britain, France, Italy, the United States, and Japan, appealed for help to Herbert Hoover and the Food Section of the Supreme Economic Council. In turn, Hoover approached the National Red Cross Societies, but because funds and personnel and supplies were not forthcoming from the great powers, the Red Cross was unable to take on the job of combating the spread of typhus in Poland.

Taking matters into his own hands, Hoover received permission from President Wilson to request that the United States Liquidation Board furnish the Polish Ministry of Health with the required equipment on credit. This included sanitary supplies valued at $6.5 million: steam sterilizers, mobile steam laundries, motorized bath plants, portable bathing plants, mobile machine shops, motor trucks, towels, and a hundred tons of soap. Hoover went one step further and convinced the boards in charge of disposing of supplies of the Allied armies to supply Poland with equipment on credit.

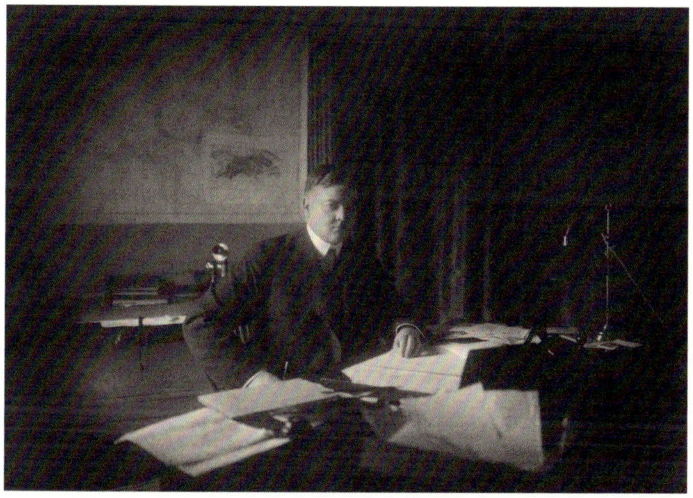

Herbert Hoover in Paris, 1919. Photograph by Studio Isabey.
World War I Pictorial Collection

It was the first step taken by America and European countries to create a "cordon sanitaire" to protect Poland and other neighboring countries from the westward spread of typhus. As Hoover explained in a letter to President Wilson at that time:

> One of the gravest questions before the Supreme Economic Council relates to the sanitation of Central Europe. A typhus epidemic is raging throughout eastern Poland. The disease is most easily controlled during the summer and displays its worst ravages during the winter. If the infected area is not cleaned of vermin during this summer, we must anticipate a dreadful epidemic during the coming winter with the great danger of spreading westward.

Equipment without experienced men to operate it was of little use, Hoover pointed out, requesting of Wilson and General John J. Pershing the services of Colonel Harry L. Gilchrist, Medical Corps, US Army, along with a detachment of officers for service with the Polish Ministry of Health.

During the war, Colonel Gilchrist had organized and led the highly successful effort to keep the American troops louse-free. At war's end he was stationed in Paris to oversee research on gas warfare, but in July 1919 he found himself back in the business of lice eradication when he assumed command of the American Typhus Relief Expedition in Poland. In August 1919, together with over five hundred enlisted volunteers and nearly thirty officers who were stationed in Paris, Colonel Gilchrist went to Poland, where his team worked for over a year installing and operating the steam laundries and bath plants for the populace, and disinfecting railway cars and quarantine stations, which often housed refugees. The work was arduous, and infection was always a real danger. But they maintained the "cordon sanitaire" up until the time when Russia invaded Poland in May 1920, at which point the anti-typhus campaign in Poland came to an abrupt halt.

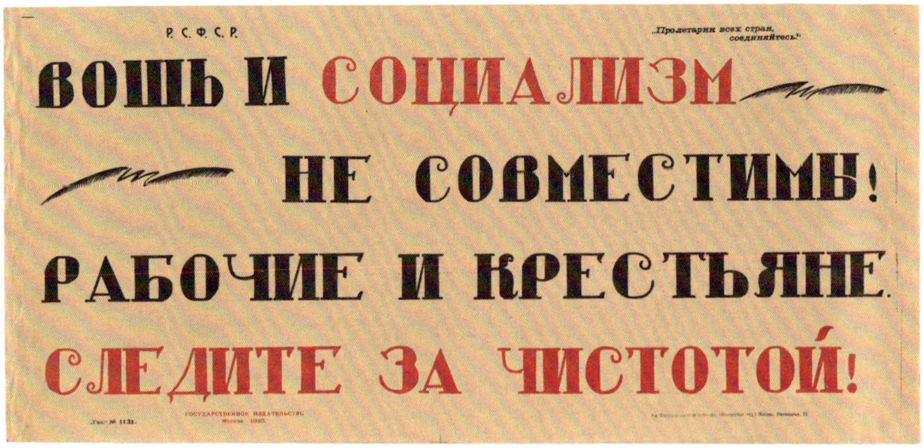

Soviet typhus poster, Вошь и социализм не совместимы! Рабочие и крестьяне—следите за чистотой! [The louse and socialism are not compatible. Workers and peasants–keep clean!], 1920.
Poster Collection RU/SU 1587

Only when the Russian Civil War wound down in 1920, and fewer people were moving about the country to participate in or flee the fighting, did the level of typhus in Russia actually dip, and Russian epidemiologists recorded a steady decline during the first ten months of 1921. The reprieve was destined to be brief. By the autumn of 1921, as a consequence of the famine, the disease recrudesced in another wave that peaked in summer 1922 and accounted for 1,402,683 official cases. Most diseases thrive on social disruption and human physiologic stress, conditions that were widespread and acute in famine-ravaged Russia. What had earlier been a "typhus of war" now became a "typhus of famine."

The Vector Identified

The exact method of transmission of typhus had been discovered only years earlier. In 1900, researchers determined that yellow fever was spread by a particular species of mosquito that carried the virus. This finding encouraged scientists to consider other insects as vectors, and in 1906 it led Howard Ricketts to identify the tick as the source of Rocky Mountain spotted fever. In 1909, he proposed that the human body louse—*Pediculus humanus corporis*—was the agent of infection for typhus. Ricketts died of the disease in 1910 before he could confirm his hypothesis. A contemporary of Ricketts, French bacteriologist Charles Nicolle, succeeded in proving that the human body louse did indeed spread typhus fever. This discovery, made in 1909, earned him the 1928 Nobel Prize in Physiology.

Working at the same time as Ricketts, Czech parasitologist Stanislaus von Prowazek had confirmed Ricketts's identification of the human body louse as the vector—and he, too, died of the disease, in 1914. In honor of these two dedicated researchers, pathologist Henrique da Rocha named the bacterium that causes the disease *Rickettsia prowazekii.*

The ability to identify a pathogen and a vector at the turn of the twentieth century marked a revolution in bacteriology. Before the 1880s, Russian doctors had correctly observed that typhus was associated with poverty, filth, and overcrowding. In the age of miasmatic thinking, however, they assumed it lingered in the air around those ill with the disease. Thus the physicians caring for the sick were at high risk of contracting the disease, and yet, oddly, so too were the laundresses who cleaned the louse-ridden clothing and bedding. In 1908, Russian bacteriologist N. F. Gamaleia, working at the esteemed Bacteriological Station in Odessa (today Odesa), observed another key feature associated with the occurrence of the disease: the presence of lice.

Typhus is derived from the Greek word *typhos*, meaning "smoky" or "hazy," in reference to the delirium that is a symptom of the disease. It is part of a group of diseases that are differentiated by the insect vector. Epidemic typhus is spread by the human body louse; scrub typhus is spread by chiggers (mites); and murine typhus is spread by fleas. Typhus in Russia was entirely the louse-borne Epidemic type and was also called typhus exanthematicus, or spotted typhus, in reference to the common symptom of body rash.

The ARA physicians in Soviet Russia filled out medical forms every month in which there was a category for the number of cases of what was at that time classified as the "Three Types of Typhus: Exanthematicus; Recurrens; Abdominalis." At best, this grouping reveals a lack of understanding about the causative agent of each disease; at worst it is misleading, because typhus recurrens was, in fact, relapsing fever, a louse-borne infection but of a spirochetal nature, like syphilis. Both relapsing fever and syphilis were successfully treated with the antimicrobial drug Neosalvarsan. Even more confusing was the term *typhus abdominalis*, which was in fact an entirely different disease—namely typhoid, which was a waterborne disease. And there was a vaccine to combat typhoid. A correct diagnosis identified with the accurate name of the disease meant the possibility of a curative treatment in the case of relapsing fever, or a preventive vaccination for typhoid.

Pediculus Humanus Corporis

By 1918, the human body louse had become the vilified mascot of soldiers in the Great War. The insect lived in clothing, especially rough seams, and flourished in the physical proximity of humans huddled together for warmth in trenches, in railway cars, or in cramped living quarters, all without the ability to maintain cleanliness. During winter and spring months when people were unlikely to bathe or even change clothes because of the cold, the temperature-sensitive louse nested and fed securely against human skin, driven out only if the person spiked a fever (too hot) or died (too cold). In fact, the louse was as much at risk from the typhus pathogen as was its host. It acquired the infection during its natural blood meal taken from an infected human, and it was destined to die within one or two weeks, turning bright red just before its demise. Until that time, however, it simply lived as a parasite, ingesting human blood, and defecating its bacteria-laden feces on its host's skin.

Typhus develops slowly, during an incubation period of about a week. After that the onset of symptoms is sudden and rapid: severe headache, fever rising to 104 degrees, full body aches. Around the fifth day, a rash may appear on the upper trunk, spreading all over the body except on the face, palms, and soles of the feet. The color of the rash turns from bright red to deep purple. A dry, barking cough adds to the discomfort. Bouts of mental confusion, hallucination, and delirium are often severe and prolonged.

By 1921, vaccines against cholera, typhoid, paratyphoid A and B, and smallpox were available worldwide. Antitoxins, made using serum taken from animals deliberately infected with a specific disease, existed for rabies, diphtheria, and tetanus. But there was no treatment, either preventive or curative, for typhus. That made the disease an object of terror and also the subject of high-priority

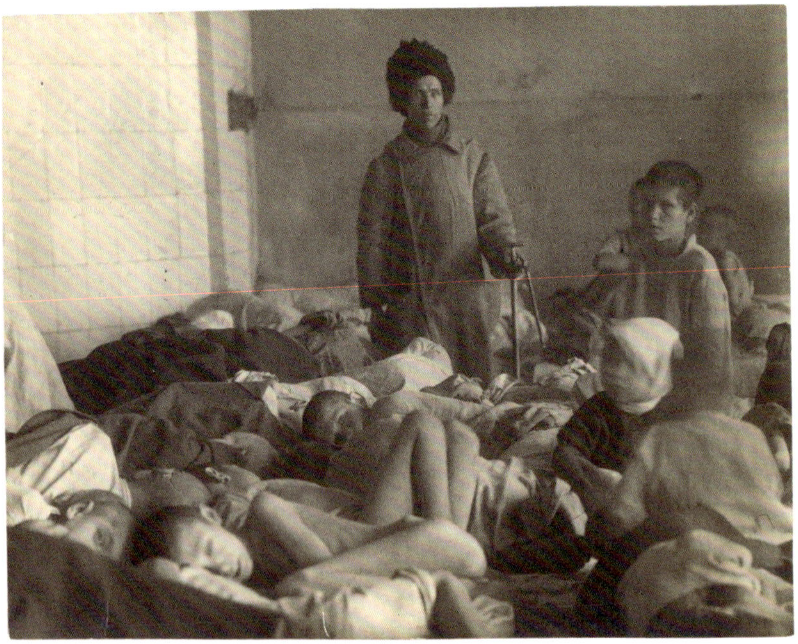

Children's home, Saratov, winter 1922.

research worldwide. In 1922, a commission organized by the League of Red Cross Societies to study typhus in Poland established that the human body louse was, in fact, the sole vector for typhus, and published its findings in *The Etiology and Pathology of Typhus*. The new book was made available to all the ARA physicians working in Russia and was included in the supply of medical literature donated to Russian medical schools. It was considered an example of cutting-edge research and science.

The Etiology and Pathology of Typhus endorsed a treatment for typhus that began with admitting the patient into an isolation hospital. The patient was shaved of all hair, bathed in soap and water, and rubbed all over with "light-wood oil" mixed with kerosene. A cloth cap was placed on the head to retain this oil mixture on the scalp. Digitalis or strychnia was given "for supportive effect" and camphor or caffeine in case of "collapse." All these addressed the low blood pressure (hypotension) and sluggish blood flow characteristic of the disease. Codeine was dosed for the cough, and a morphine shot worked to delay exhaustion from the cough, insomnia, and delirium. The scientific report noted candidly that none of the above treatments showed "any manifest advantage." Enemas were administered every second day, and cool sponge baths given for high fevers. Caregivers tried to relieve pressure points and resulting bedsores on the comatose body by turning the patient and adjusting with pads. Upon recovery, and with no complication such as gangrene, patients remained in the isolation hospital for an additional five to fifteen days.

The intensive and laborious care of typhus patients inevitably put caregivers at high risk for contracting the disease if infected lice were still present. The precautions they took included wearing special louse-proof gowns with closed stocking-footed trousers and full cloth head-coverings. Rubber gloves, tight-fitting at the wrists, and a spray of cedarwood oil at the wrists and neck-opening of the gown completed the armor. Gowns were deloused at the end of each day by placing them in galvanized iron cans with a generous sprinkling of naphthalene over each gown. Success of delousing was confirmed each morning when the boxes that had been placed among the gowns in each can revealed only dead lice.

The Campaign to Combat Typhus

In the early weeks of the medical campaign, Stephen Venear, an ARA medical staff member, made inspections of hospitals and children's homes in Kazan. He noted that each institution was "swarming with lice" and did not think that only smoke from sulphur and formaldehyde would work well enough to lessen the insect invasion. In one collecting home, with 900 children, 112 were sick with typhus. "All of them were lousy, many were picking them as we entered and there was not the slightest means of delousing these much worn out and filthy clothings," Venear wrote to Beeuwkes on November 1. Alarmed at the number already infected, a number that would likely only increase with colder weather, Venear asked for big guns in the form of delousing and disinfecting apparatuses to fight the epidemic.

On November 29, Beeuwkes inquired of Dr. Walter Davenport, who was out in the field inspecting conditions in Samara and Ufa, as to how best to approach typhus prevention. "Do you think our scheme looking forward to the preparation of baths and delousing stations practicable in Samara?" Davenport's bleak assessment of the state of hospitals he had inspected in Samara, which lacked fuel, food, clothing, medicines, and bathing and toilet facilities, "let alone some of the refinements as delousing, disinfecting and ventilating and laundry facilities," was a resounding answer in the negative. In other words, the fire was already out of control.

It became increasingly apparent to the ARA Medical Division during the autumn months of 1921 that conditions for any mass-scale disinfection campaign against typhus in Soviet Russia would differ significantly from the major effort undertaken during the world war, as well as the smaller one carried out in Poland in 1919. Delousing a population and disinfecting clothes had been practiced and nearly perfected by the Western armies during World War I. It was one of the basic techniques for disease control and was at the heart of all public health. And it was missing on a grand scale in Russia, allowing diseases with a louse vector to spread like wildfire. During the winter months of 1921–1922, each of the American district physicians conveyed to Beeuwkes the same message: there was positively no systematic delousing going on anywhere.

The infrastructure in large areas of Soviet Russia was in ruins. To fight a civil war against the White armies, the Red Army under Leon Trotsky had requisitioned nearly every useful item from the civilian population, often including so much of the plumbing equipment that cities, towns, and villages were left without the operating water pumps and plumbing needed for basic water supply or for sanitation systems. The local governments had no money to buy fuel to run the water pumps and furnaces for the bathhouses or to pay attendants; the bathhouses, which were in a state of disrepair, could not be fixed for lack of funds and parts; and there was no soap for washing or disinfectants such as sulphur, creosol, or formaldehyde for killing lice in clothing. Only the largest hospitals in the major cities could set aside rooms for disinfecting clothes, usually using sulphur fumes, which required no water. Where a bathhouse did exist and was operational, it was private and too expensive for the average person. It became incumbent on the ARA physicians to convince the district boards of health that bathing was not a luxury, but a basic sanitary necessity and one of the keys to effective public health.

The ARA physicians in the famine districts eventually and independently were confronted by the fundamental shortage of fuel needed to operate the pumps and provide water, which rendered the option of using the kind of efficient mobile steam laundries and bath plants that had served so well during the war, and later in Poland, moot from the start. Instead, the ARA medical team resorted to using massive amounts of fumigating disinfectants, which did not require water: 800,000 pounds of sulphur; 200,000 pounds of creosol; 200,000 pounds of formaldehyde; 60,000 bottles of carbolic acid; and 55,000 bottles of corrosive sublimate (mercuric chloride) for use in hospitals, institutions, and disinfecting chambers. Finally, 2,400,000 pounds of soap made their way into the hands of the Russian people. Soap would be made available in most ARA kitchens, where children arriving to receive their daily meal would be made to wash their hands and face before receiving their food.

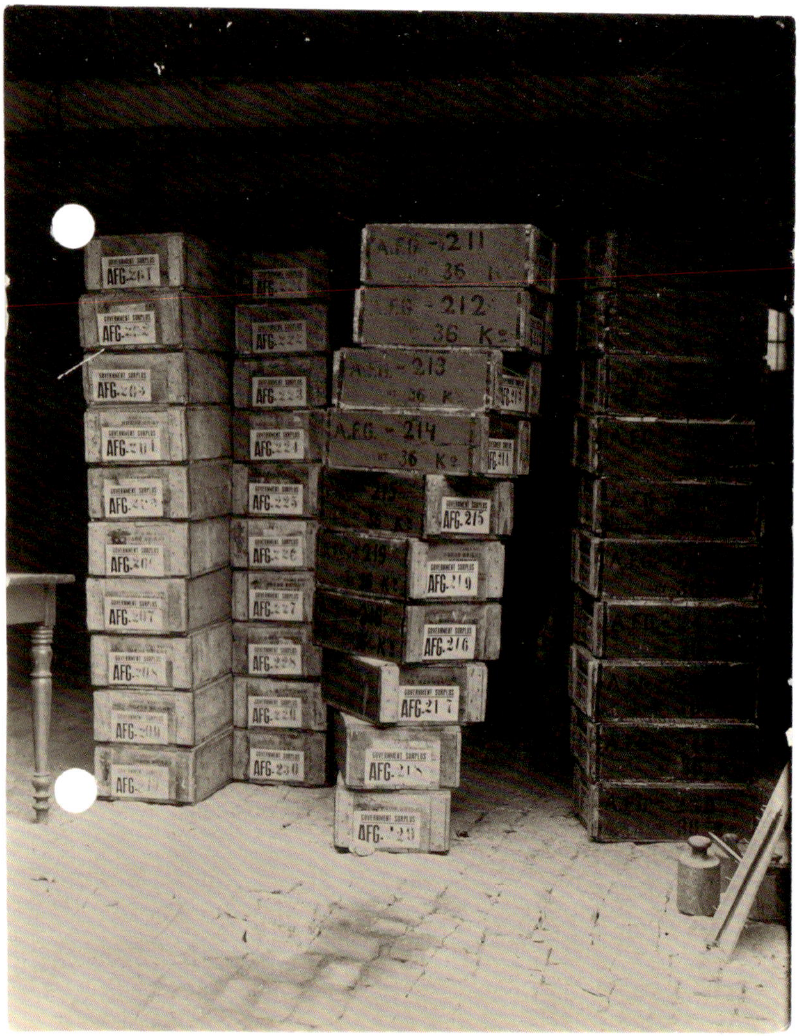

Armed with medicines and hospital supplies, each district physician laid plans to address the diseases prevalent in his district, beginning with personal inspections of hospitals, children's homes, and other medical institutions. The American physician assessed the needs and supplied the materials. It was a practical, curative plan that was theoretically achievable, that is, until each district physician grasped the fact that underlying the spread of disease was a more fundamental problem, one that would nullify therapeutic relief efforts unless it was addressed first.

The sanitary practices in most Russian towns and villages bordered on primitive; by 1921, they were nearly nonexistent. Dr. Raymond McKnight Sloan reported his disbelief at the state of affairs in Ufa: "The population were appallingly ignorant of personal hygiene and sanitation and the various Governmental Departments failed to properly cooperate in this work." Dr. Otto Beck in Orenburg concurred: "the people, uninstructed in the rules of sanitation[,] are guilty of a mode of life contrary to the cardinal rules of health." Treating disease with medicine under such conditions was like putting a Band-Aid on a gaping gash.

Most of the ARA doctors reached their posts in the famine zone by January 1922. It was prime typhus season, driven by overcrowding in unheated homes, a massive refugee movement in search of food, lack of fuel for water pumps and for any bathing, a lack of clothing, and a complete absence of disinfectants. Soap was "the commodity most called for," emphasized Dr. Beck in an April 20, 1922, letter from Orenburg. "We can use all the soap that the A.R.A. possesses." The first steps in bringing provincial Russia back into a modern sanitary age would start with the 2,400,000 pounds of soap provided by the ARA.

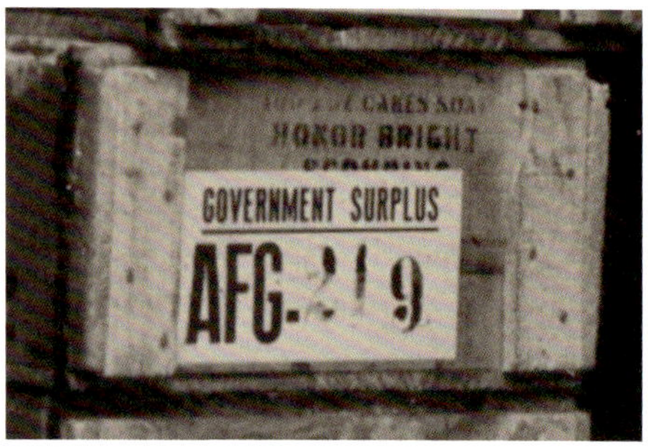

Crates containing soap, among the surplus US Army supplies provided to the ARA in Soviet Russia from the stocks of the American Forces in Germany (AFG), in Coblenz, Germany, 1922.

DETAIL: Honor Bright Soap lettering visible on shipping crate.

Refugees

The approach to delousing a local, stationary population centered on bathing and disinfecting, seemingly achievable by the ARA medical relief efforts. But these local populations, especially those situated along the major railroad lines, were continually exposed to the greatest disseminator of typhus: the refugee. When thousands of displaced people camped in railway stations, or in local cellars and hallways, crowded human conditions persisted, lice proliferated, and typhus remained an epidemic threat. The situation presented the district physicians with a logistical puzzle and the question of where best to direct their efforts.

Dr. Frederick Foucar in Samara, a major railroad junction, made refugees a priority and pressed to have them removed from the railway stations and segregated into barracks where they could be properly inspected for disease, isolated, and hospitalized if necessary. It was a "filtration" process, as Foucar called it, straight out of army practice. The ARA supplied materials for bathing refugees, disinfected their clothing, and fed them once a day. Nutrition was considered an important tool to combat disease. But the gradual success of the program came with a price.

Russians employed by the ARA to screen the refugees were often exposed to infected lice, and too often they succumbed to typhus within a mere three weeks of contact. Consequently, the ARA medical care that was available to the Americans was also extended to all Russian employees and their families.

In Ufa, Dr. Sloan recognized a similar threat to railroad employees who herded refugees daily away from the stations. Knowing how critical the railroads were to the entire medical relief effort for transporting supplies and medicines, Sloan made sure to keep the hospitals that served the railroad workers well supplied with disinfectants. A sprinkling of chloride of lime on the station platforms or the odor of ARA-supplied Lysol inside the railroad stations indicated successful sanitary efforts. While these sanitary measures curtailed the spread of lice and disease from refugees, most of the Americans realized that the larger goal was to stem the tide of refugee travel altogether.

As spring approached, typhus naturally lessened its hold on the population. The warmer weather enabled people to shed layers of clothing and bathe outdoors in the rivers. Many Russian refugees headed home to their villages in anticipation of summer work in the fields. The remaining refugees, mostly from other

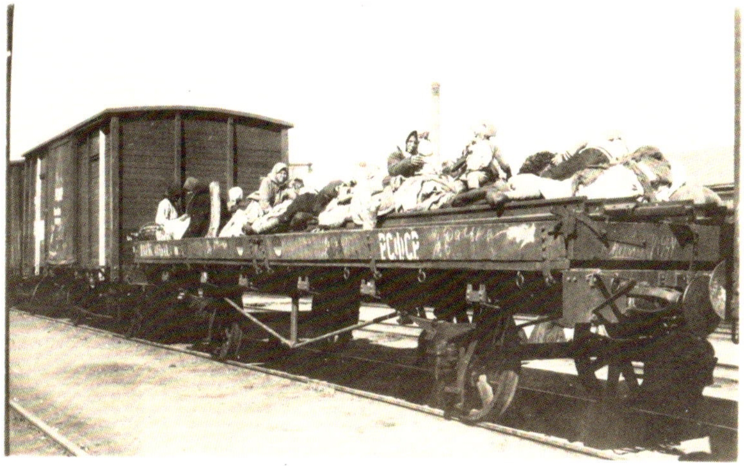

ABOVE: Refugees in flight from the famine, autumn 1921. American Relief Administration European operational records

BELOW: Map made by the ARA in Moscow showing refugee movements in Soviet Russia, ca. 1922.

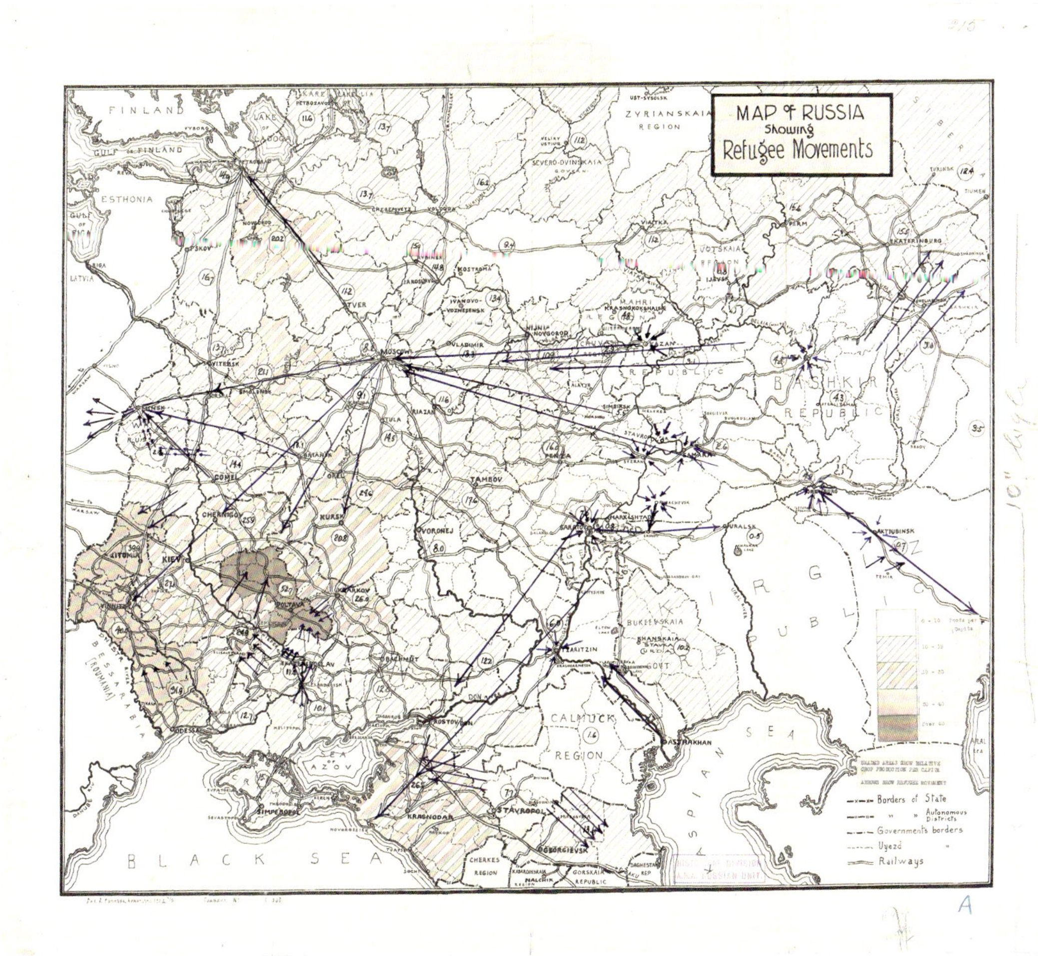

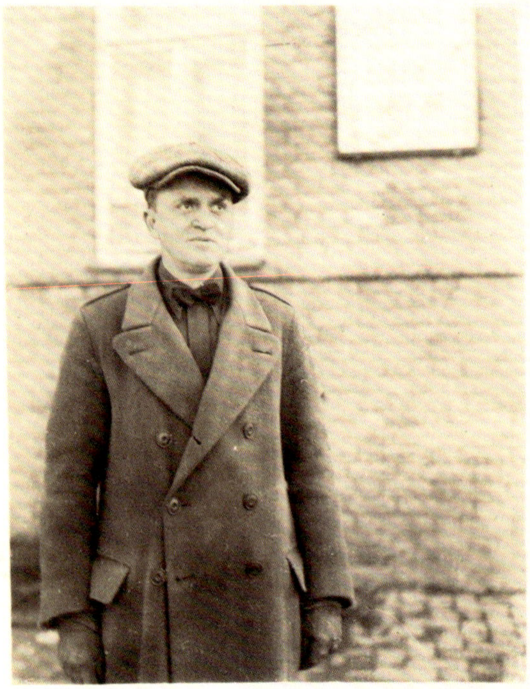

countries, and former POWs continued to migrate westward and homeward to Poland, Latvia, Estonia, and Lithuania. The Soviet government further reduced the numbers of displaced persons traveling by rail and boat when they increased the cost of travel, placing the option out of financial reach for most people.

Russian Baths

Dealing with refugees was a first line of attack on the louse-borne diseases of typhus and relapsing fever. The next step in the campaign involved attention to the equally needy local populations. They, too, deserved basic sanitary services, but they were at the mercy of the local governments that were helpless to provide sufficient resources—physical or financial—for sanitary improvement. Dr. Foucar in Samara, ever the man to take on a problem directly, proposed the model of an ARA free bathhouse for the poorest and neediest, a plan that worked around the fee required by most local establishments. The ARA would shoulder the expense of the bathhouse, starting with the repairs necessary for its function: installing windows, repairing plumbing and furnaces, and getting the steam disinfecting autoclaves in working order.

The local workers doing the repairs and the personnel assigned to run and maintain the baths would be paid with ARA food packages or corn rations. Only the supply of fuel needed to pump the water and heat it remained unaccounted for, and Foucar, to his delight, managed to secure the agreement of the local Samara board of health to provide this.

On January 3, 1923, the first ARA bathhouse opened in the city of Samara: the Chaikovsky Bath House, purposed to bathe 2,000 people a day and at the same time disinfect clothing in a steam-formalin chamber. The bathing groups included

ABOVE: Dr. Frederick Foucar, ARA district physician in Samara, 1922. A native of New York City, Foucar received his medical degree from Columbia University and served as a major in the US Army Medical Corps before joining the ARA in Soviet Russia.

BELOW RIGHT: Children queue up outside an ARA bathhouse, Samara, winter 1922.

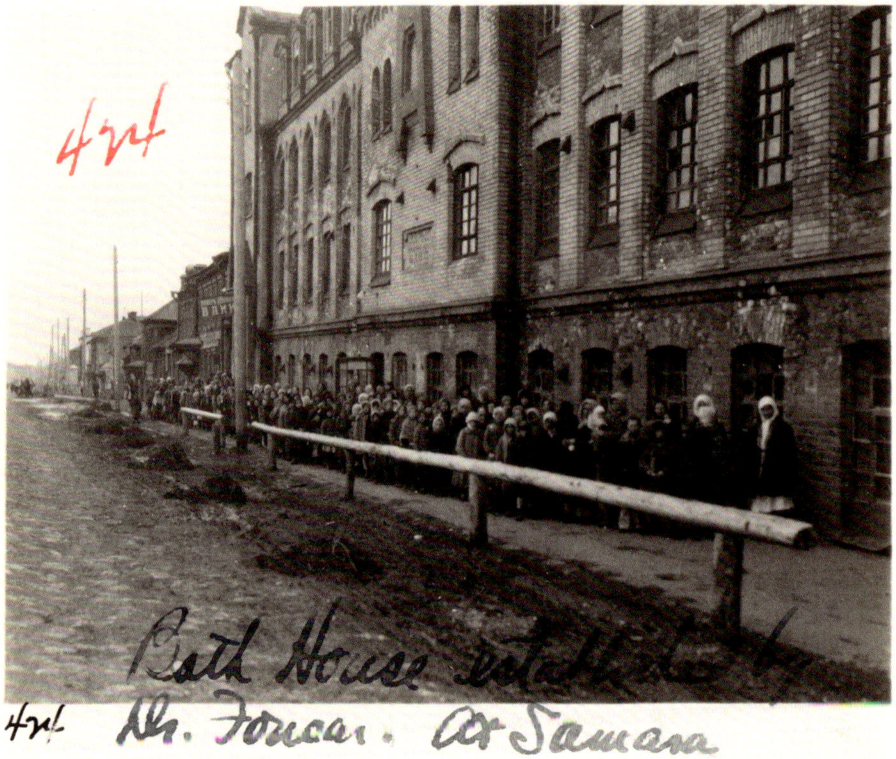

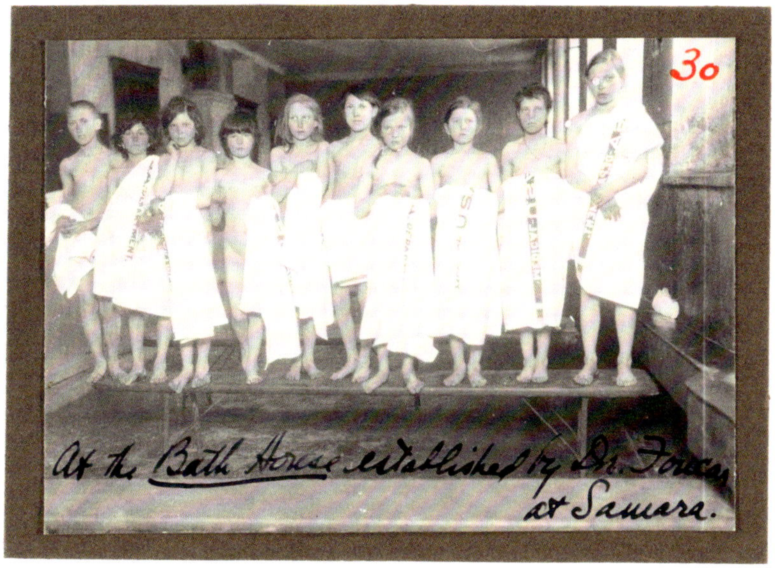
30
At the Bath House established by Dr. Foucar at Samara.

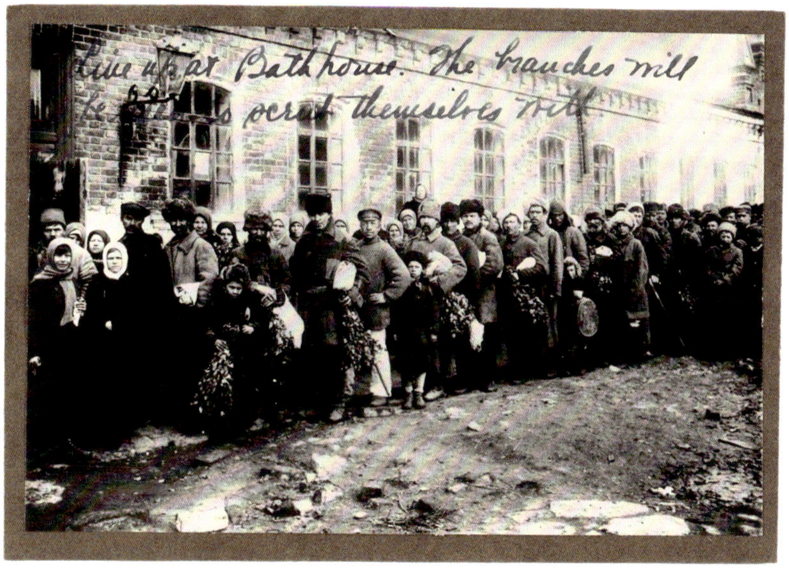
Line up at Bathhouse.

children from children's homes; the poor and unemployed; union workers; Samara University students; and Gubzdrav (Board of Health) employees. Tickets to the bathhouse were given to hospitals for distribution to needy patients. Staff workers at the bath provided bathers with a cube of soap cut from a larger bar and a towel.

ABOVE LEFT: Children inside an ARA bathhouse, Samara, winter 1922.

ABOVE RIGHT: Adults queue up outside an ARA bathhouse, Samara, winter 1922.

BELOW: Children at an ARA bathhouse, Odessa, 1922.

Typical Russian baths involved two steps: the first in a steaming room in which bathers beat their skin with a switch of twigs to enhance circulation and force dirt from skin pores; they then moved to the washroom to wash with soap and water. Children were given a pail of warm water and a small cube of soap in the steaming room. Working together, the children would lather each other, then dump the pail of soapy water over their bodies, followed by a rinse from a pail of clean water. Once free of dirt and lice, and most often with hair newly clipped or shaved, bathers then reclaimed their disinfected clothing.

After a total of 23,896 locals used the Samara facility in just the first twenty-one days, Dr. Foucar relished the success, knowing that the ARA had significantly reduced the incidence of typhus among an impoverished population. And within the month the effort multiplied when the ARA opened another free bath in the city, and the local board of health joined the sanitary campaign by opening three more.

Other districts had equally successful free baths. In Odessa, Dr. W. R. Smith complained to Beeuwkes that the local government had increased the tax on water such that the poor were unable to pay it and the city simply shut off their water supply. Once again, the Americans engineered a work-around. On August 1, 1922, a free ARA bathhouse for children opened in Odessa. On the first day, 2,600 children from the twenty-one ARA feeding stations were bathed and had their clothes disinfected; on the eighth day the number had reached 6,300. In addition, nearly 2,000 children from other homes enjoyed the bath, and one day was set aside for students from the University of Odessa and employees working for the ARA. A disinfecting chamber disinfected clothing placed in individual bags within 20–25 minutes while the bathers were cleansing.

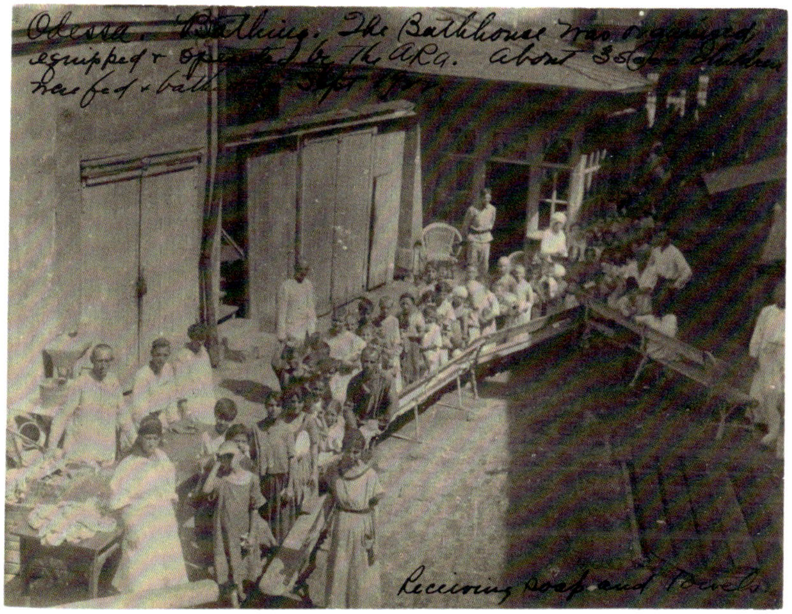
Odessa. Bathing.
Receiving soap and towels.

In Moscow, newly washed children standing in line at an ARA food kitchen greeted Dr. William Nickelsen with an exuberant "*Bani—bolshoe spasibo!*"—meaning "Baths—many thanks!"

The Great Equalizer

Probably the greatest single threat to the physical well-being of the American relief workers in Russia was typhus. For protection against other forms of infectious disease, such as cholera, which was widespread in the summer of 1922, the relief worker could be vaccinated; but typhus was the great equalizer.

Many ARA workers had already made the acquaintance of the typhus louse, dubbed the "cootie," during the Great War, but they had seen nothing like what the Russian setting had to offer. An ARA feeding instruction manual stated the danger plainly, calling the louse the "greatest enemy to mankind today in Russia." There are numerous depictions of refugees at train stations engaged in mutual delousing, an activity described by more than one American as "the favorite indoor and outdoor sport in Russia."

Although the Americans of the ARA were not nearly as exposed to the dangers as were their beneficiaries or even their local employees, the fear of infection was a continuous source of anxiety among them. This did not prevent the louse from becoming, as it had been among the doughboys in recent years, an object of black humor. The weekly ARA newsletter produced in Moscow, the "Russian Unit Record," brought to light a good-natured difference of opinion among the personnel as to the most effective preventive measures for stopping the cootie in his tracks: some, dubbed "smooth roaders," advocated the wearing of silk underwear; the rest of the crowd were "rough roaders."

When ARA publicity chief George Barr Baker returned from his February visit to Soviet Russia, he released a statement to the press on the mode of operations of the Russian louse. As reported in the "New York News Letter of the A.R.A.," under the title "*Pediculus vestimenti muscovitus*," Baker had "recently returned from a first hand observation of this versatile vermin on its native Russian heath." Mr. Louse, according to Baker, took three working days to accomplish his deadly mission. "On the first day, he takes up his position on the human frame and devotes himself to exquisite and diabolical meditation; on the second day, he discharges his cargo of fatal juices and retires to his thoughts until the third day, when he buries his obnoxious cargo beneath the epidermis of his victim." Soap and water were said to be the "pet abominations" of Sir Louse, and it was found that frequent revolving of one's underwear hampered his progress. "First allow him to work his way through the strands of your balbriggan; then turn the garment inside out forcing him to repeat the digging-in process. By constantly reversing the garment, M. Louse will become utterly exhausted." Evidently Baker was a "rough roader."

That the cootie had penetrated the consciousness of everyday life in Moscow is illustrated in ARA representative Harold Fleming's description of a ride on a streetcar, a means of transportation that doubled as vehicle for the spread of typhus. The scene Fleming recounts involves a car typically overcrowded with passengers, not all of them of the human variety.

> Now having gotten all the dirty ones into this means of common intercourse, you push them up against each other as far as they can go till they hang on

the outer doors, and compel them to rub themselves against each other as much as possible. Having gotten them well rubbed, you then required them to leave the car by the forward door, instead of the rear door by which they came in, and when they hesitate, you push them on and say, "Go on up there and get infected!"

The Americans stationed in the capital could better afford such levity, for as compared with their colleagues in the famine districts they were hardly at all in danger of infection. But as soon as they climbed on board that train departing Moscow for the provinces they left behind their relative invulnerability. The Russians who worked for the ARA as couriers and whose job involved nearly continuous train travel fell victim in large numbers, with nearly one-third of their number becoming infected during the first year of the mission.

New American arrivals to Moscow had the danger impressed upon them and anticipated their rail journey into the famine zone with considerable trepidation. Dr. George Cornick, setting out from Moscow by train for Tsaritsyn on Christmas Eve 1921, confided to his diary that he was "trusting to insect powders, luck and the Lord on high to protect me from Typhus and recurrent fever this trip." William Kelley left Moscow for the Volga the following day, and he shared in the paranoia: "Last night I refused to take off a single garment. I stretched out with the flannel lining of my trench coat on me and the coat itself as a cover. The equipment of the wagon-lit is limited to a mattress and a pillow, both under suspicion. I was not aware that I was sleeping for very long intervals but morning came soon enough."

Often the only space available on a train was in a car packed with refugees. Dr. Mark Godfrey, en route to his assignment as district physician in Simbirsk in December 1921, recounted in a letter to Beeuwkes his reception by his fellow train travelers:

> When the peasants learned that I was an American Doctor they cleared off and gave us an entire seat about eight feet long and observed me with great respect. One fearing that my feet were cold dug out some carpet and came and wrapped them up for me. I slipped in some naphthalene and hoped for the best. A little later another fellow seeing that I still looked cold outdid his friend by giving me a big buffalo skin to wrap up in. Not only did he give it to me but he actually wrapped me up. . . . Of course I pulled out more naphthalene and besprinkled myself with it.

Despite the genuine risk of being infected with lice, Godfrey saw the generosity in the Russians' gestures, telling Beeuwkes: "I am for these people. They are a good people I am sure."

Shortly after Freddie Lyon arrived in Orenburg in November 1921 to open up ARA headquarters there, he dashed off a letter to a Moscow colleague describing his journey, which brought his train into Orenburg at 1:30 a.m. He bunked down in the train station hoping to get some shut-eye, but as he tells it, the local citizens kept him occupied by walking on his feet and spitting the shucks of sunflower seeds in his face. And there was more. "Any desire that I may have had for sleep was taken away after witnessing the wild gesticulations of my fellow travelers in

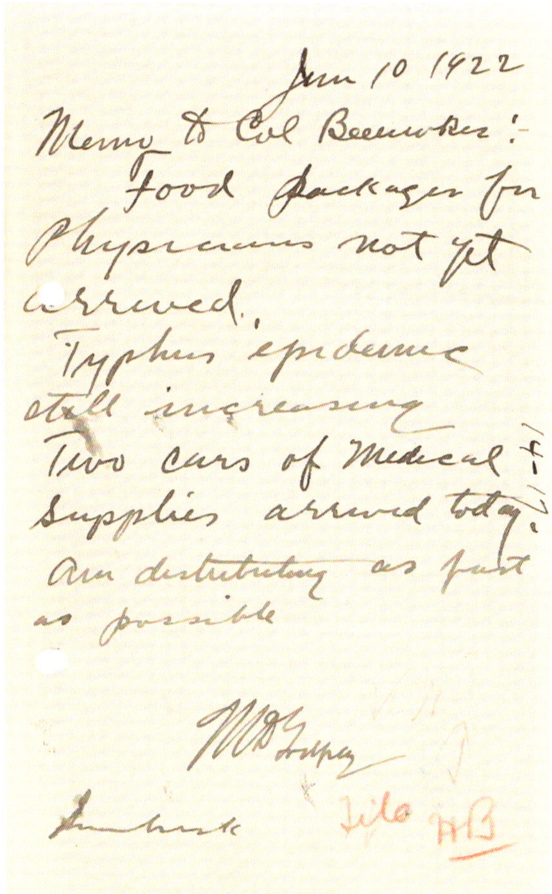
Jan 10 1922
Memo to Col Beeuwkes:-
Food packages for Physicians not yet arrived.
Typhus epidemic still increasing
Two cars of Medical Supplies arrived today.
Are distributing as fast as possible
MDGodfrey
Simbirsk
File
HB

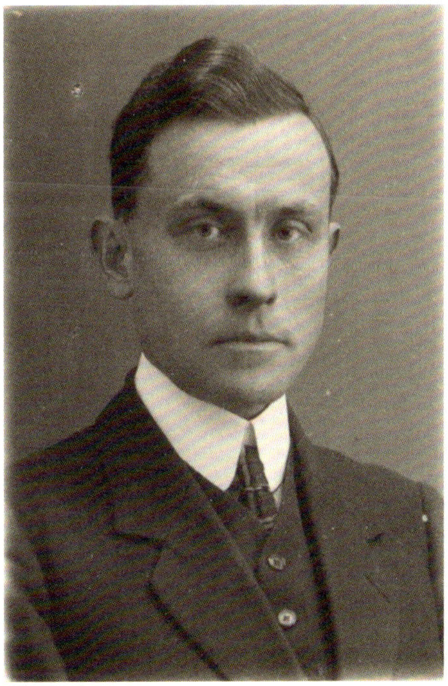

TOP: Handwritten memo from Dr. Mark Godfrey, ARA district physician in Simbirsk, to Henry Beeuwkes in Moscow, January 10, 1922.

ABOVE: Dr. Mark Godfrey, ca. 1921.

their pursuit of the ever present insect, the flea or louse." At Lyon's outpost in Orenburg the threat of typhus was substantial: at one time as many as a quarter of the ARA's local Russian employees across the district were stricken.

It is remarkable that out of three hundred Americans in the mission only eight relief workers contracted typhus while in Russia, and of them there was only one fatality.

This was not simply a result of the preventive measures taken by individuals but was partly a reflection of the ARA's modus operandi. An American's contracting typhus in the famine region was considered a serious affair, with consequences extending beyond the health of the particular individual. American manpower was spread thin in the districts, and the loss of one relief worker for several weeks, especially a district supervisor, increased the already enormous burden on his colleagues and threatened the efficiency of ARA operations. Still, beyond that, there was something more at work. An American laid low by typhus was regarded within the organization as a threat to its reputation as a smooth-running machine. It was the American's duty to take all preventive measures in order to keep himself in good health and on the job. To be outwitted by Mr. Louse was to fall short of being a clever and efficient relief worker.

The ARA district physicians worked louse-free in their respective headquarters, warehouses, and living quarters by following strict precautions. They were well armed with soap, water, naphthalene, and sulphur. But their duties included periodic inspections of hospitals, children's homes, even refugee centers located far and wide in their districts, and, depending on the time of year, sometimes requiring a three-day journey in a railway car packed with refugees, and, when traveling by sleigh, perhaps an overnight stay in a peasant dwelling.

One such trip by sleigh involved James Rives Childs, ARA district supervisor in Kazan. To pass a few hours while waiting for a change of horses for his sleigh, he was conducted into a peasant hut, which he described as "one of the filthiest homes into which it has ever been my lot to be introduced. . . . I was worn out and I desired to lie down, but when I saw bugs crawling about the floor, I changed my mind. I took my seat on a bench alongside the wall and was about to put down my

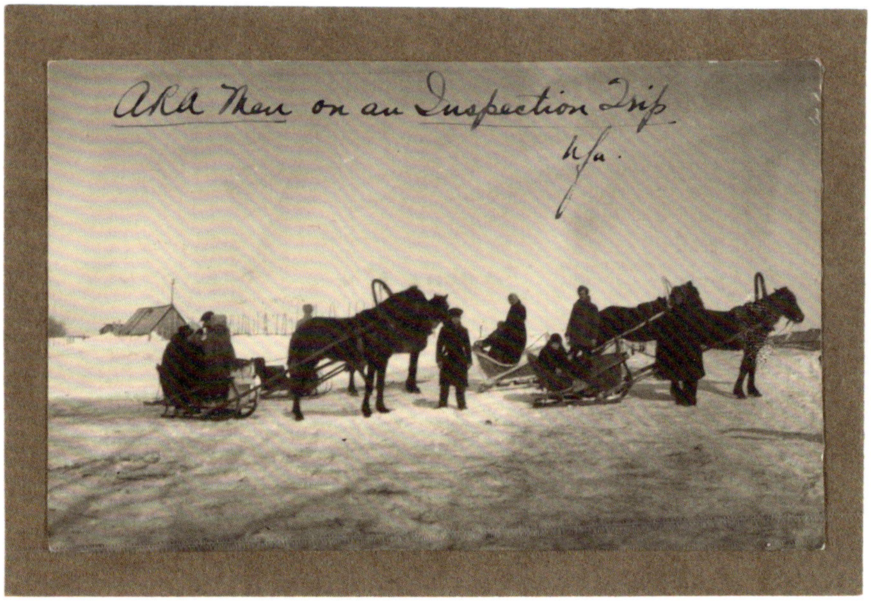

ARA men on an inspection trip in the district of Ufa, winter 1922.

coats and lie upon these on the bench, when I took one look at the wall and felt my skin creep at the sight of the hundreds of bugs which were disporting themselves behind me."

Some travelers brought along a folding cot, thus solving one problem, although it could do nothing to improve the air. After a frustrating day's journey by sleigh, Stephen Martindale's only refuge for the night was a cottage that was so filthy and malodorous that he retreated outside into the sleigh and, under two fur coats, went to sleep. In the morning, his interpreter found him half-frozen and had to apply a snow massage to thaw him out. While Martindale's experience was not unusual, more typically, with the temperature outside dipping to thirty degrees below zero, the decision to retire to the sleigh was arrived at only after a few fitful hours spent in the close air of the peasant's hut conjuring up terrifying images of the invisible typhus carrier within.

It is likely that the precautionary measures they took against typhus contributed to the Americans' reputation for being cold and aloof. "We never think of picking up the kids or even patting them on the head for fear of infection." This is Kelley writing about Ufa, but the statement could well have come from almost any of the Americans in the famine zone. Cornick wrote to his parents on January 19, 1922, describing the outdoor ceremonies in Tsaritsyn marking "one of the big Church holidays," where "the crowd got too thick and we like to avoid crowds on account of the filth and vermin." He relates that on this religious holiday the waters of the Volga River were said to have "healing properties" and that "every man woman and child had a bucket or pail with which they dipped some of the water from this common bathing hole and drank. Instead of healing them I of course feel that this will help to further spread the Typhoid, cholera, and dysentery, but religious customs can not be changed."

In November 1921, Colonel Walter Bell, district supervisor in Ufa, known as the gateway to Siberia, was out on an inspection in the town of Belyi Bey when he felt the onset of fever and chills. He dropped into delirium on the three-day sleigh ride back to the ARA headquarters in Ufa, regaining full consciousness three weeks later. Dr. Davenport, traveling from Samara, attended to Bell during the entire period. "This was a blessing from the Gods," wrote Bell's translator, Boris Elperin, "for Bell's condition was so serious that none of the Russians held out any hope for him."

When Davenport arrived, Bell had already been ill for five days, at which point the telltale rash appeared and verified the diagnosis of "typhus exanthematic" or spotted typhus. He was delirious, with a temperature of 104 degrees Fahrenheit. After seventeen days, Davenport assumed Bell had passed the crisis and was on the mend but the patient was still extremely weak and had severe bronchitis. Davenport informed Beeuwkes that the local medical care had been first-rate, employing the standard treatments of camphor in oil, caffeine, digitalis, strophanthinum (all for cardiac stimulation), along with sodium benzoate (perhaps used like sodium bicarbonate). The physicians caring for Bell were attuned to cardiac exhaustion from the prolonged high fever; hence the use of all the stimulants.

Chicago Daily News reporter F. A. Mackenzie, arriving in Ufa at this juncture, seemed to hold out no hope for the colonel. His book *Russia Before Dawn*, published in 1923, leaves the impression that Bell had given up the ghost: "The list of deaths among relief workers was soon to grow." In fact, while members of the

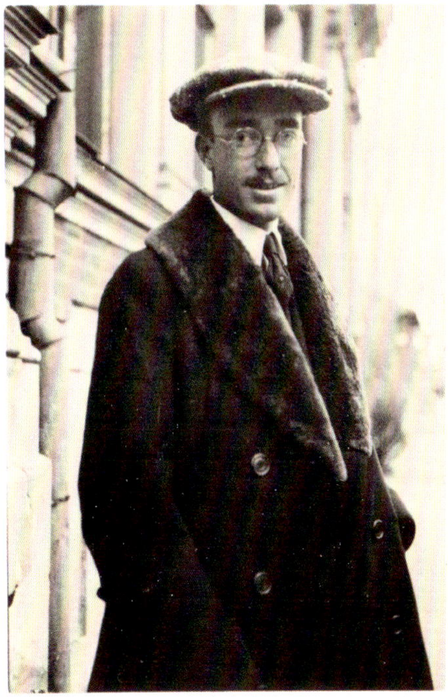

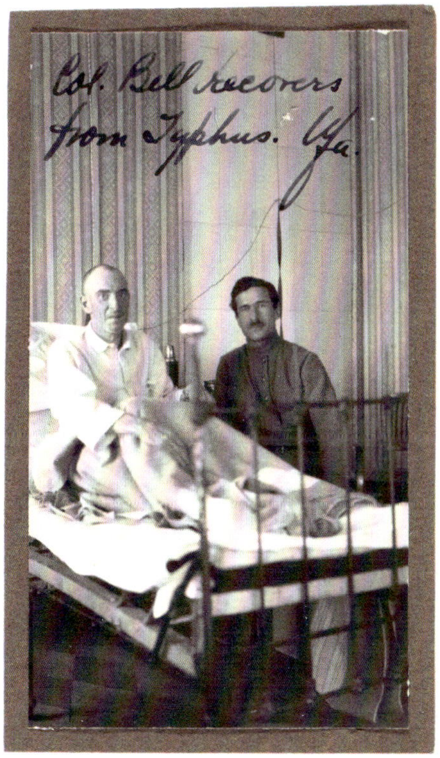

TOP: Dr. George Cornick, ARA district physician in Tsaritsyn, 1922. Frederick Dorsey Stephens papers

ABOVE: Colonel Walter Bell recovering from typhus, Ufa, December 1921.

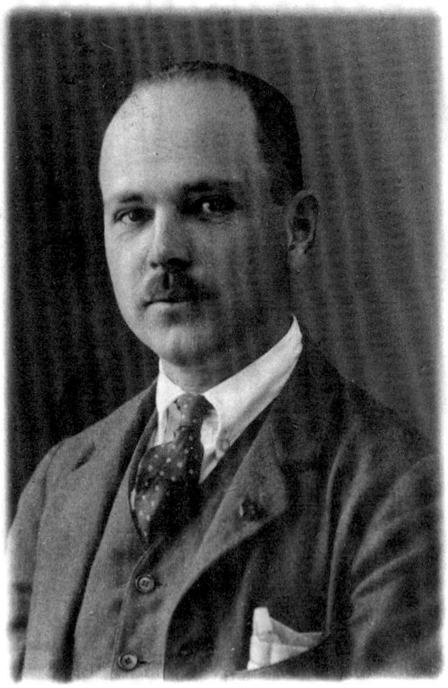

James Rives Childs, ca. 1921.

other foreign relief organizations had recently succumbed, Bell was the first ARA worker to be stricken. He proved Mackenzie wrong and was soon once again hard at work, having refused an order by Colonel Haskell to recuperate on the Riviera.

The American physicians working for the ARA in Russia knew well enough how to avoid contracting typhus. But inspired by Davenport's recent trip to oversee care for Bell, Beeuwkes thought it prudent to send out a memorandum to all relief workers on the prevention of diseases. This circular, sent out very early in January 1922, reminded the Americans to avoid crowds, keep hair cut short, and opt for smooth fabrics such as trench, leather, or rubber for outer clothing, and silk for undergarments, because these nap-free surfaces provided less of a foothold for lice. He prescribed naphthalene—the main ingredient in mothballs—and insect powder made from the plant extract pyrethrum, which is toxic to insects but safe for humans, for liberal use on clothes and bedding, and sandalwood oil to be sprinkled on underwear. Rubbing the neck, arms, and legs with an ointment of 5 percent naphthalene mixed into petroleum rounded out the regimen. Kerosene and gasoline also found their way into anti-typhus mixtures. By World War II, naphthalene was replaced by DDT; neither was safe for human use.

Beeuwkes's memo advised that should lice or nits be found in clothing, especially in seams, underclothing should be boiled, whereas outer garments should be baked or ironed with a very hot iron. Ideally, a room should be set aside in any home for disinfection of clothing and bedding using sulphur fumes.

James Rives Childs, in Kazan, became the first well-known ARA typhus case when the Associated Press reported it in the American newspapers in January 1922, which he says made his parents "desperate with anxiety." A special prayer service for him was held in a Kazan church. Childs had traveled by train from Moscow to Kazan, where he arrived with a temperature of 102.5 degrees, prompting Venear, of the medical staff, to put his chief to bed. Thinking it was a bad cold, Venear gave him calomel and magnesium sulphate, since a laxative purge to treat a cold (and almost anything else) was a standard practice of the day. But the high fever persisted. Venear called in a Russian specialist who immediately diagnosed typhus. For the next five weeks, Childs remained bedridden, passing in and out of periods of delirium and unconsciousness, until finally he was able to rise from his bed and begin to learn how to walk again before making his way out to Berlin for convalescence.

The high fever of the typhus patient lasted at least several days, with most of that time spent unconscious. The delirium induced in some the most creative kinds of hallucinations, not all of which seem to have been unpleasant. Childs was left "fully convinced that my parents had died during the Christmas holidays and it was not until I had actually received letters from them dated in the month of January that I could be assured that they were alive."

When Dr. A. B. Musa in Orenburg contracted typhus in late January 1922, Dr. Foucar was asked to travel from Samara to care for his fellow physician. The two men had journeyed together from New York to Moscow. Foucar, who had seen his very first case of typhus just a month earlier in Moscow, worried that he did not have the camphor or olive oil to treat Musa. Camphor—and digitalis—were used for "cardiac stimulation," the assumption being that the heart became exhausted after eight or nine days of fever hovering around 104 degrees. As prescribed by *A Handbook of Useful Drugs*, published in 1914, camphor should be

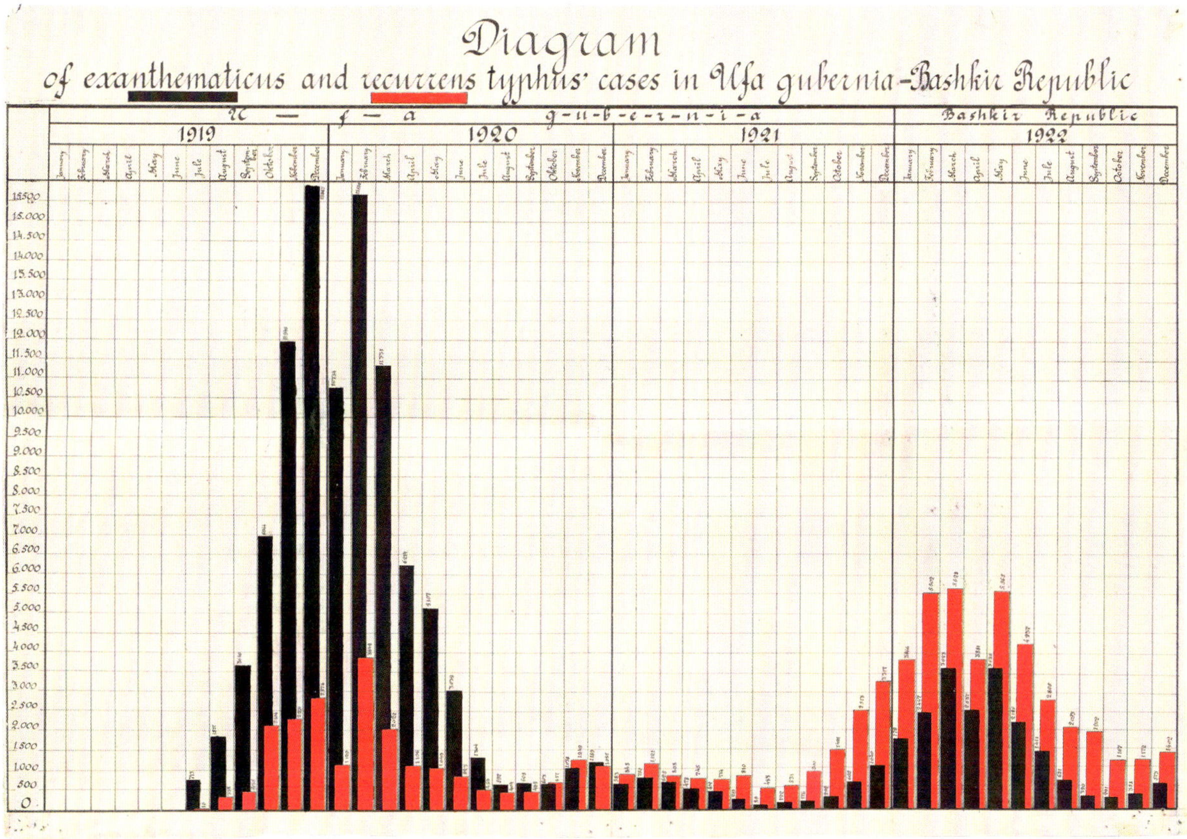

Diagram of exanthematicus and recurrens typhus cases in Ufa gubernia and the Bashkir Republic, 1919–1922.

"mixed in a solution with olive oil to be administered hypodermically . . . every fifteen minutes for four doses if needed" until the "crisis" at about day thirteen to sixteen when the fever subsided.

When he arrived at Musa's bedside, Foucar noticed body lice on the patient's blankets and ordered the blankets and all of Musa's clothing baked in the oven. He consulted with the Russian physicians, who, Foucar conceded, had "vast typhus experience, while I had none." This was not an admission of shortcoming on his part, but rather was a reflection of the fact that in most Western countries, sanitation, hygiene, and modern systems of public health had decades earlier eradicated most diseases of filth, including typhus.

Foucar took issue with the local doctors over the recovery diet. While they assumed a hearty appetite for all manner of food, Foucar knew a patient weakened by disease required a special diet and oversaw the preparation of "orange-albumen-water, beef juice, ice cream, poached eggs, and fricasseed chicken." Russians, he noted, had heard of none of these, "excepting the ice cream." Musa eventually recovered and Foucar was able to return to Samara, reporting to Beeuwkes in a letter of February 6 that Musa was making a rapid recovery, running a normal temperature for four days before Foucar left, and having had a "typical course of *typhus exanthematicus*"—or spotted typhus, in reference to the telltale body rash.

Joseph Brown, a relief worker in the Crimea, became the next ARA typhus victim, in March 1922. With the sudden onset of chills, Brown suspected that he had another bout of malaria, a disease he experienced episodically all his life. He went to bed and drank hot liquids and quinine. The chills subsided and a fever started, all in keeping with a typical course of malaria except for the fact that he did not start to sweat. At 103 degrees, the temperature worried Brown, who called for a

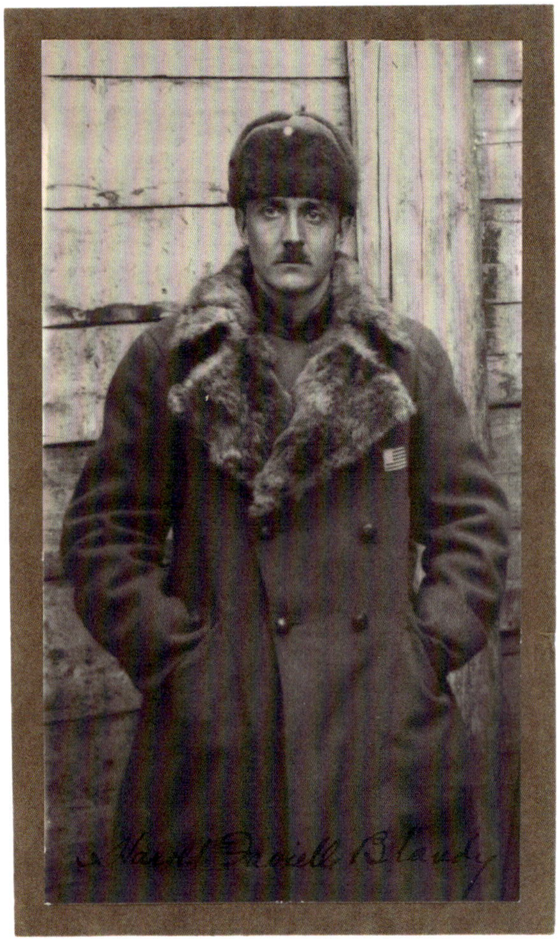

ABOVE: Harold Blandy, Ufa, winter 1922.

BELOW RIGHT: Harold Blandy (at center) among abandoned children in Sterlitamak, in Ufa province, winter 1922.

local doctor since no other American physician was stationed there. Still unable to make a diagnosis, Brown called for another Russian doctor, who arrived the next day. This physician suspected early typhus, with the rash yet to erupt. Brown says he felt "like a person who had received his death sentence." He had seen the ravages of "spotted typhus" during his work in Theodosia (today Feodosia) and throughout the Crimea.

Still febrile, Brown instructed his assistant to send a radiogram to the chief of the ARA's port operations at Novorossiysk requesting that he send a US destroyer with an American physician to Theodosia. The response arrived a day later that the USS *Fox* was en route from Odessa with Dr. Jesse McElroy on board. It is unclear if Brown was made aware of this before he slipped into unconsciousness. The ship arrived in port the following day. His medical chart documented a fever of 105 degrees for days at a time and a pulse rate of 150 beats per minute. In between hallucinations, Brown tried to get out of bed, creating a danger to himself that required a large man to sit on him until his agitation and restlessness subsided.

True to the peripatetic spirit of the ARA personnel, Brown did not spend these two weeks idly. "I was under the impression that I had fallen from an airship, and that was the reason I was in bed; for during my period of unconsciousness I had made regular trips around the world in a big Zeppelin and discharged passengers at such places as Shanghai, San Francisco, Chicago, New York and Paris." Accounts of air travel among the American typhus sufferers were not uncommon. Anna Louise Strong, who worked with the American Quakers, also made productive use of her period of unconsciousness, "escaping from Samara in a soft, warm airplane." For years she traveled the world, visiting London, Chicago, crossing the Arctic Circle, until finally, seven days later, she landed safely back in Samara.

Brown regained consciousness after sixteen days. "There was a terrible buzzing sound in my ears and my head was full of boilershop noises. I discovered I was unable to move my right leg and when I spoke it was hardly above a whisper." On May 1, he was able to hobble around using a cane, aware of the weight he had lost and how exceedingly hungry he was.

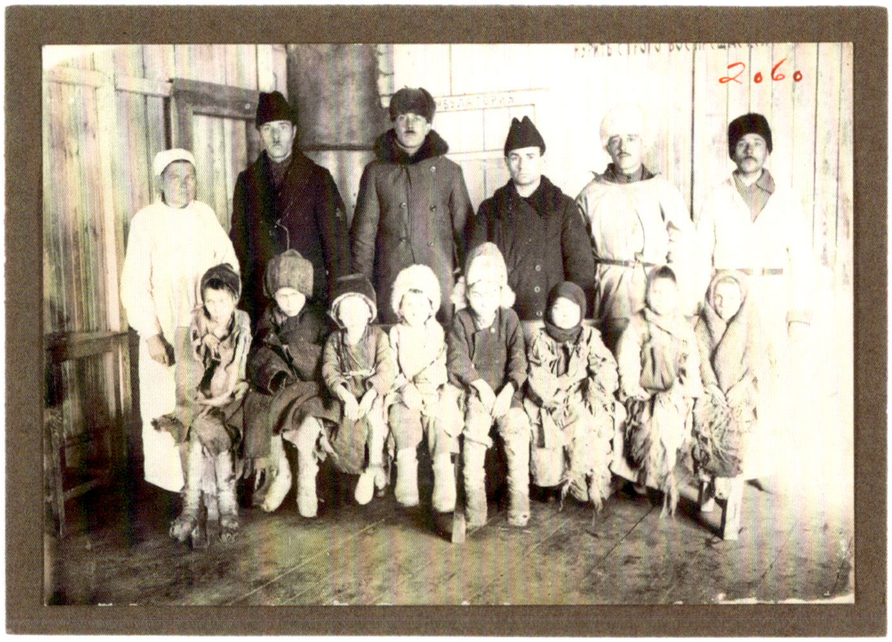

American relief worker Harold Blandy did not survive his bout with typhus. He died in Ufa on May 17, 1922. These were difficult days for the ARA in Ufa. At the time of Blandy's death, sixteen of the city's Russian staff were infected with typhus. "Its ravages have been terrific here lately," William Kelley testified. Fifty-seven of the Russian personnel in the Ufa office would contract typhus during the first six months of 1922, and fifteen of them would die. The threat of typhus was so severe in Ufa that the ARA maintained the services of two Russian physicians and one nurse on its payroll. There, Piet Hofstra had joined the ranks of typhus patients after he returned from an inspection trip to Chelyabinsk in the first week of April. Both Hofstra and his interpreter, Willig, were forced to stay overnight in a peasant hut in the area. Willig died within days of returning to the Ufa headquarters, likely having contracted typhus in the peasant hut; shortly after, Hofstra showed severe symptoms, and although Dr. Sloan was aided by two of the best local doctors, he sent for Dr. Foucar of Samara. Hofstra ran a temperature for about twenty-five days, a length of time that Foucar classified as a severe, "protracted course" of typhus. Hofstra was still recovering at the time Blandy succumbed.

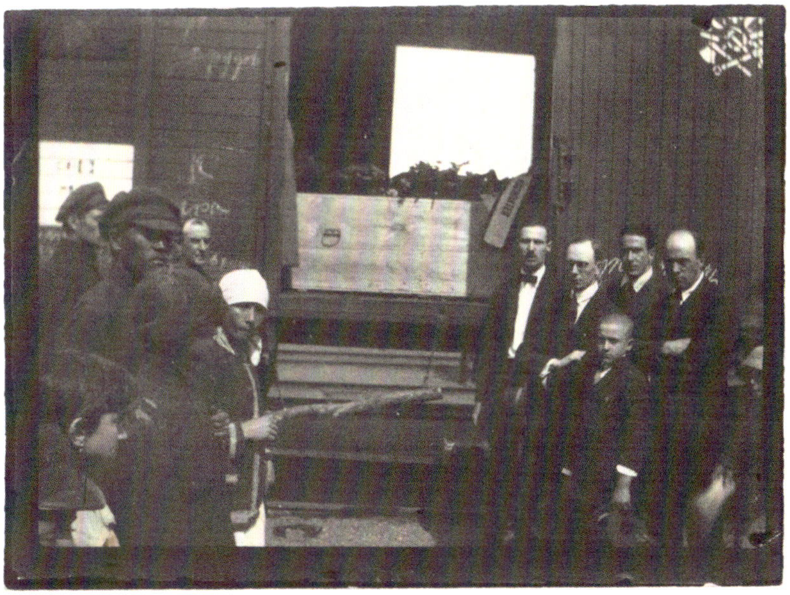

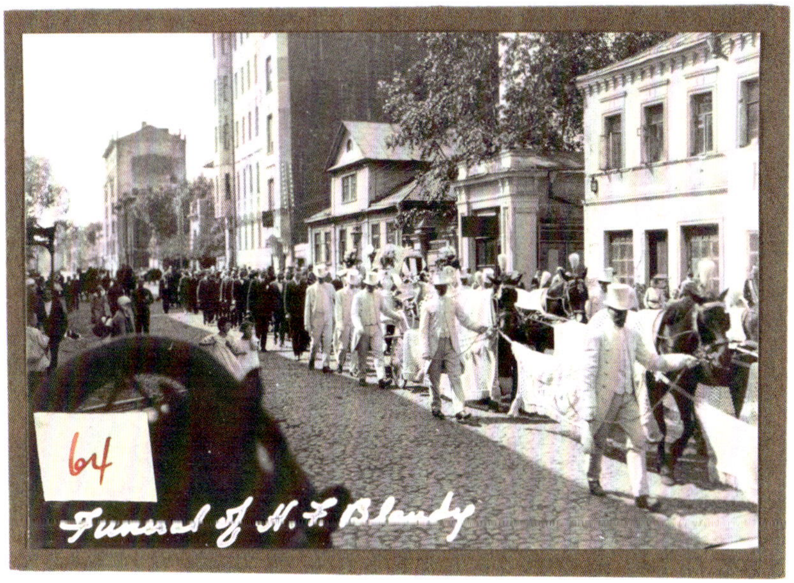

Colonel Bell eulogized Blandy, recalling his "intense sympathetic nature," for which he was beloved by the ARA Russian personnel and Russian citizens throughout the district. This is confirmed by the letters received by the ARA in Ufa in the subsequent days. The Russian staff members wrote of Blandy that they had "learned to love him for his sensitive heart always ready to respond to human affliction." A letter signed by "Beeshev" observed that Blandy had worked "not for fear, but for love, not even caring for his life," and that "the memory of him will live for a long time in the hearts of the Bashkir people." A letter written by Blandy's interpreter, Gorin, told of Blandy's "great sympathy" for the starving people, whom he "sincerely and greatheartedly" assisted.

Gorin recalled how Blandy visited the sick "never thinking of the possibility of getting the infection"—in fact, he "often laughed at the danger of death from typhus." Maybe so, but when he fell ill, Blandy was fully aware of the seriousness of his case. A sketch of Blandy's final days written by one of the Russian staff remarks, "The moment Blandy knew that he had typhus he lost all heart and decided that he was bound to die."

Blandy had returned to Ufa on April 12 after a six-week inspection tour and complained that he felt ill. Out in the district a Russian physician had diagnosed pleurisy and treated Blandy with a purge of calomel and magnesium sulphate. On April 29, Blandy and his interpreter went by boat to Sterlitamak 400 miles away to oversee the unloading and warehousing of a shipment of corn. Feeling sick the entire time aboard the boat, Blandy reached Sterlitamak in such bad condition that he wired headquarters of his decision to return immediately.

TOP: Harold Blandy's casket loaded onto a boxcar at the Ufa railway station for transport to Moscow, as the American staff looks on, May 1922. To the right of the door, with moustache, is the ARA medical doctor Raymond McKnight Sloan; to the left of the door is the district supervisor, Colonel Walter Bell. Raymond McKnight Sloan papers

ABOVE: Scene from Harold Blandy's funeral procession in Moscow, beginning outside ARA headquarters and ending at the train station, May 1922.

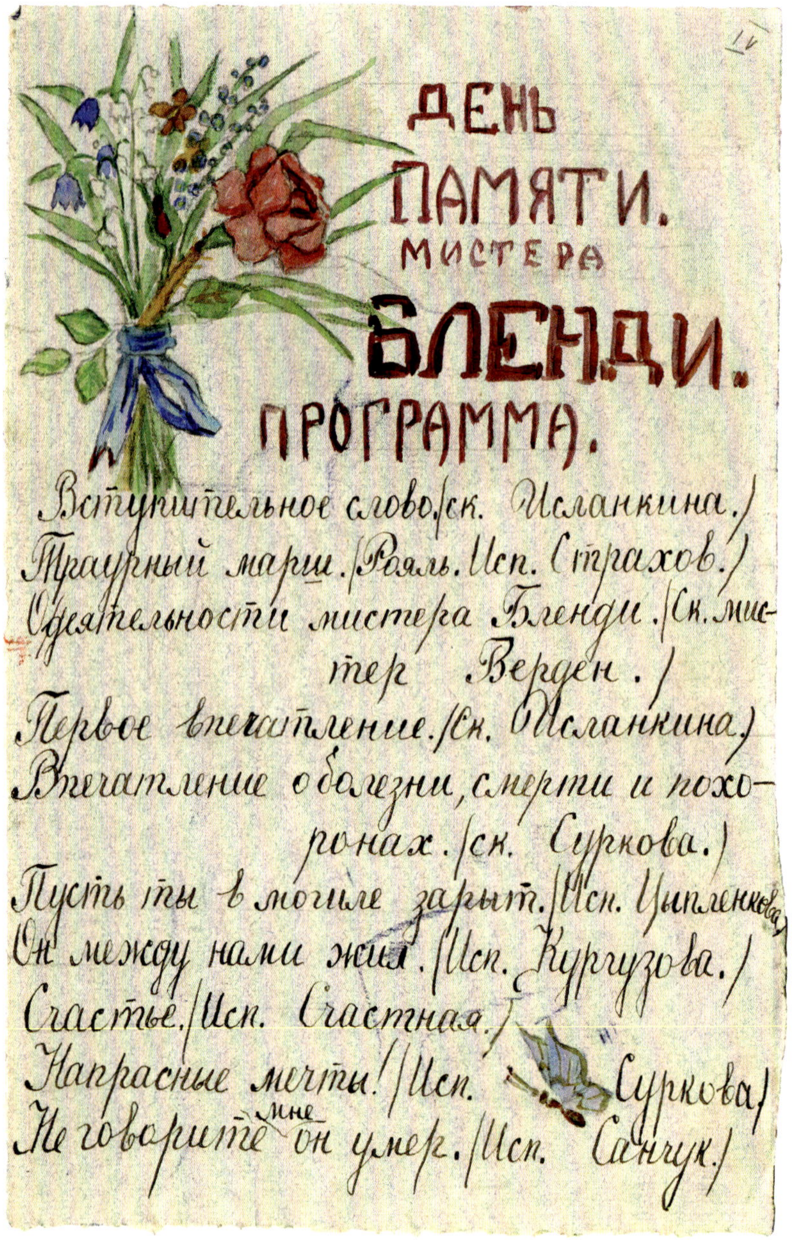
ДЕНЬ
ПАМЯТИ.
МИСТЕРА
БЛЕНДИ.
ПРОГРАММА.
Вступительное слово. (Ск. Исланкина.)
Траурный марш. (Рояль. Исп. Страхов.)
О деятельности мистера Бленди. (Ск. мистер Верден.)
Первое впечатление. (Ск. Исланкина.)
Впечатление о болезни, смерти и похоронах. (Ск. Суркова.)
Пусть ты в могиле зарыт. (Исп. Цыпленкова)
Он между нами жил. (Исп. Кургузова.)
Счастье. (Исп. Счастная.)
Напрасные мечты! (Исп. Суркова)
Не говорите мне он умер. (Исп. Санчук.)

Program for a memorial service in honor of Harold Blandy, Ufa, May 1922.
Belgian-American Educational Foundation Records, Herbert Hoover Presidential Library and Museum

Dr. Sloan had taken up his post in Ufa in April just as Hofstra was down with typhus. Sloan received Blandy when he returned on May 6 and from then on rarely left his bedside. Blandy's fever began to rise, and with his history of feeling poorly for the past month, Sloan at first suspected typhoid, the waterborne disease that was prevalent in the district. But by May 9, the telltale rash appeared, and Sloan knew the disease was typhus exanthematicus. When the rash became hemorrhagic, the spots turned purple, and Blandy's heart "rate and force" remained irregular. Even the cardiac stimulation, whether by camphor or caffeine, failed to make an improvement. In a state of exhaustion, Blandy suffered from low blood pressure that led to shock and finally heart failure. He died on May 17, 1922. "Everything that could be done was done for him," Sloan wrote to Beeuwkes, "two of the best physicians in Ufa were called in for consultations, and continued to visit Mr. Blandy daily during his illness, and for the last four days were with him continuously." Kelley tells us that Sloan was "much cut up about the loss of his patient," while Hofstra "received quite a shock from Blandy's death. His recovery may be retarded."

In Moscow, Blandy was given the equivalent of a state funeral by the Soviet government. Of this latter event there are several journalists' accounts, numerous photographs, and a motion picture as well. Blandy's body lay in state at ARA headquarters. The casket, provided by the Moscow soviet, was draped with a large American flag and a blanket of blue forget-me-nots and wreaths. The American Lutheran minister Dr. J. A. Morehead conducted the service, during which he read aloud from a telegram Blandy had sent his mother a few days before his death, telling her he could not come home "till my work is finished." In his eulogy, Morehead told the congregation that Blandy had performed his work not only with efficiency but with sympathy. Perhaps, ultimately, that was Blandy's undoing.

The formal ceremony was followed by a grand procession, seven miles in length, two hours in duration, through the sun-drenched streets of Moscow to the train station. Participants included the ARA's local American and Russian personnel as well as a good number of curious Muscovites. The casket, escorted by ushers in white formal attire, was borne on an open white hearse pulled by eight impressive horses. "Moscow must have been searched to find them," wrote a foreign journalist. The ARA was forbidden to fly Old Glory in Russia and the appearance of the stars and stripes on the casket lends a further disorienting note to the surviving images of the occasion. At the railway station the casket was loaded onto a special train destined for Riga.

Hoover sent a telegram of condolence to Blandy's mother, assuring her that her son had made the supreme sacrifice for a gallant cause "on the battlefield of famine." President Harding wrote to her: "He has died in the service of America."

In September, American newspapers reported the founding in Ufa city of the Harold Blandy Memorial Hospital, a former surgical hospital recently repaired by Russian workmen who were receiving ARA corn rations. There was also an announcement of the intention to erect a Blandy Memorial Monument in Ufa's central square.

+ + +

Typhus was historically a disease of war, nurtured by the amassing and movement of troops and the lack of sanitary systems. But by the time the ARA arrived in Soviet Russia, typhus had also become associated with both dire poverty and widespread famine, both of which forced people to wander in search of food and live in immensely crowded and unsanitary conditions. Beeuwkes and all the ARA district physicians and medical workers first fought to stem the tide of typhus in the famine zones by reconstructing public baths and rehabilitating water systems (pumps, plumbing) for large-scale disinfecting campaigns. The ARA feeding program fortified Soviet citizens and enabled them to better fight infection. Over months in 1922, the ARA efforts gained traction and began to reduce the spread of the disease.

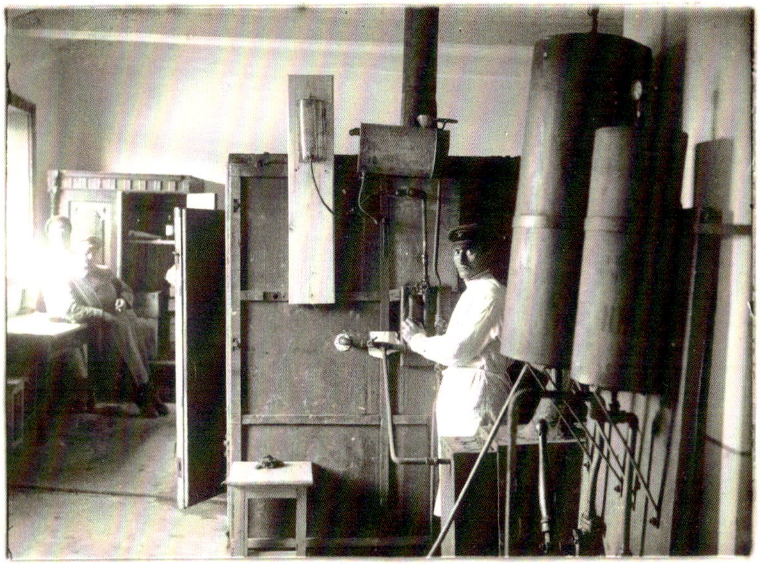

Disinfecting chamber, refugee camp, Minsk, ca. 1922.

Nevertheless, Soviet Russia's typhus and other epidemics threatened to spill out along the Western frontier, carried by the migrations of refugees and POWs trying to return home from Russia. Russian epidemiologist Lev Tarassevitch had written in a report delivered to the Health Section of the League of Nations: "The entire epidemic constitution of Europe, which is only now reestablishing itself after the great influenza pandemic, may become entirely changed by what is happening now on the Volga." The largest evacuation points for POWs and refugees traveling west into Europe were in Kiev (today Kyiv) and Minsk, locations that were not initially part of the ARA famine and medical relief districts.

Beeuwkes wrote in his Medical Division report for June–July 1922: "We can not assume responsibility for the protection of Western Europe but, realizing the importance of the work on the western frontier, we are extending every assistance possible." He was referring to the fact that in April 1922 the ARA opened medical relief districts in Kiev (Ukraine) and Minsk (Belorussia), and ARA supplies of soap and disinfectants were arriving in vast quantities at the evacuation points through which passed thousands of people displaced by war and exposed to disease. Six large French disinfecting cameras (chambers), funded by the American Red Cross, disinfected tons of louse-ridden clothing, and physicians triaged those with diagnosed illness to an ARA-equipped hundred-bed isolation hospital or to a dispensary stocked with ARA medicines. Refugees who had previously camped in trains, railroad station grounds, empty lots, or ruined buildings transferred to an ARA-organized refugee camp in Minsk built to accommodate fifteen thousand people. The entire effort was reminiscent of the disease triage and containment of the "cordon sanitaire" organized in Poland three years earlier with the help of Herbert Hoover.

ПРОЛЕТАРИИ ВСЕХ СТРАН, СОЕДИНЯЙТЕСЬ!

ХОЛЕРА

БОЛЕЗНЬ ЗАРАЗНАЯ,

ОНА ПОРАЖАЕТ ПРЕИМУЩЕСТВЕННО ЛЮДЕЙ, ЖИВУЩИХ СКУЧЕННО, НЕОПРЯТНО и БЕДНО.

Великий ученый Роберт Кох открыл, что заболевание холерой вызывается особыми микробами.

Микробы—это мельчайшие живые существа, которых можно рассмотреть лишь

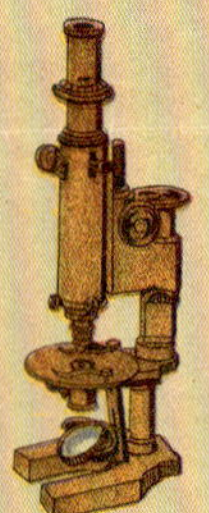

при помощи микроскопа. Называются они холерными вибрионами.

Легкое заболевание холерой выражается поносом, иногда рвотой; тяжелое заболевание—поносом, рвотой, сильным исхуданием и похолоданием всего тела, синюхой, остановкой мочи и судорогами.

В 2–3 дня, а иногда в несколько часов оно может окончиться смертью.

Выздоровевшие от холеры люди еще долго носят в себе заразу и могут передавать ее другим.

Мухи нередко переносят холерных вибрионов с испражнений больных на пищу и предметы домашнего обихода.

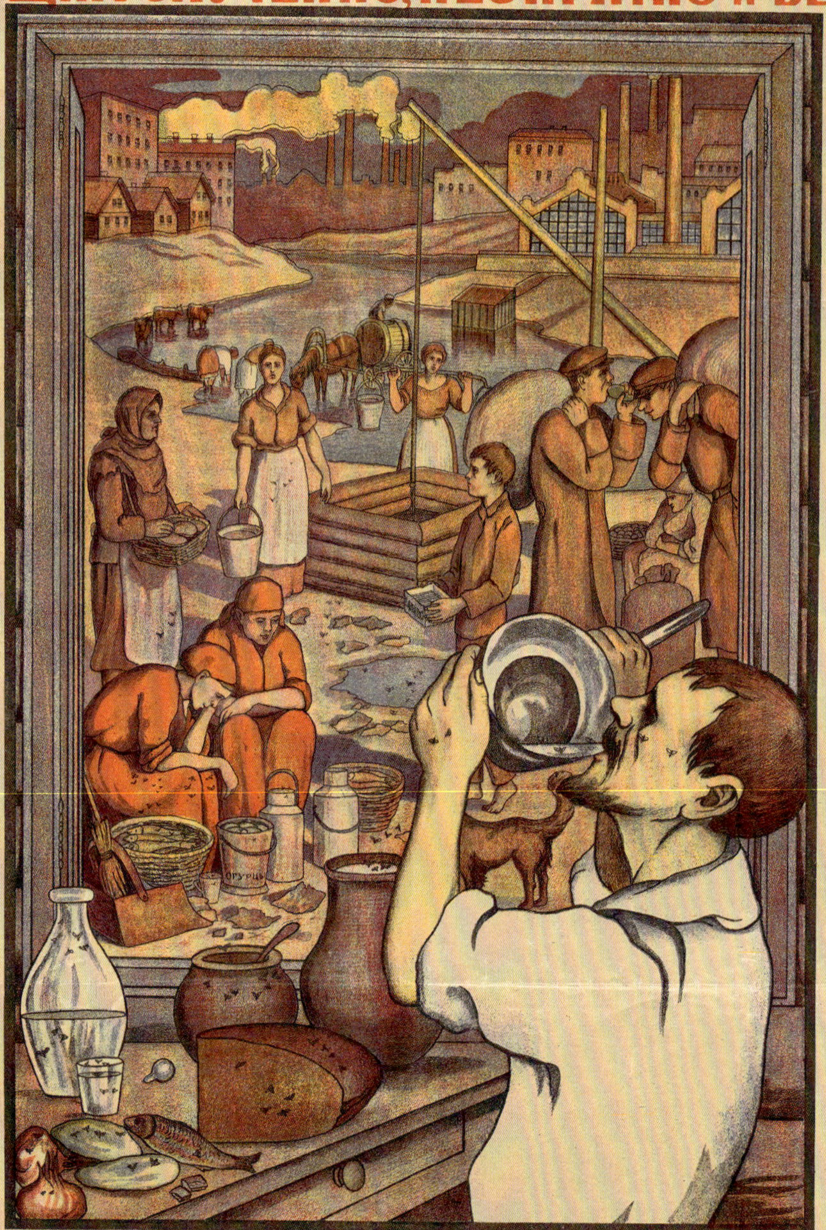

Особенно опасно попадание холерного вибриона в источники питьевого водоснабжения: это вызывает среди населения, пользующегося источником, массовые заболевания холерой.

. Холерные вибрионы вызывают заражение человека только тогда, когда микробы попадают в его кишечник через рот с пищей и питьем или с немытых рук.

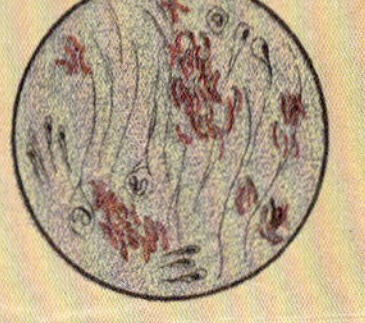

Покупаемые на рынках или у разносчиков продукты (молоко, овощи, фрукты) могут оказаться зараженными холерой.

Вместе с испражнениями, содержащими холерные вибрионы, зараза попадает в почву, может попасть на одежду, на предметы домашнего обихода, в пищу и питьевую воду, через них зараза может передаваться другим людям.

Открытый водоем нельзя надежно защитить от загрязнения.

Воду из него следует употреблять лишь после предварительной очистки или кипячения.

В случае заболевания холерой, спешите лечь в больницу, только там вы получите всю необходимую помощь. Помещение холерного больного в больницу устраняет опасность передачи болезни его близким и окружающим.

НАРОДНЫЙ КОМИССАРИАТ ЗДРАВООХРАНЕНИЯ

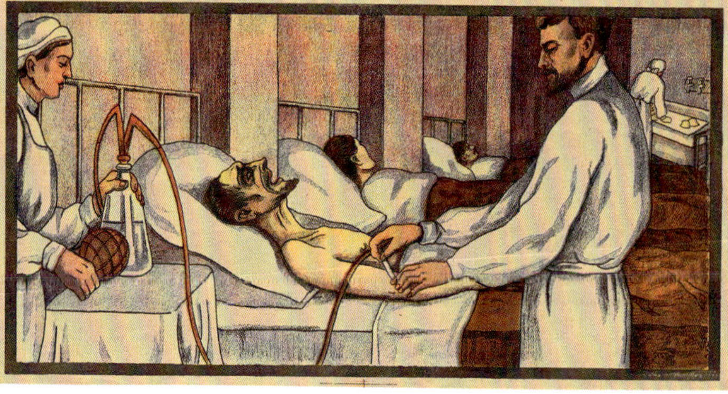

—ОТДЕЛ— САНИТАРНОГО ПРОСВЕЩЕНИЯ

CHAPTER 4

The Ghost of Cholera

"Cholera was the name of the ghost lurking behind the corners of the filthy streets, the railroad stations, all homes—everywhere."

—*American relief worker in Tsaritsyn, May 1923*

As the seasons changed in Soviet Russia, so too did the diseases. Typhus waned as people shed layers of lice-infested clothing, spent more time outdoors, and even bathed in the rivers. Lice were banished from their human hosts. While most American relief workers took satisfaction in the seasonal demotion of typhus, Orenburg district supervisor Walter Coleman anticipated another health impact of spring. "We have cleaned kids for weeks only to have them now use the 'cholera-infected' Ural River," he wrote to ARA Moscow headquarters in June 1922. With the breakup of winter ice on the rivers, water transport resumed, and barges and steamships carried cargo, refugees, and, inadvertently, the disease of cholera up and down the Volga, the Ural, and the Kama rivers.

Dr. Henry Beeuwkes, head of the ARA's Medical Division, knew that cholera typically remained latent in rivers during the winter months but then reappeared each spring, primarily in southeastern Russia, with the algae blooms. He expected high numbers of cases in the Samara, Saratov, Tsaritsyn, Ufa, and Orenburg districts. Early in January 1922 he issued Medical Memorandum No. 5 to all the district physicians to alert them to the coming threat posed by waterborne diseases: cholera, typhoid, and paratyphoid A and B. All four were contracted by ingesting water or food contaminated with the specific bacterium associated with each disease (*Vibrio cholerae*, *Salmonella typhi*, and *Salmonella paratyphi* A or B). Of the four bacterial diseases, cholera was the most severe, infecting the gastrointestinal tract and causing diarrhea and acute dehydration, which was often fatal. By orders from ARA headquarters in Moscow, all American personnel in Russia received inoculation against the four intestinal diseases; eventually this practice extended to all local ARA staff workers and their families.

Beeuwkes asked district physicians to gather initial information on the sources of drinking water and the conditions (or existence) of the sewer systems in their respective districts. In this request, he followed the prescribed practice of every epidemiologist since John Snow had solved the mystery of a cholera outbreak in London in 1854. Snow's "ghost map" of a neighborhood infected with the disease ultimately zeroed in on a single water well at 40 Broad Street as the source of the infection: contaminated human waste had seeped into the well water. Once the pump handle was removed and the well inactivated, cholera disappeared from the area. Snow's finding ushered in a revolution in the understanding and prevention

Department of Sanitary Enlightenment, People's Commissariat of Health, Холера болезнь заразная [Cholera is a contagious disease], ca. 1920.
Poster Collection RU/SU 1322

of cholera: water carrying a "toxin" was identified as the source of disease instead of the conventionally suspected miasmic or bad air. It was also a critical moment in the advent of proper sewer systems, engineered to be separated from sources of drinking water.

Today, physicians treat patients with cholera using rehydration therapy and antibiotics. But neither of these was available in 1922, two decades before the introduction of antibiotics. Nevertheless, Beeuwkes developed a practical and effective plan of attack based on two fundamentals of preventive medicine: ensuring a supply of safe drinking water and inoculation against waterborne diseases. These became hallmarks of the ARA's medical relief campaign in Soviet Russia.

Cholera in Russia

By the mid-nineteenth century, the lenses of modern microscopes had become powerful enough for researchers to see microscopic entities, a development that would pave the way for the germ theory of disease. In 1854, Italian physician Filippo Pacini saw curved particles in feces samples under the microscope during a cholera outbreak in Florence, a discovery for which he was credited only posthumously. The more renowned German scientist Robert Koch observed similar shapes in 1883 during his research on cholera in India. He identified the shapes as *Vibrio cholerae* bacteria and established the source of infection as contaminated water. Spanish physician Jaime Ferrán, who had studied under Louis Pasteur, developed a vaccine against cholera in 1885. By 1896, vaccines against cholera and typhoid were available worldwide, practically eliminating the diseases.

There had been eight cholera epidemics in Russia since 1823, when it first arrived from India via Persia. The number of cases fluctuated dramatically over the years, reaching a high of over 600,000 in the famine year 1892, prior to the availability of the vaccine. Refugees from Tashkent flooding into the Volga valley stoked the epidemic of 1921, when there were over 93,000 cases reported in the Volga region, with a 50 percent mortality rate reported during the first three months of the year. The Russian epidemiologist Lev Tarassevitch cited 182,722 total cases in Russia for 1921, a number he later amended to 202,948. And as he knew, the actual number of cases was likely significantly higher because many peasants never sought medical help.

Soon after their arrival, the American physicians inquired about and inspected the waterworks in their districts, interrogating the local water authorities on the potability of the water. Prior to World War I, the Government Hydrotechnical Bureau used dedicated funds to maintain the water purification systems in most cities; people in rural areas used private wells. The disruptions caused by the war, the revolution, and the Russian Civil War took a steep toll on basic utilities. Individual responses to Beeuwkes's query about water conditions were disturbingly similar, with most relief workers reporting a complete breakdown of the local water systems. Dr. Glenn Jones in Saratov informed Beeuwkes that the "people of this district are living in a most primitive manner—the result of complete collapse of practically all utilities . . . without adequate water supply (and that available not potable) and without sewerage systems." Dr. A. B. Musa in Orenburg reported in April 1922 that the city's piping system to deliver clean, safe drinking water had been built in 1864; the pumps had been replaced in 1888 and again in 1907, but since then there had been no repairs.

When Dr. Frederick Foucar arrived in Samara in January 1922, he had bacteriological analyses done on water samples, and all showed, as he wrote, a high bacterial count "according to American standards." Other physicians reported similarly unnerving discoveries: that city water came directly from the Volga with no filtration, or that it was pumped from the Ural River near where the city sewer emptied. As an intestinal disease, cholera was transmitted by human feces in a fecal-oral cycle. Having the source of drinking water anywhere near the sewer outlet was inviting disaster. Beeuwkes concluded from the district reports that while most provincial cities once had operating water purification plants, they had become dangerously deteriorated from neglect, abuse, and disrepair. If a water treatment plant was still intact, as in Petrograd and Moscow, it still lacked the chemicals necessary to purify water.

Spring Cleaning

Inspections of hospitals and children's homes revealed the horrifying consequences of the lack of basic sanitary systems. During the winter, when it was too cold to go outside, institutions set aside a room in which buckets of human excreta were dumped. In an early report from Saratov, Dr. Jesse McElroy informed Beeuwkes that he came upon one room in a children's home in which the accumulated excreta was two feet high. In March 1922, Dr. William Dear in Kazan wrote of inspecting children's homes in which "barefooted little children have to paddle over a feces covered floor in a room which is often located on some exposed back porch." The sight compelled him to propose a cheaply constructed commode in which the bucket was easily extractable and able to be carried on a yoke stick. Private homes either used existing cesspools in their backyard, or, when those were full, committed the entire backyard to piles of human waste. The horses or camels ordinarily used to cart away the waste on a monthly basis were no longer available, being either too exhausted or dead.

With the spring thaw, rivers swelled, and water spilled over the banks often for miles in all directions. When it receded, it dragged back into the river human waste that had overflowed from the backyard cesspools or had been hidden under snow elsewhere, revealing how commonly people had relieved themselves in town and village streets. Or the contaminated water invaded local wells built only with porous, earthen walls. Any filth left behind—human excrement, decaying organic material—then became a breeding ground for flies, which transmitted disease, especially by depositing pathogens on food sitting out in kitchens, which had no screening over the windows. Dr. Musa in Orenburg observed children playing in cesspool runoff in the streets and men in the markets washing their hands in the same streams.

The critical accelerant in this dangerous mix was the circulation of refugees via river and railroad transportation. These people, an American relief worker in Tsaritsyn remarked, had simply "become unused to live like human beings." He observed the mass of refugees passing through Tsaritsyn on their way to the imagined "golden south": "There was nothing human-like in them," he remarked. "They were a severe violation of the most innocent and most rudimentary laws of cleanliness and hygienics. This is the least to be said about them." Despite the harshness of the observation, all ARA medical workers knew that the Soviet government, and by extension the local boards of health, provided

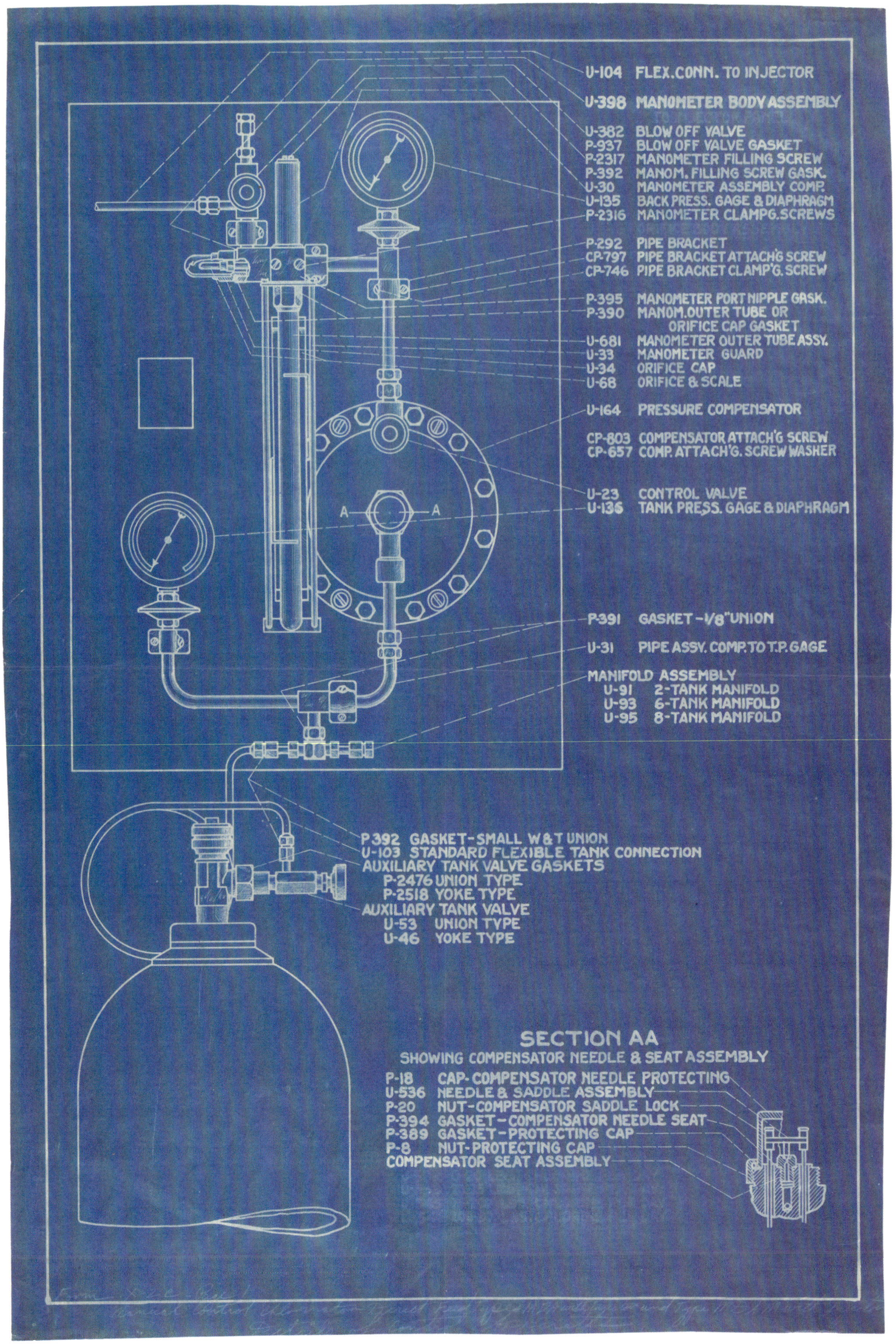
U-104 FLEX. CONN. TO INJECTOR
U-398 MANOMETER BODY ASSEMBLY
U-382 BLOW OFF VALVE
P-937 BLOW OFF VALVE GASKET
P-2317 MANOMETER FILLING SCREW
P-392 MANOM. FILLING SCREW GASK.
U-30 MANOMETER ASSEMBLY COMP.
U-135 BACK PRESS. GAGE & DIAPHRAGM
P-2316 MANOMETER CLAMPG. SCREWS
P-292 PIPE BRACKET
CP-797 PIPE BRACKET ATTACH'G SCREW
CP-746 PIPE BRACKET CLAMP'G. SCREW
P-395 MANOMETER PORT NIPPLE GASK.
P-390 MANOM. OUTER TUBE OR ORIFICE CAP GASKET
U-681 MANOMETER OUTER TUBE ASSY.
U-33 MANOMETER GUARD
U-34 ORIFICE CAP
U-68 ORIFICE & SCALE
U-164 PRESSURE COMPENSATOR
CP-803 COMPENSATOR ATTACH'G SCREW
CP-657 COMP. ATTACH'G. SCREW WASHER
U-23 CONTROL VALVE
U-136 TANK PRESS. GAGE & DIAPHRAGM
A
A
P-391 GASKET - 1/8" UNION
U-31 PIPE ASSY. COMP. TO T.P. GAGE
MANIFOLD ASSEMBLY
U-91 2-TANK MANIFOLD
U-93 6-TANK MANIFOLD
U-95 8-TANK MANIFOLD
P392 GASKET - SMALL W & T UNION
U-103 STANDARD FLEXIBLE TANK CONNECTION
AUXILIARY TANK VALVE GASKETS
P-2476 UNION TYPE
P-2518 YOKE TYPE
AUXILIARY TANK VALVE
U-53 UNION TYPE
U-46 YOKE TYPE
SECTION AA
SHOWING COMPENSATOR NEEDLE & SEAT ASSEMBLY
P-18 CAP - COMPENSATOR NEEDLE PROTECTING
U-536 NEEDLE & SADDLE ASSEMBLY
P-20 NUT - COMPENSATOR SADDLE LOCK
P-394 GASKET - COMPENSATOR NEEDLE SEAT
P-389 GASKET - PROTECTING CAP
P-8 NUT - PROTECTING CAP
COMPENSATOR SEAT ASSEMBLY

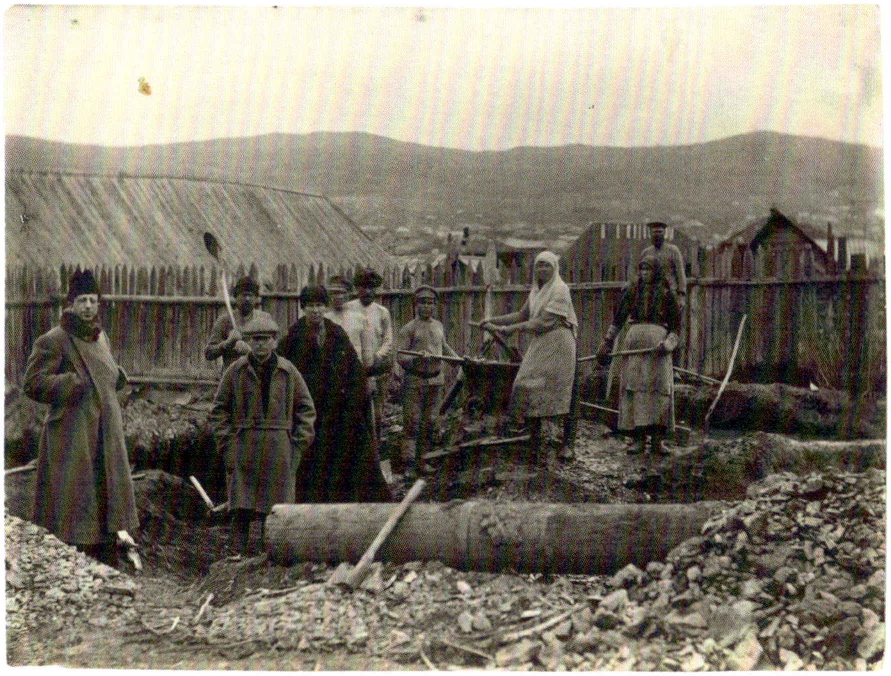

FACING: Chlorinator blueprint, ca. 1922.

LEFT: Laying a new sewer line, Ufa, ca. 1922.
Raymond McKnight Sloan papers

BELOW: Chlorinators of the Samara Water Works installed by the ARA, ca. 1922.

nothing for refugees in the way of shelter, food, safe drinking water, or, above all, sanitation.

Every American physician in Soviet Russia confronted the fact that, as one of them in Saratov put it in March 1922, "every means that operates for the safeguarding of health and prevention of disease has reached a state of demoralization." They saw no recourse but to take upon themselves the responsibility for improving sanitation, and each of them devised a plan for providing safe drinking water first and foremost.

The primary step involved a citywide and sometimes district-wide cleanup campaign, employing able-bodied local and refugee men and women. As American corn began to arrive in the famine zone in spring 1922, various relief workers took the initiative to use some of the corn as remuneration for those enlisted in the cleanup operations. This particular use of corn was not inspired by a central directive from Moscow headquarters; rather, several district supervisors and physicians hit upon the idea independently at roughly the same time. The chief goal was to promote sanitation and thereby prevent epidemic disease, but the end result was also an improvement in psychological health. It is a prime example of how these relief workers, several of them engineers by profession back home in the United States, were efficiency-minded problem solvers like Herbert Hoover, their role model, eager to take on the assignment of bringing order out of chaos.

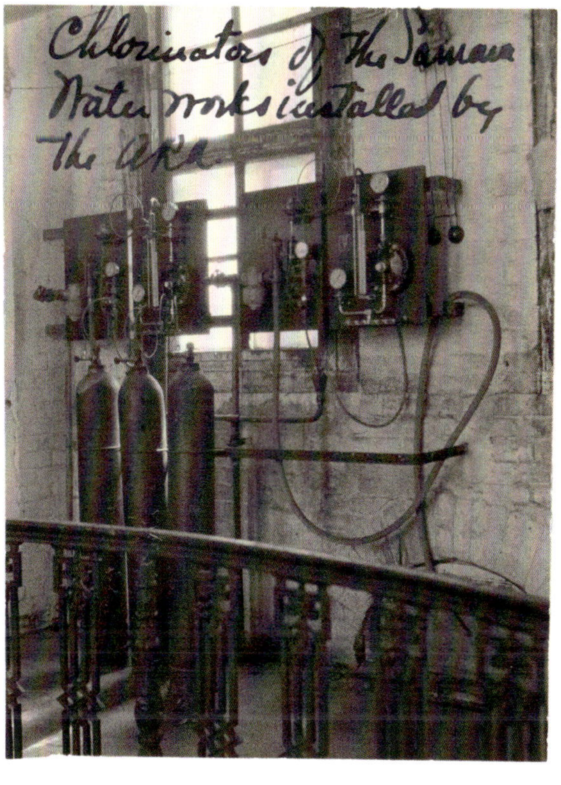

Corn rations served as wages for the so-called corn gangs, typically composed of refugees, that were mobilized to clean city streets of the filth that had accumulated over the previous five years and was now laid bare by the melting of the snow. Corn gangs were employed for a variety of projects, including the repair of railways, roads, and buildings, and the construction of bridges and dams. These proto–public works projects were organized in the provincial capitals and subdistrict cities and towns. The corn gangs of Orenburg city gave employment, at their peak, to some one thousand refugees. Coleman, the district supervisor there, channeled a portion of the first corn shipment to men repairing a water tank, men digging graves, men engaged in cleaning night houses, and employees of the sewerage disposal plant. The success of this initial venture encouraged him to

THE ROUX LABORATORY IN SAMARA

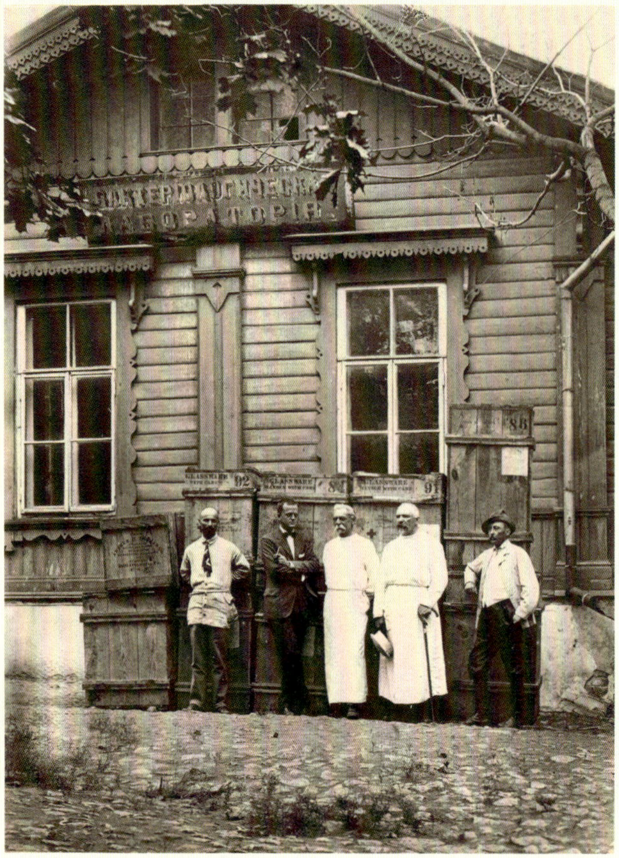

Dr. Frederick Foucar (second from left) and doctors from the Roux Laboratory in Samara, standing in front of crated laboratory supplies shipped from the United States, July 7, 1922.

Laboratories and bacteriological institutes in Soviet Russia facilitated the ARA vaccination campaign by supplementing the ARA tetra vaccine. This cooperation was critical, especially in May 1922, when Beeuwkes warned the district physicians of a delay in the shipments of the vaccine because trainloads of American corn were making their way from the Baltic and Black Sea ports to the famine zone, straining the capacity of the railways. In order to avoid losing momentum in the campaign, he advised the ARA physicians to meanwhile make use of the Russian-made mono-vaccine for cholera.

Like most institutions, medical laboratories in Russia had been hollowed out during the years of war. Devoid of almost all equipment, a few labs in government hospitals nevertheless managed to produce some serums, especially for the treatment of rabies from wolf bites, which were not uncommon during the famine. In Samara, Dr. Frederick Foucar was generous in his praise of the Microbiological Institute and the University Laboratory, recognizing them as "fine institutions, managed by self-sacrificing and deserving men." Foucar was not alone in his appreciation of the work of Soviet Russia's bacteriological institutes. In their prewar prime, they rivaled any of their peers in Europe. Dr. Francis Rollins in Ufa and Dr. William Dear in Kazan were similarly appreciative, and both men informed Beeuwkes that their local institutes of bacteriology could make bivalent vaccines for cholera and typhoid as soon as they were properly outfitted with the essential equipment and other supplies needed to operate a working lab.

Foucar took a special interest in the Roux Laboratory in Samara. Indeed, it is no exaggeration to say that it became his passion project during the famine year. The provincial government intended to close it down; Foucar was determined to get it back on its feet. The Roux Laboratory was named for Émile Roux, a colleague of Louis Pasteur's and cofounder of the Pasteur Institute in Paris, which he now directed. Foucar deemed the Roux Laboratory "the most important of its kind in Europe" after the Pasteur. Foucar informed Beeuwkes in early January 1922 that although scientists in the lab "were loath to make a polyvaccine," they would be quite capable of making a monovalent cholera vaccine, a monovalent typhoid vaccine, and a bivalent vaccine for cholera and typhoid by the spring—but only if the ARA provided the lab with needed supplies, including flasks, glass ampoules, cotton, microscopes, chemicals, syringes, and a large quantity of stains. In addition, the laboratory horses (for making serum) needed straw for bedding, oats and hay for food, and currycombs and brushes. In their current emaciated state, these animals could serve no medical purpose.

Foucar began to badger the local authorities to supply the Roux Laboratory with fuel and water and to make repairs to the building. In exchange, he promised that the ARA would provide the needed laboratory equipment and assist the personnel with a monthly food package. He sent Moscow an itemized list of desired laboratory equipment, and a dedicated order for these supplies was placed in the United States. In time, the building's water pipes were repaired and the aged water tank was replaced, so that the lab had adequate water pressure and running water at all times. Foucar arranged for each of the lab's twenty-four staff members to receive a monthly ARA food package. In April, Foucar reported triumphantly to Beeuwkes that the lab was functioning once again: "gas on tap, under good pressure and the burners all working in good shape," "rooms all freshly painted, clean and all apparatus brightly polished," "morale of the personnel excellent," and so on. The bulk of the laboratory supplies promised by the ARA was still to come, but a corner had been turned.

Beeuwkes's history of the ARA medical program states: "The importance of our aid to laboratories can scarcely be overestimated. The Roux Laboratory at Samara was completely supplied by a special purchase made in America and was continuously assisted throughout the operation. Through American aid it was converted from a paralyzed and demoralized organization, producing nothing, into a most active and effective institution manufacturing all varieties of vaccines and sera in quantity, and carrying out important bacteriological work for surrounding hospitals."

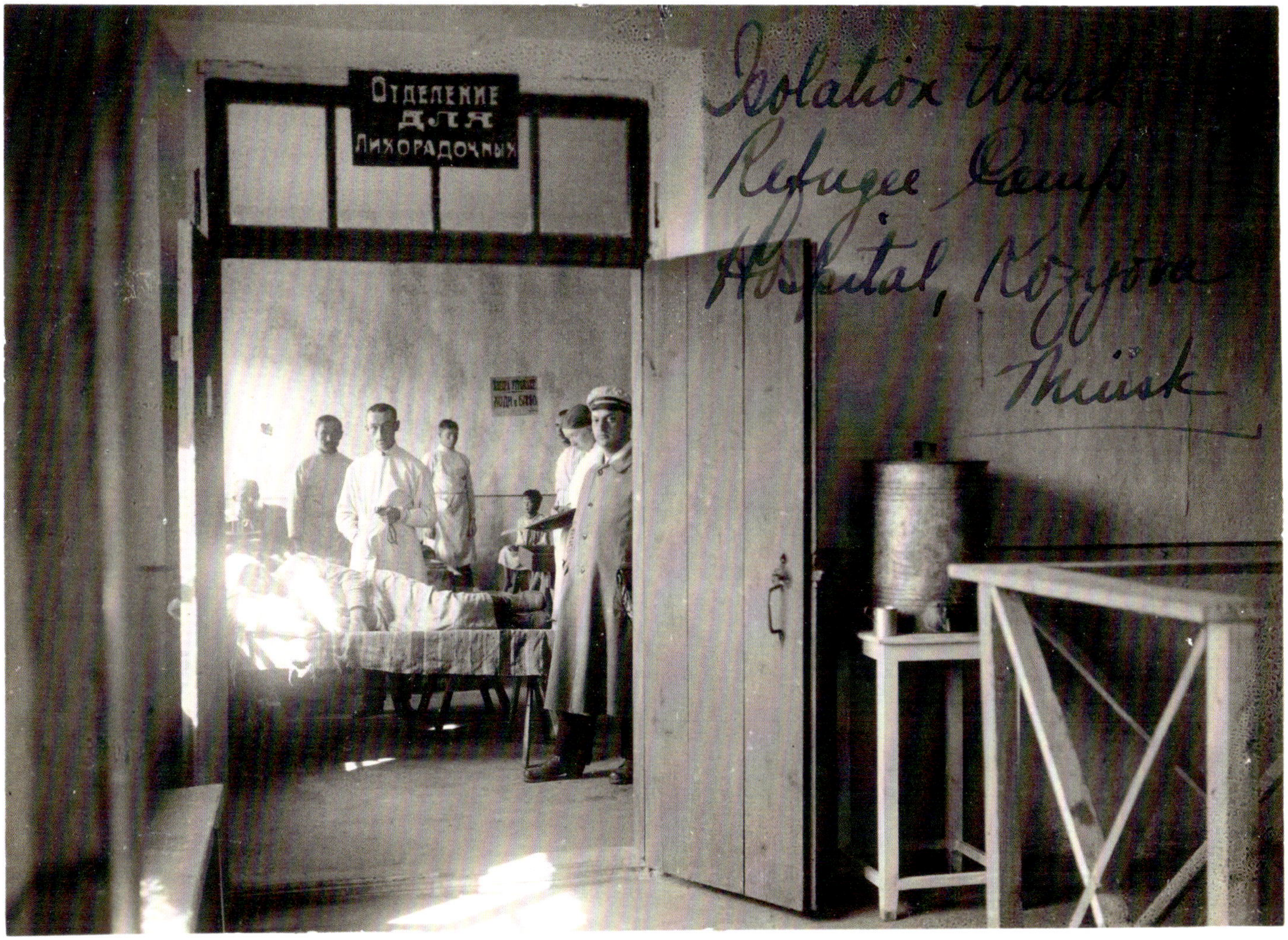

Isolation ward, refugee camp hospital, Kozyova, Minsk, ca. 1922. Sign above the doorway reads (in Russian): "Department for the feverish," sign visible on back wall: "Kholera ugrozhaet. Khodi v Baniu." [Cholera threatens. Visit the bathhouse (*bania*).]

continue the cleanup campaigns of these corn gangs through the summer months. Initially weak from hunger, they worked slowly, just two hours a day. In time and with added physical strength, their endurance increased to six hours of work per day. Using picks and shovels, they dislodged a two-year accumulation of utter filth on Orenburg's streets; cleaned out the sewer system with the ARA-supplied chloride of lime; dug graves for the remains of the dead; and repaired the filter beds, pumps, and trenches for the water plant. Before they were disbanded for harvest season, Orenburg's corn gangs repaired three city streets using stones they carried from nearly two miles away.

The Ufa district, under the resourceful district supervisor Colonel Walter Bell, engaged in a variety of such "reconstruction" activities carried out by what the ARA designated as "City Improvement Committees." Workers in Ufa constructed a new cesspool for the city's Infection Hospital, with cemented—not porous earthen—walls and a flyproof lid. The same crew also designed wire nets for the hospital windows to keep out the flies. Again, the ARA provided the workers with a corn ration.

In the mining town of Zlatoust, Colonel Bell arranged the employment of 2,142 refugees to engage in various cleaning and construction projects in return for one meal a day in regular kitchens or in mobile "military" kitchens when the work site was out of town. In this way, 270 road bridges were built and 160 repaired, ninety-four drinking fountains constructed, and two large schools completely restored. The flower of this enterprise was the construction of a drainage canal nearly eight hundred meters long and one and three-quarter meters wide and deep. It seems that such a canal had been discussed for over seventy years, but only the extraordinary circumstance of the American famine relief could bring the idea to life.

The various ARA-sponsored cleanup campaigns provided some sanitary relief and reinforced for their beneficiaries what the Americans expected in terms of sanitary standards. Beeuwkes parceled out hundreds and thousands of pounds of chloride of lime to districts with rebuilt water-purification systems. Dr. Foucar in Samara, drawing on his experience doctoring in France, requested of Beeuwkes two complete sets of Wallace & Tiernan Chlorine Control apparatuses to be attached to the water mains that supplied water to the city of Samara. In February 1922, Coleman suggested the same system for Orenburg, where, as he informed Beeuwkes, the main pumping station "has no filtering plant. It pumps dirty water direct from the Ural River near where the sewer empties to all parts of the city. This very important source of cholera must be combatted at once; otherwise the death toll will be so high that there will be very few living left here."

Letter from E. J. Swift, American Red Cross, Paris, to M. C. Bryant, ARA Paris, April 29, 1922, concerning an order placed with the Pasteur Institute for tetra and cholera vaccines for the ARA in Moscow.

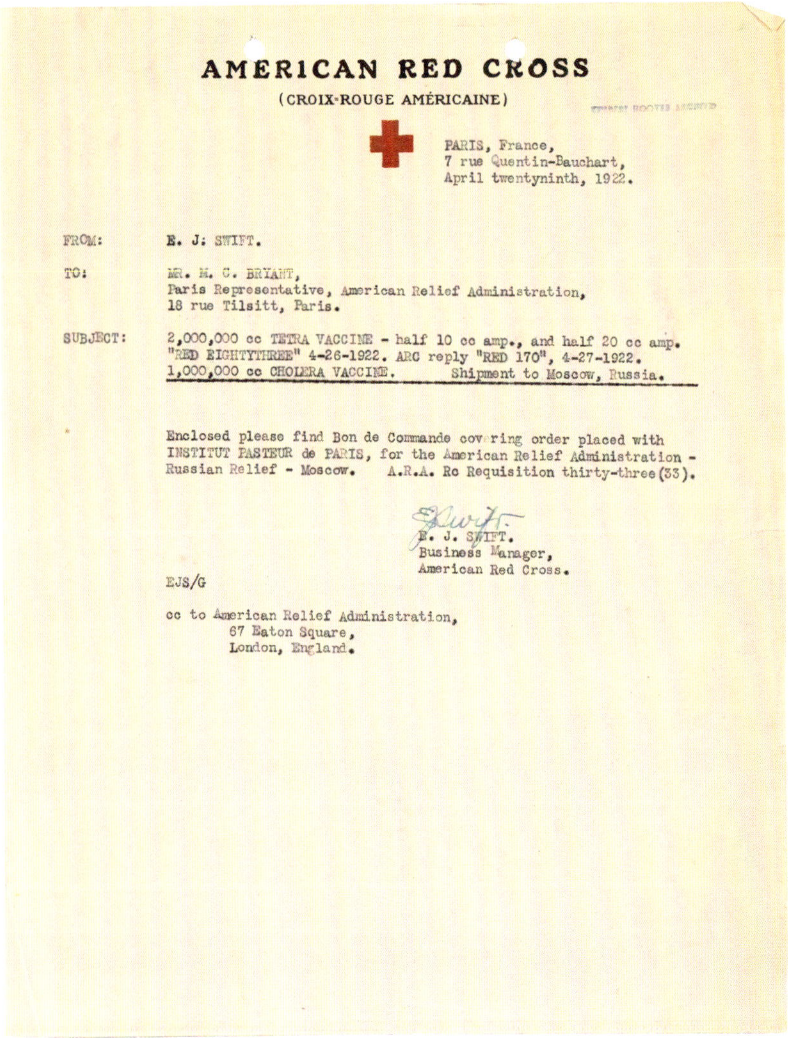

AMERICAN RED CROSS
(CROIX-ROUGE AMÉRICAINE)

PARIS, France,
7 rue Quentin-Bauchart,
April twentyninth, 1922.

FROM: E. J. SWIFT.

TO: MR. M. C. BRYANT,
Paris Representative, American Relief Administration,
18 rue Tilsitt, Paris.

SUBJECT: 2,000,000 cc TETRA VACCINE - half 10 cc amp., and half 20 cc amp.
"RED EIGHTYTHREE" 4-26-1922. ARC reply "RED 170", 4-27-1922.
1,000,000 cc CHOLERA VACCINE. Shipment to Moscow, Russia.

Enclosed please find Bon de Commande covering order placed with INSTITUT PASTEUR de PARIS, for the American Relief Administration - Russian Relief - Moscow. A.R.A. Rc Requisition thirty-three (33).

E. J. SWIFT.
Business Manager,
American Red Cross.

EJS/G

cc to American Relief Administration,
67 Eaton Square,
London, England.

In the summer of 1921, before the ARA's arrival, the entire Volga region was the scene of what Dr. Walter Davenport characterized as "an almost explosive epidemic of cholera." Davenport heard about this raging cholera outbreak, which was estimated to have carried off twenty thousand people in Samara province alone, during his initial inspection trip to the Volga in November 1921. "Owing though to very energetic steps taken by the military authorities through obligatory vaccination of all soldiers, organization of isolation barracks for both soldiers and refugees, forced bathing and a strict sanitary control of the food markets, this epidemic practically over the whole of the Volga was under control by the middle of September."

Lyster bags, a staple of military camps since their invention in 1910, were provided to larger hospitals, children's homes, refugee camps, railroad stations, and along the rivers where dockworkers served arriving and departing barges and steamships. These thirty-six-gallon linen bags were hung from a tripod and fitted with six faucets around the base. The water inside each bag was purified with chlorine ampoules and served about a hundred people. The campaign to eradicate dirty, contaminated water included educating the public to the dangers of drinking unboiled water and eating raw foods. Yet a lack of the fuel required for boiling hampered the drive for safe drinking water.

Isolation of cholera patients, once a standard medical practice in Russia when hospitals were properly supplied and staffed, became the next preventive tool encouraged by the ARA. A June 1922 article in *Petrograd Pravda*, the organ of the local Communist Party, cited a recent congress of bacteriologists and epidemic specialists who warned that a "considerable part [of transmission of cholera] was played by cholera bearers, i.e. persons, who being apparently in perfect health, carry germs of this disease and are a dangerous source of infection." The warning echoed the story of "Typhoid Mary," an American cook who, in the first decade of the twentieth century, was identified as a symptomless carrier of typhoid. The cholera carriers in Russia were unknowingly transmitting cholera by the fecal-oral route. Isolation had been the key to disrupting disease transmission by Typhoid Mary, and now the method served again in Russia, thanks to the supplies, medicines, and food rations that the ARA provided to the isolation hospitals. In Kazan, cholera receiving stations were established aboard boats and steamships moored on the Volga and equipped with personnel to screen people with cholera-like symptoms before they were sent to city isolation hospitals.

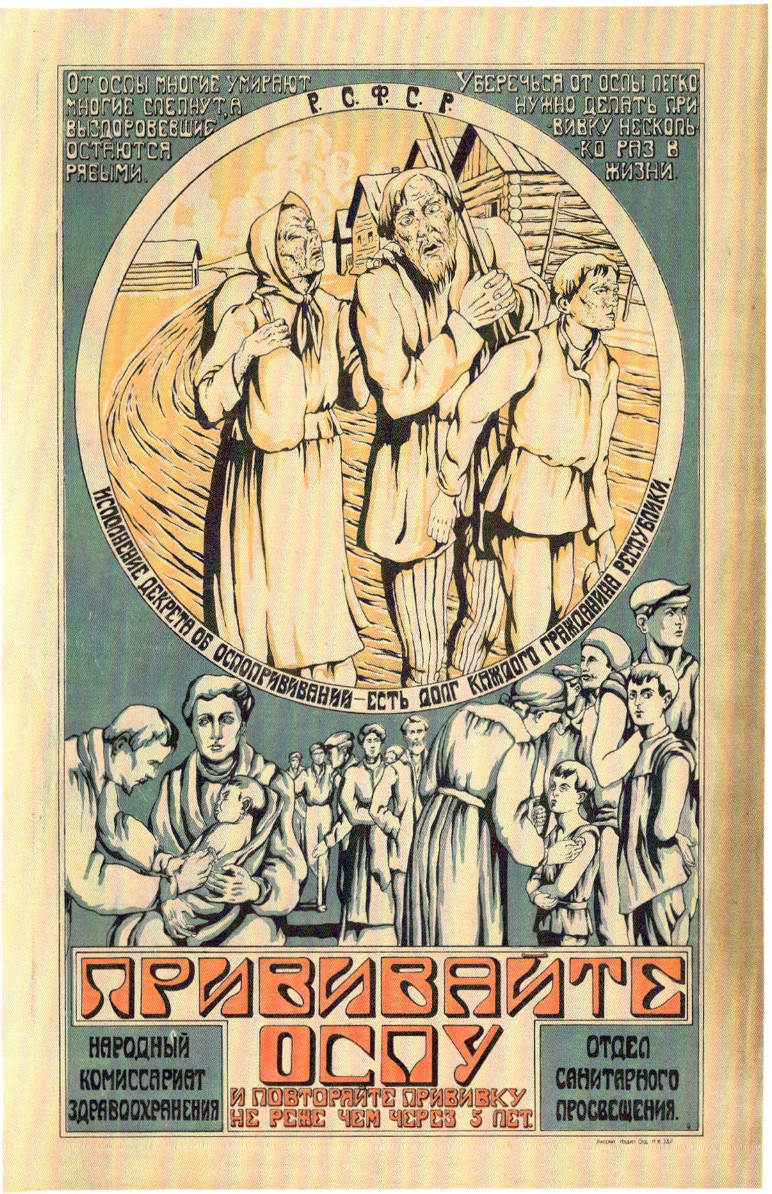
От оспы многие умирают многие слепнут, а выздоровевшие остаются рябыми.
Р. С. Ф. С. Р.
Уберечься от оспы легко нужно делать прививку несколько раз в жизни.
Исполнение декрета об оспопрививании — есть долг каждого гражданина республики.
Прививайте оспу
Народный комиссариат здравоохранения
и повторяйте прививку не реже чем через 5 лет.
Отдел санитарного просвещения.

Unidentified artist (Russian), Прививайте оспу и повторяйте прививку не реже чем через 5 лет." [Inoculate (against) smallpox and repeat the vaccination at least every five years], ca. 1920.
Poster Collection RU/SU 1589

State-of-the-Art Preventive Medicine: Vaccination

With summer approaching and cholera threatening, the ARA initiated a vaccination campaign against waterborne diseases. ARA publicity man Farmer Murphy, based in Moscow, conveyed a sense of the ambitiousness of the effort in an April 24 cable he sent to ARA publicity chief George Barr Baker in New York:

> A.R.A. through Medical Department beginning what probably most extensive sanitary prophylactic program ever attempted. Plan proposes inoculation every individual both adults [and] children to whom ARA affording relief and to all others who may volunteer. This means that 8 million and more probably 10 million will be inoculated against 5 communicable diseases Typhoid, Paratyphoid (A and B) Cholera and Smallpox.

Dr. Davenport, Beeuwkes's assistant in Moscow, in a May 1922 letter to Dr. John Toole, district physician in Saratov, characterized the vaccination campaign as "the most constructive piece of work in preventive medicine we have attempted." Beeuwkes, writing at about that same time, spelled out the rationale for the undertaking in his more matter-of-fact style: "We are carrying out this measure upon refugees and others of the poorest and most ignorant classes; those most liable to contract and disseminate infectious diseases. We believe the immunization of these classes against cholera, typhoid fever, paratyphoid A and B, and Small Pox to be of inestimable value in prevention of epidemics and protection of the general population." The cholera inoculation would provide protection for six months or longer, while the typhoid inoculation would last at least three years.

The vaccination campaign first came into focus in February 1922, when Beeuwkes sent a letter to all district physicians announcing the plan to use a tetra vaccine—made of a "saline suspension of killed bacilli (of cholera, typhosus, paratyphosus A and B) prepared in the Pasteur Institute in Paris." The ARA

АМЕРИКАНСКАЯ АДМИНИСТРАЦИЯ ПОМОЩИ.

Русский Отдел.

Медицинский Отдел.

Москва, 21 апреля 1922 года.

Распоряжение по Медицинскому Отделу № 6.

ПРОГРАММА ПРЕДОХРАНИТЕЛЬНЫХ ПРИВИВОК.

В качестве практической и действенной профилактической меры против 5 заразных болезней, а именно: тифоида, паратифоида „а“ и „б“, холеры и оспы, которые безусловно появятся в эпедемической форме среди той части населения, которой Американская Администрация Помощи стремится предоставить помощь продовольствием и медикаментами, если не будут приняты решительные меры к предотвращению таковых болезней, принята программа проведения предохранительных прививок, которая должна быть выполнена по всем районам Районными Уполномоченными при содействии районного врача.

ПЛАН ПРОВЕДЕНИЯ ПРЕДОХРАНИТЕЛЬНЫХ ПРИВИВОК.

План этот предполагает производство прививки всем лицам, которым мы предоставляем продовольствие и помощь, как взрослым, так и детям, а равно и другим лицам по их желанию.

Центральное Правительство и местные Отделы Здравоохранения обещали свое содействие и помощь в этом вопросе прикомандированием персонала, широким оповещением в прессе и предоставлением всех существующих помещений для производства прививок, как то: больниц, амбулаторий, лечебниц и приемных пунктов. Районные уполномоченные и врачи должны использовать все эти возможности для того, чтобы предохранительные мероприятия могли быть быстро выполнены. Так как условия различных районов, где мы работаем, могут быть различны, настоящим Главная Контора наша не желает предписывать подробностей, каким образом должен быть выполнен весь этот план.

ТЕТРАВАКЦИНА.

Для Медицинского Отдела Американской Администрации Помощи были изготовлены институтом Пастера в Париже вакцины, содержащие следующее количество микроорганизмов в кубических сантиметрах:

Холера	4.000.000.000
Тифоид	1.800.000.000
Паратифоид „а“ . . .	1.250.000.000
Паратифоид „б“ . . .	1.250.000.000

Вакцина эта даст иммунитет против указанных болезней на значительный период времени и вполне равноценна тетравакцине, с успехом употреблявшейся во французской армии на Востоке и в Армени „Помощью Ближнему Востоку“.

Прививка этой вакцины для взрослого производится в два приема с промежутком от 7 до 10 дней. В первый раз впрыскивается 1 кубический сантиметр, во 2-й раз—2 кубич. сант. Прививка женщинам и детям должна быть произведена в дозах, соответствующих весу тела, причем средним весом для взрослого принимается вес в 150 фунтов.

Местом прививки выбирается рука около прикрепления дельтовидного мускула. Если по каким либо причинам нельзя сделать прививку в этом месте, иглу можно ввести в спину над нижней частью лопатки или в грудь под ключицей. Прививка должна быть впрыснута **под кожу** и никак не в мускул или в самую кожу. Руку необходимо вымыть как перед всякой операцией. Считается достаточным смочить до и после впрыскивания место такового, протерев кожу досуха, настойкой иода или спиртом.

Ампулы должны быть чистыми, а вакцину из таковых надлежит доставать шприцем. Шприцы и иглы должны быть стерилизованы или кипячением или опуская иглы предварительно в раствор фенола, а затем в чистый спирт. Для каждого человека желательно употребление свежей иглы.

Вакцинация не может быть произведена при нездоровьи пациента или повышенной его температуре. Если температура или другие симптомы указывают на болезнь, вакцинация должна быть отложена.

В день прививки не следует пить никаких алкогольных напитков. При вакцинации наиболее удобным временем для производства таковой следует считать время около 4 часов дня, така как тогда значительная доля вызываемых вакцинацией последствий проходит до следующего утра. Обычно она вызывает некоторую головную боль и плохое самочувствие, а также в месте прививки появляется покраснение и болезненность размером с ладонь, и иногда боль в подмышечной железе. Желательно недопускать после прививки никакого физического напряжения. Редко случаются более тяжелые последствия, выражающиеся в головной боли, спинной боли, тошноте, рвоте, сыпи на губах и повышенной температуре с появлением белка в моче и потере веса. Случаев таких последствий очень немного и обычно они, независимо от степени своей, проходят через 48 часов.

ПРОТИВООСПЕННЫЕ ПРИВИВКИ.

После прививки первой дозы тетравакцины каждому пациенту будет привита оспа в ту же или другую руку. Указанная прививка не будет произведена тем, у кого имеются явные следы перенесения означенной болезни или недавно принявшейся прививки оспы.

ПЕРСОНАЛ.

Районные врачи должны сделать все, чтобы об'яснить нашему персоналу всю важность и необходимость предохранительной прививки и вакцинации, а равно предоставить все нужное для осуществления таковых.

ОТЧЕТНОСТЬ.

Районные врачи должны заставить весь персонал, участвующий в этой работе, представить список всех произведенных прививок. В списке должны быть указаны имена, рост, возраст, местожительство пациента и число произведенных прививок тетравакцины и оспы. Районный врач должен проставлять на оборотной стороне ежемесячного медико-санитарного отчета (бланк Медицинского Отдела „А“) количество прививок тетравакцины и оспы, произведенных за месяц.

МАТЕРИАЛЫ.

Тетравакцина и оспенный детрит, шприцы, перевязочный материал будут предоставлены Медицинским Отделом в Москве всем районам, где мы производим операции, за исключением вакцин для тех районов, где имеется в достаточном количестве правительственных запасов холерной вакцины, дивакцины и др. подобных. Как тетравакцина, так и детрит должны храниться в холодном и сухом месте. При таком способе хранения они не портятся втечении 4-х месяцев.

ОБЩИЕ САНИТАРНЫЕ МЕРОПРИЯТИЯ.

Хотя прививки считаются вполне достоверным способом предохранения от болезней все же в случаях кишечных заболеваний они не дают всех 100% иммунитета; поэтому для того, чтобы вообще улучшить санитарные условия в районе, особенно в больших городах, Районный Уполномоченный по своему усмотрению может при содействии местных Здравоотделов организовать санитарные отряды или кампании из среды местных взрослых беженцев, которые за свой труд будут получать взрослый паек кукурузы или беженскй паек.

Работа их должна происходить по указаниям районного врача и местных Здравоотделов и заключаться в выполнении мероприятий общественного характера, которые приведут к общему улучшению положения в смысле чистоты и санитарии, и могут состоять из чистки улиц, грунтовых дорог, дворов, водостоков и т. под., чем будут уничтожены очаги распространения мух и комаров.

По распоряжению полк. *ХАСКЕЛЛЬ.*

К. Д. К. Квинн
Пом. Управл. делами

Д-р *В. П. Девенпорт*
И. о. Нач. Медицинск. Отдела.

Зак. № 366.

Medical Memorandum No. 6, issued on April 21, 1922, by the ARA Medical Division in Moscow, instructed district physicians in the "how-to" of the ARA's vaccination campaign.

would also provide the smallpox vaccine to be given at the same time as the tetra vaccine. Anticipating resistance to the campaign from the local medical community, Beeuwkes decided to rely almost exclusively on vaccines produced by the Pasteur Institute in Paris. Vaccines could be procured from the United States at cheaper cost, but local physicians held the Pasteur Institute in especially high regard, which would boost the credibility of the vaccines and thus facilitate the campaign.

Although vaccination was not compulsory before the revolution, in 1920 the People's Commissariat of Health responded to the 158,505 registered cases of smallpox by decreeing the smallpox vaccination mandatory, especially for the many children who had not been vaccinated for the disease in the years since the start of the war in 1914. It was impossible to carry out the order, however, because of the dearth of physicians in the rural areas and the unreliable quality of the Russian-made vaccine, which did not always produce a "take," or positive reaction, evident in the pustular lesion and eventual scab on the arm. "Non-takes" resulted from improper administration or from a vaccine that had lost its potency. Not until the ARA procured a reputable smallpox vaccine from the Pasteur Institute in Paris in 1922 was the 1920 Soviet decree fulfilled.

The excellent reputation of the Pasteur Institute notwithstanding, Beeuwkes, anticipating resistance to the immunization campaign from local health workers, instructed district physicians to query local government authorities and Russian physicians about conditions on the ground: Local cooperation? Facilities? Popular sentiment about vaccines? Newspaper publicity? Beeuwkes proposed that the ARA would provide all vaccines and inoculations, syringes, sterilizing material, and instructions, if the local boards of health agreed to organize physicians, feldshers, nurses, and medical students to staff the vaccination squads. In addition, the ARA would provide food and clothing packages to the Russian physicians and an adult corn ration to the other health care workers for their efforts.

Medical Memorandum No. 6, issued on April 21, 1922, from Beeuwkes's office in Moscow, instructed district physicians in the "how-to" of the campaign. The adult course of the tetra vaccine consisted of two doses (first dose: 1 cc; second dose: 2 cc) at seven-to-ten-day intervals. Children received reduced dosages dependent on age, body weight, and health. The elderly, feeble, and undernourished received a half dose. Injections were to be given in the arm, the back over the scapula, or in the chest over the clavicle. On the other arm, physicians would score or scratch the skin and then dab the opening with the smallpox vaccine. All vaccinations were to be registered on official cards and include name, height, age, residence, and date of vaccinations.

\+ + +

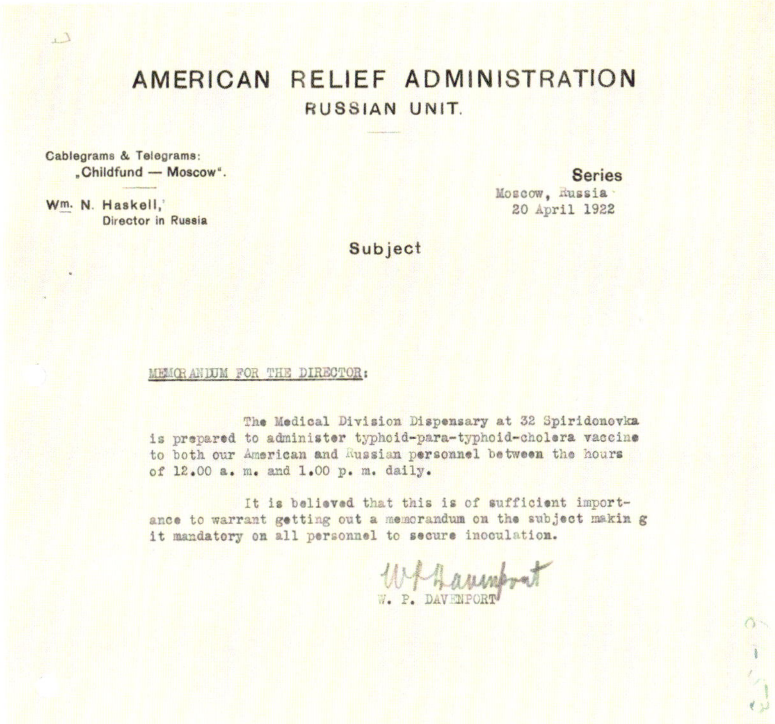

AMERICAN RELIEF ADMINISTRATION
RUSSIAN UNIT.

Cablegrams & Telegrams: „Childfund — Moscow".

Wm. N. Haskell, Director in Russia

Series

Moscow, Russia
20 April 1922

Subject

MEMORANDUM FOR THE DIRECTOR:

The Medical Division Dispensary at 32 Spiridonovka is prepared to administer typhoid-para-typhoid-cholera vaccine to both our American and Russian personnel between the hours of 12.00 a. m. and 1.00 p. m. daily.

It is believed that this is of sufficient importance to warrant getting out a memorandum on the subject makin g it mandatory on all personnel to secure inoculation.

W P Davenport
W. P. DAVENPORT

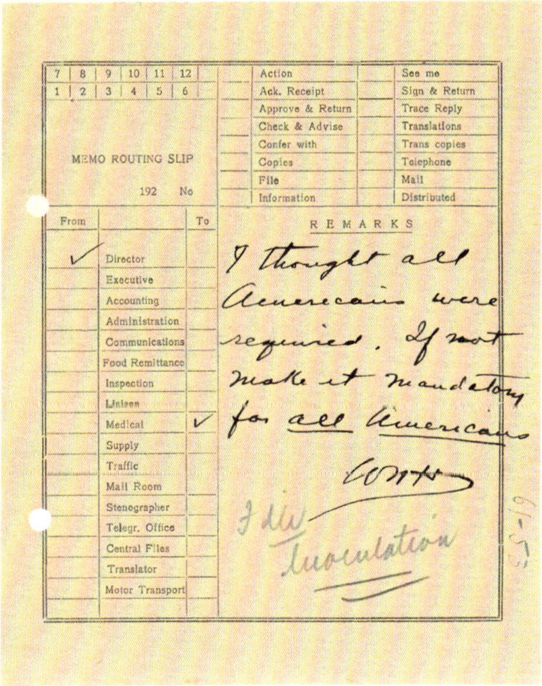

MEMO ROUTING SLIP

192 No

Action	See me
Ack. Receipt	Sign & Return
Approve & Return	Trace Reply
Check & Advise	Translations
Confer with	Trans copies
Copies	Telephone
File	Mail
Information	Distributed

From / To: Director ✓; Executive; Accounting; Administration; Communications; Food Remittance; Inspection; Liaison; Medical ✓; Supply; Traffic; Mail Room; Stenographer; Telegr. Office; Central Files; Translator; Motor Transport

REMARKS

I thought all Americans were required. If not make it mandatory for all Americans
WNH

File
Inoculation

Memorandum from Dr. Walter P. Davenport to Colonel William Haskell, April 20, 1922, regarding the vaccination of the ARA's American and Russian personnel at Moscow headquarters. Vaccination of ARA staff, both American and local, was made mandatory, as Colonel Haskell's note appended to Davenport's memo makes plain: "I thought all Americans were required," Haskell wrote. "If not make it mandatory for all Americans. WNH."

Unidentified artist (Russian), Граждане! Делайте себе противохолерные прививки. Только против прививки бессильна смерть [Citizens! Get your cholera vaccinations. Only against vaccination is death powerless], ca. 1920. Poster Collection RU/SU 985

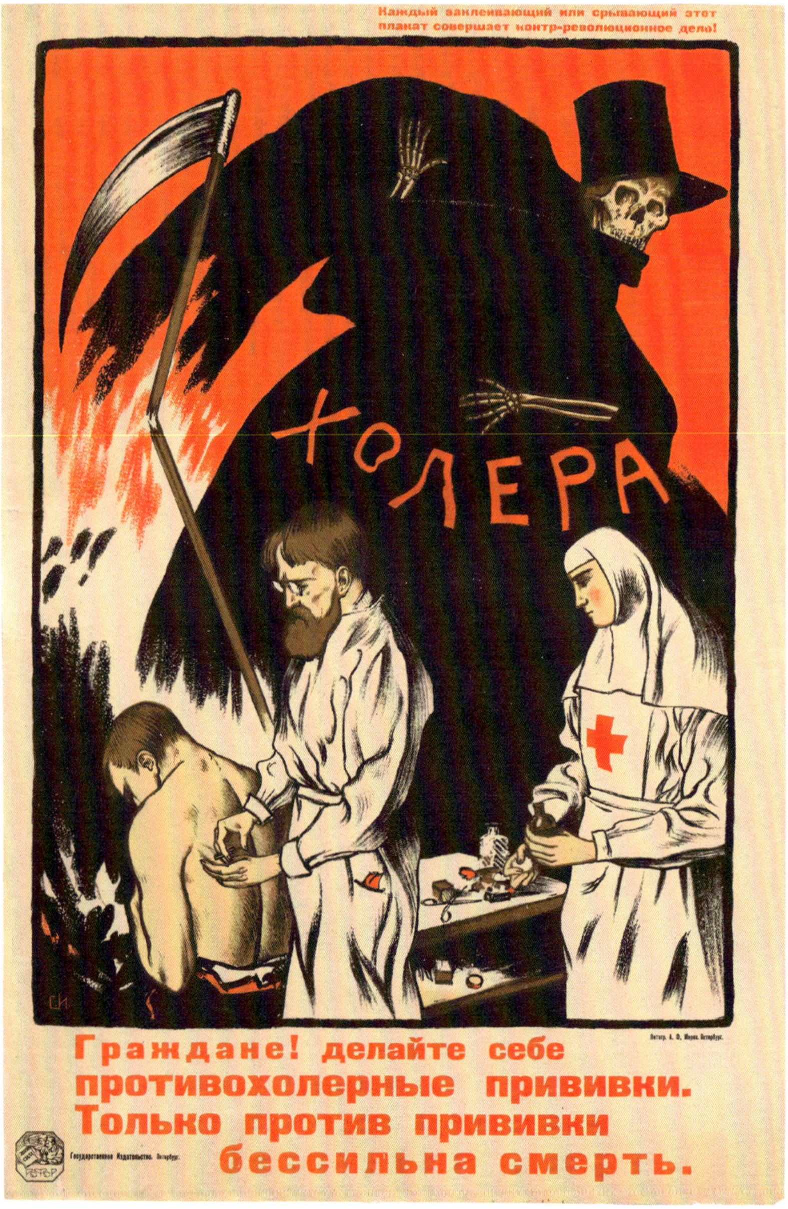
Каждый заклеивающий или срывающий этот плакат совершает контр-революционное дело!
ХОЛЕРА
Граждане! делайте себе противохолерные прививки. Только против прививки бессильна смерть.

On March 28, 1922, Dr. Foucar in Samara wrote to Beeuwkes to convey the local outlook for the vaccination campaign then in preparation: "Sentiment of the *general population*: in this country, it is safe to assume that the sentiment will be decidedly against it (vaccination) as it also would in America or anywhere else: knowledge of a trifle immediate discomfort always outweighing fear of future possible, though much greater, evils. However, thru aid of active propaganda, aided by the contrôle thru the distribution of food, the vaccination campaign will succeed."

There was plenty of anecdotal evidence suggesting that popular suspicion, and therefore the potential for resistance, ran deep. With luck, the medical teams were on the heels of some positive publicity done by the local authorities in the newspapers, or, for a largely illiterate public, through the distribution of pictorial posters. One movie theater in Kiev promised to advertise on screen the prophylactic benefits of the inoculations administered in the ARA dispensaries. In Saratov, the local *Sickle and Hammer* praised the medical work of the ARA and encouraged readers to adopt a progressive mindset with regard to medicine: "We understand perfectly well that the time of cholera-mutinies on the part of ignorant peasants has passed, that our village has made great progress during the revolutionary period. Vaccinations are the achievement of high culture! Peasants of our uyezd [county], avail yourselves of the relief of ARA." From Kazan, Dr. Dear assured Beeuwkes that "there would be no problem getting the populace to submit to vaccination," that "their love and respect for Americans is such that they will virtually do anything which we may advocate or initiate."

Whatever the influence of the official enlightenment campaign or the local affinity for all things American, as Dr. Foucar made clear, when it came to persuading the skeptical masses of the wisdom of vaccination, the ARA possessed the ultimate leverage in the form of food. As the vaccination "squads," or "companies," each composed of a Russian physician-inspector and in some cases fourth- and fifth-year medical students, fanned out across an assigned territory, they began by vaccinating children arriving for meals at ARA kitchens and adults receiving ARA corn rations. Food proved to be a powerful inducement, decisive in overcoming any hesitancy about short-term pain and superstitions about the inoculation site leaving the "antichrist's seal" or the letters "ARA."

Among those requiring some enlightenment in the benefits of prophylaxis were local health workers, including doctors. From Tsaritsyn, Dr. George Cornick, of San Angelo, Texas, complained in July 1922 that "the vaccination program was moving slowly because little cholera has appeared and it is difficult to force vaccination when fear of the disease is not present." Dr. Mark Godfrey, writing from Simbirsk that same month, echoed the complaint: "Russians can't understand the prophylactic/preventive role of tetra vaccine. They must see deaths and evidence of it first." A medical report from Tsaritsyn observed that local

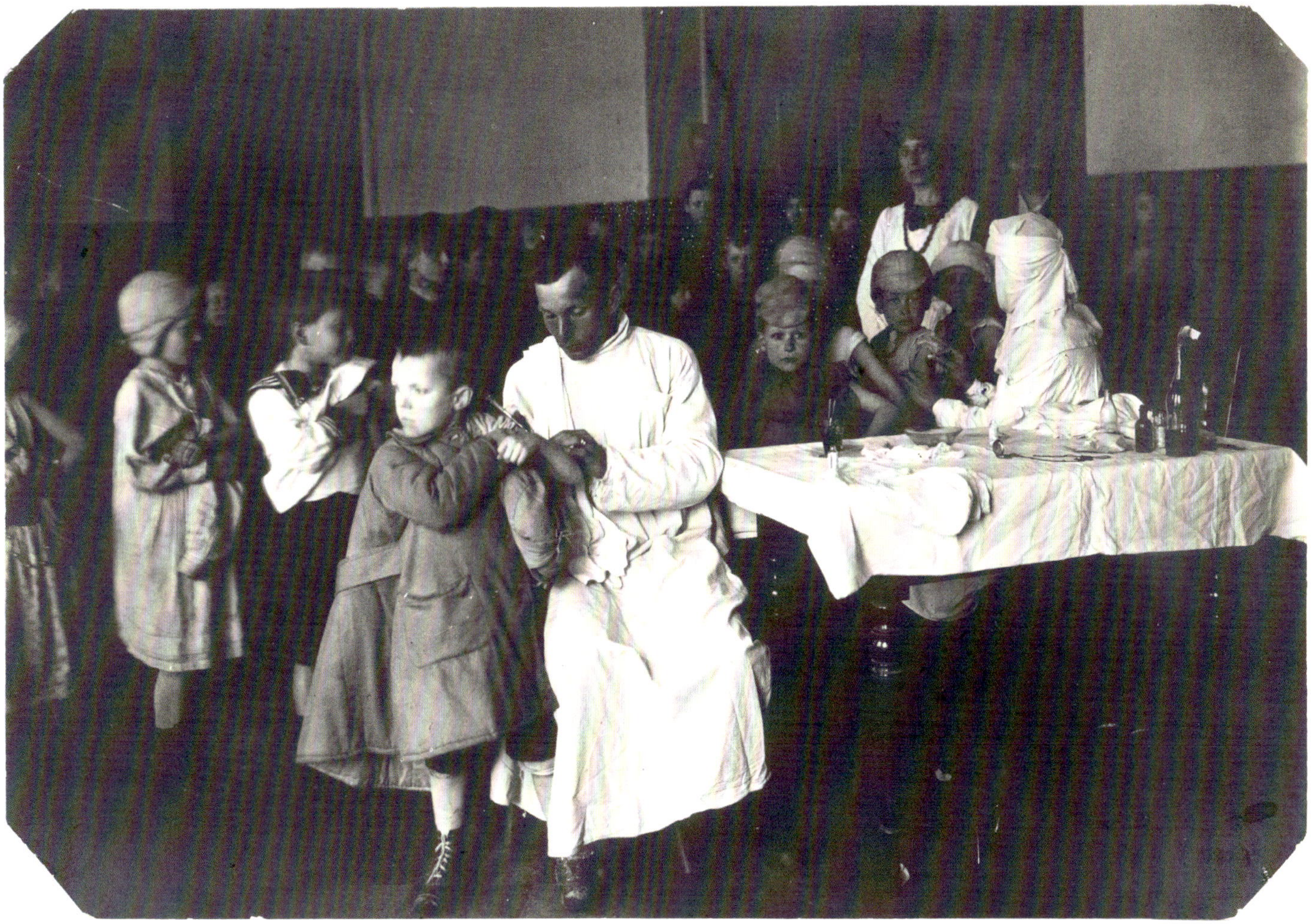

Inoculation of children with the tetra vaccine at the ARA kitchen on Gagarin Street in Petrograd, spring 1922.

physicians were inclined to stop vaccinating for cholera as soon as there was any sign that cases of the disease were lessening. "It constantly had to be shouted at them . . . that tetra-vaccine was not only a prophylactic specificum against the cholera but also was of great value for the prevention of three types of typhus fever, wherefore it was called 'tetra-vaccine' and not simply 'anti-choleric-vaccine.' " Local physicians in Odessa, expressing concerns about some of the components in the tetra vaccine, argued that the paratyphoid A and B vaccines were unnecessary since neither disease had been detected in Odessa. Perhaps some of them were worried that possible adverse physical reactions to the injection—fever, headaches, body aches, weakness—would make the general population even more vaccine averse.

For refugees, if the threat of withholding their daily meal was not inducement enough, the knowledge that a certificate of vaccination was required to purchase a railway ticket usually served to overcome any resistance. And for those travelers heading to countries on the western border of Soviet Russia—Poland and the Baltic states—the stakes grew higher: only the certificates for inoculations given with the ARA vaccines were acceptable; those given with the Soviet government bivalent vaccine for cholera and typhoid, often made in quantity in Moscow or Petrograd, were considered inferior and the corresponding certificate not valid for travelers leaving Soviet Russia.

The ARA's vaccination campaign was carried out from June to September 1922. The general plan having been laid out by Beeuwkes, each district

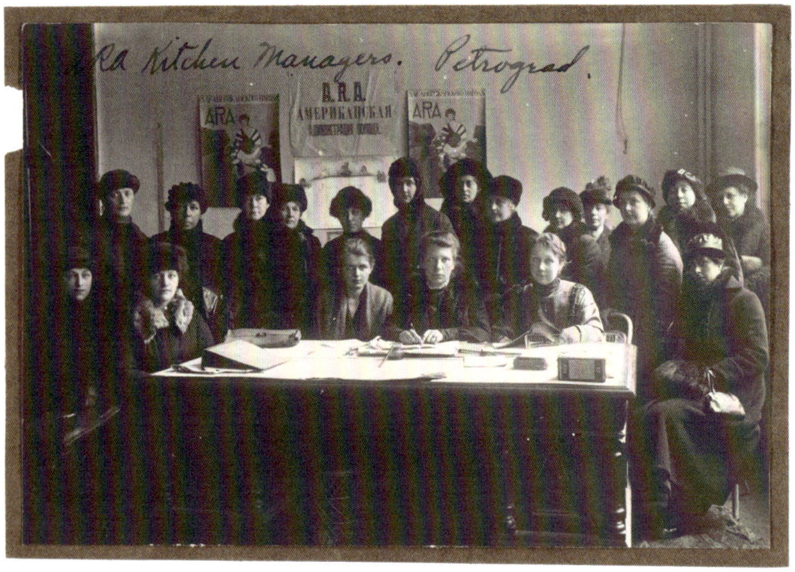

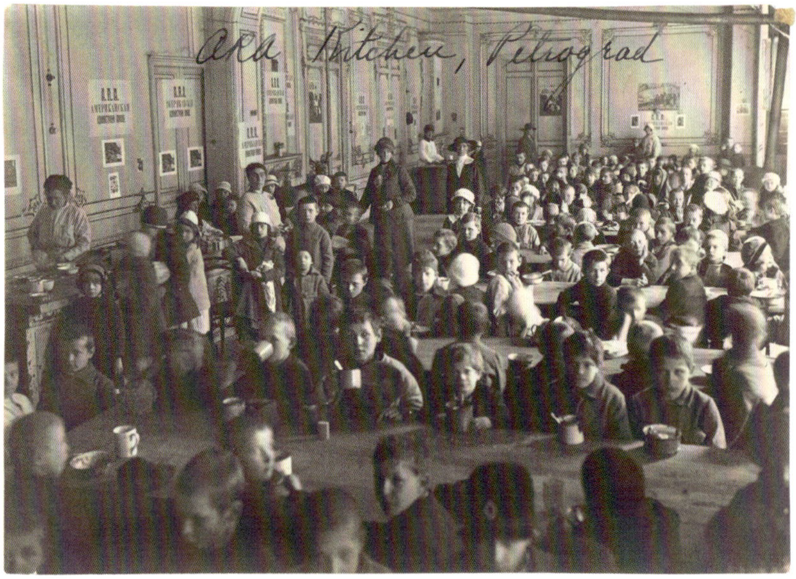

ABOVE LEFT: American Lizzie Bach, of Cornwall, Pennsylvania (seated at center), among other managers of the ARA's kitchens in Petrograd, 1922. They supervised the vaccination of children receiving a daily meal from the ARA.

ABOVE RIGHT: ARA kitchen, Petrograd, ca. 1922.

BELOW: Dr. John Toole, Moscow, 1923.
Courtesy of Bess Rattray

physician had some latitude to organize and improvise the district's campaign based on the availability of qualified personnel, the cooperation of local institutions and health workers, and the physical distances to be covered. Also a factor was the availability of the vaccine, which arrived from the Pasteur Institute in Paris in small shipments, necessarily prolonging the campaign. In Samara, Dr. Foucar recorded the campaign, "carried out by mobile vaccinating companies, each company consisting of one doctor and one assistant," as an unqualified success.

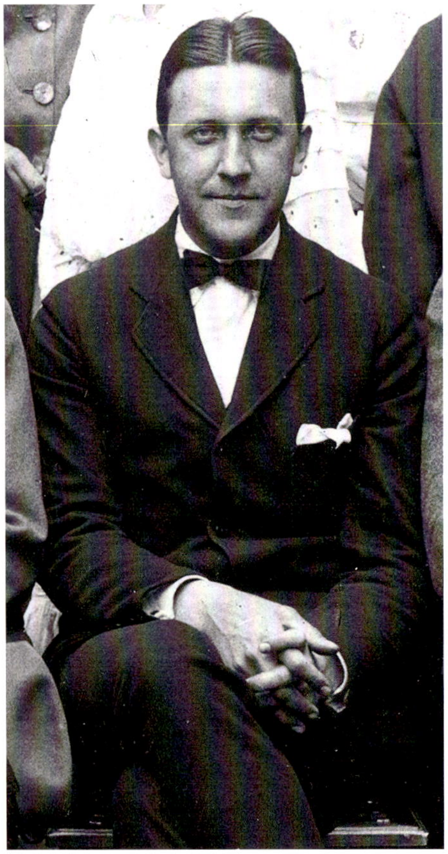

> The "companies" were supplied by us with the vaccine and with syringes, needles, tincture of iodine, gauze, clean sheets to cover tables, operating gowns, and the necessary utensils for boiling the syringes and needles and washing the hands. The personnel was remunerated for their work by being given one A.R.A. food-packet each at the termination of their work, provided they had carried this work out in a satisfactory manner. One hundred and twenty-five such companies were put into operation, and by September 1, 1922, they had completed the campaign as we had outlined it, and had given 475,488 complete courses of the vaccine. . . . In addition to the tetra vaccine campaign, smallpox vaccine was given to 10,000 adults and children who had not been previously amply protected against smallpox, a disease which is endemic throughout Russia.

Down the Volga at Saratov, Dr. Toole wrote to Beeuwkes on June 22, 1922:

> The vaccination program is progressing extremely favorably. Before the end of the month all of our feeding areas will have been completed or have received their first inoculation. This to my mind is extremely gratifying and eminently satisfactory. To have vaccinated all of the children in the A.R.A. kitchens, situated as they are all over the land and very far apart, while travel conditions have been almost impossible warrants hearty congratulations to the doctor-inspectors who have accomplished this. I am extremely pleased with the doctor-inspectors in our employ. They have done extremely fine work.

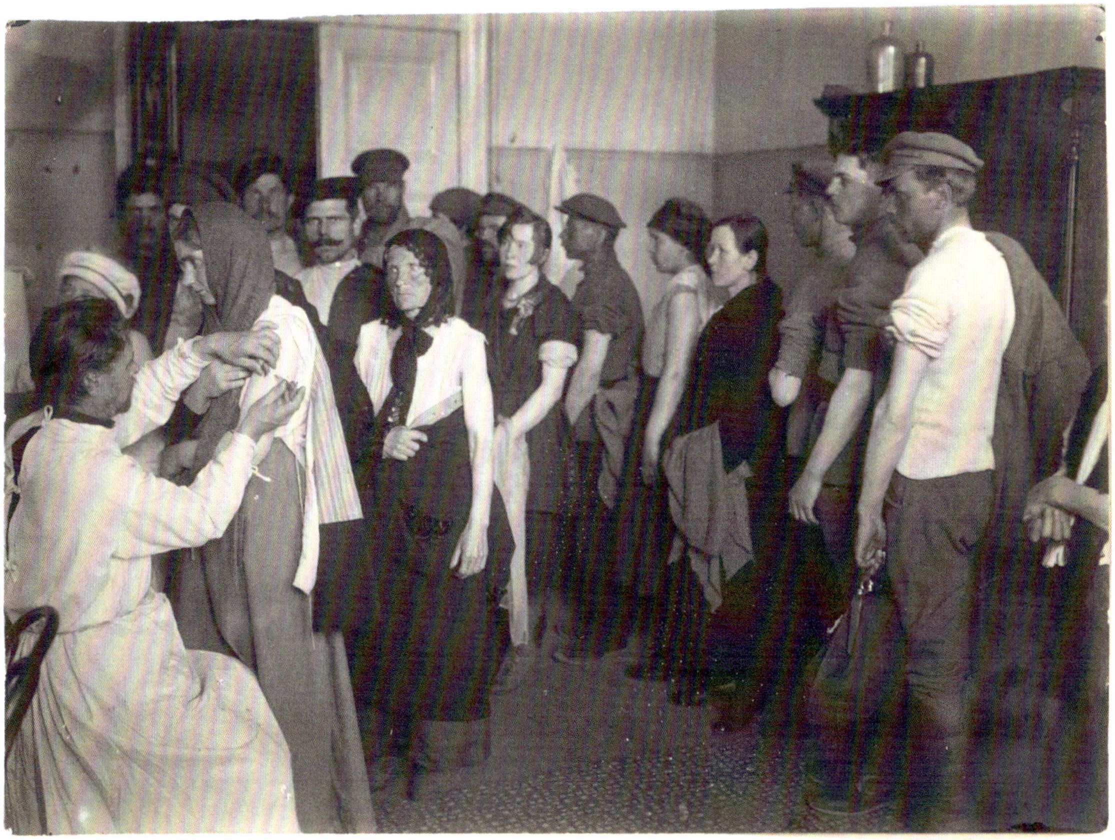

Petrograd, 1922. Vaccination of people being repatriated to the West.

Toole's summing up, in his report to Beeuwkes of August 1, noted that despite the cholera epidemic of the summer of 1921, the Soviet government seemed incapable of action to prevent a repetition of a similar outbreak that summer.

> It was therefore an act of beneficence and a tremendous undertaking in preventive medicine that the American Relief Administration undertook and accomplished in offering to vaccinate the children eating in their kitchens, and in supplying the local medical profession with vaccine so that millions of people might be provided with immunity against these dreaded diseases. It is no doubt largely due to this gift that the epidemics this year have in no way been appalling. The presence of foci of infection throughout Russia has been definitely shown by the outbreak of cholera in nearly every district and without the immunization of millions of people in these districts the outbreaks of tremendous epidemics of cholera seem certain.

Toole organized squads consisting of five to ten medical students, usually in their fourth of fifth year of medical school, and dispatched them to a designated region along with one of the ARA's inspector-physicians. "Each Vaccination Squad personnel convoyed the vaccine together with the necessary syringes, iodine, alcohol, cotton and medicine chest." After making the initial arrangements, each inspector-physician returned to his regular job and the students proceeded with the vaccinations. "Each town or village where a doctor was present, the doctor had general supervision of the work and usually examined the children concerning physical fitness etc. while the student assisted by feldsher or sisters did the actual inoculation and vaccination. Each student's area was so large that after making a complete circuit of his district, it was time to make

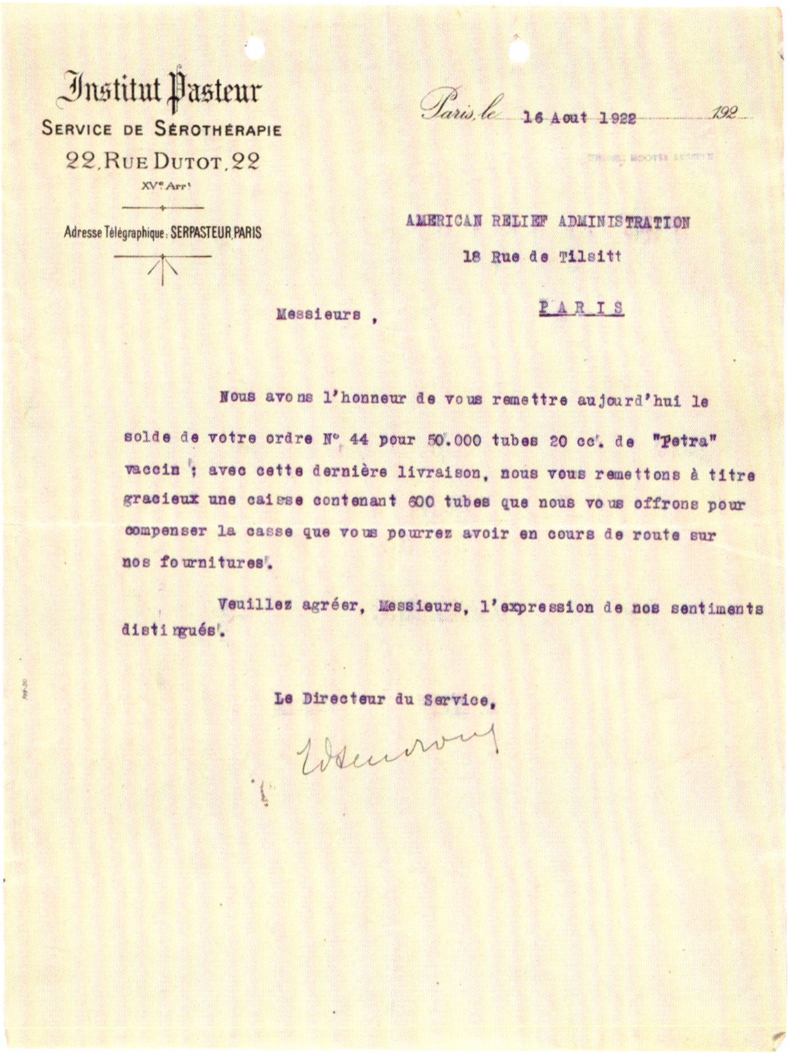

Institut Pasteur
Service de Sérothérapie
22, Rue Dutot, 22
XVe Arrt
Adresse Télégraphique : SERPASTEUR, PARIS

Paris, le 16 Aout 1922

AMERICAN RELIEF ADMINISTRATION
18 Rue de Tilsitt
PARIS

Messieurs,

Nous avons l'honneur de vous remettre aujourd'hui le solde de votre ordre N° 44 pour 50.000 tubes 20 cc. de "Tetra" vaccin ; avec cette dernière livraison, nous vous remettons à titre gracieux une caisse contenant 600 tubes que nous vous offrons pour compenser la casse que vous pourrez avoir en cours de route sur nos fournitures.

Veuillez agréer, Messieurs, l'expression de nos sentiments distingués.

Le Directeur du Service,

Letter from the service manager of the Pasteur Institute on August 16, 1922, notifying the ARA Paris office of the shipment of the balance of the ARA's order of tetra vaccine.

the second circuit for the second inoculation. So that each squad took from two to three weeks to cover its territory twice." Smallpox vaccinations, meanwhile, were administered at the same time as the first anti-cholera inoculation, and their results could be verified at the time of the second inoculation.

In cities and towns where the ARA operated, vaccinations were made available to refugees at inoculation points and dispensaries. Ufa, the largest ARA district, conducted the largest of the American vaccination drives as measured in the total number of those vaccinated and the distances covered. Some 931,928 people were successfully inoculated throughout the district. Dr. Raymond McKnight Sloan, the district physician, had to contend with the long wait times for vaccine shipments to distant Ufa. "Had we received the vaccines earlier," he noted, "I think we could have reached the million mark in total number of people inoculated." Also, the late arrival of some of the vaccines in the remote regions of the district prevented some people from getting the second inoculation. The campaign ground to a virtual halt when harvesttime arrived, and "we did not think it advisable to stop a man from work for the number of days that he would necessarily be incapacitated. And besides, by this time many were living in the fields and could not be reached[,] therefore the corn rations were not refused these people as they would have been unable to carry on their work without food."

In Ufa, too, food proved to be the ultimate inducement to getting a shot, as Sloan explained.

> When the campaign was at its height and people knew they must have [a] certificate of vaccination before they could receive corn, the ambulatories and vaccination points were besieged by hundreds of people, every one crowding the next, and it was necessary to call out special guards to preserve order. . . . The peasants at first objected to being inoculated, claiming that it was an invention of the devil. The Bashkirs particularly dislike the idea. However, with the lever of the corn ration behind it, the A.R.A. had not much difficulty in making them come round. As the villagers came in for their corn ration, they first had to be inoculated, their cards stamped and then they were allowed to get their corn. It required strong forces of militia at the various distribution points to line the people up and prevent them from crowding the doctors when they realized that their corn ration depended on their being inoculated.

By October 1922, Beeuwkes could announce that the results of the vaccination and inoculation program were "very gratifying." The numbers of cholera cases reported from the various districts in the Volga region showed a dramatic decline from 93,784 cases in 1921 to 6,671 in 1922. In Ukraine, however, where ARA operations began only in spring 1922 and where child feeding operations were

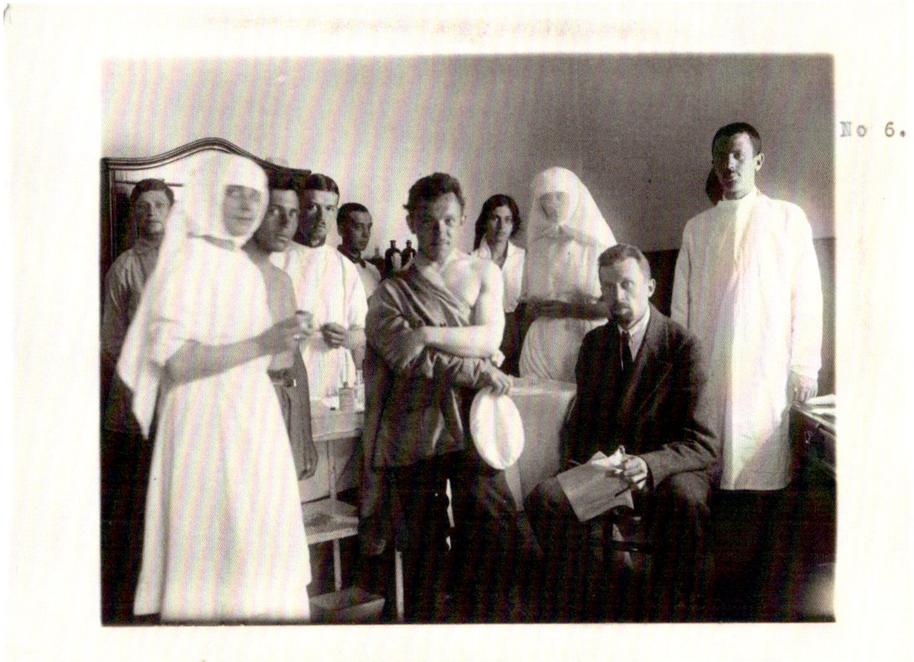

not as extensive as in the Volga region and farther east, the vaccination campaign was not as effective, and the 42,000 cases recorded in 1922 far exceeded the 10,341 cases registered in 1921.

Hundreds of squads of local physicians and medical students scratched over 1.5 million smallpox vaccines into arms and gave over six million injections of the tetra vaccine against cholera, typhoid, and paratyphoid A and B. In the summer months of 1922, the seven million cubic centimeters of tetra vaccine and three and a half million doses of smallpox vaccine purchased from the Pasteur Institute in Paris had been used to administer over eight million inoculations and vaccinations in Soviet Russia. The ARA in several districts also facilitated the production of local vaccines by restocking medical laboratories and supporting their staff members. The resounding success of the ARA campaign convinced some provincial boards of health to continue to use vaccination as a genuinely prophylactic measure in the coming year. Dr. Toole in Saratov called the vaccination program "one of the best pieces of work we have done."

ABOVE: ARA dispensary and inoculation point, Kiev, May 30, 1922. American Relief Administration European operational records

BELOW LEFT: Inoculation and wound care station for refugees sponsored by the ARA, refugee camp hospital, Kozyova, Minsk, 1922. The sign above the man at right reads (in Russian): "Cholera Threatens: Don't Drink Raw [untreated] Water." Other posted notices encourage people to wash their hands before eating and to visit the bathhouse.

BELOW RIGHT: Dr. Sloan (standing at right) and his local medical staff in Ufa, ca. 1923. Raymond McKnight Sloan papers

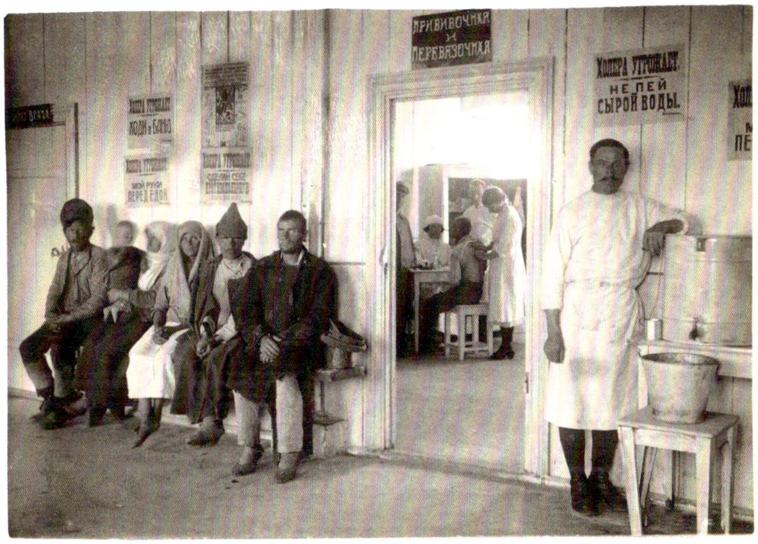

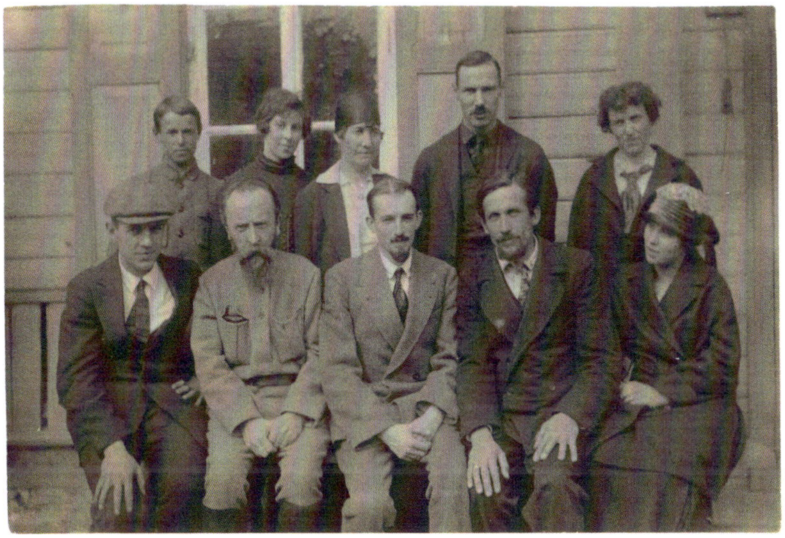

PHOTOGRAPH

Name: Dr.Otto O.Beck

Born: November 17th,1893 Grand Island Nebr.

Home Address: 2015 Warren University Place Nebr.

Nationality: American

Notify Case Emergency: G.Beck above address

Entered Soviet Russia: March 20th,1922

No.of A.R.A. Identity Card: 189

U.S.Passport No: 892

REMARKS:

[Out October 16th, 1922 Missing 656]

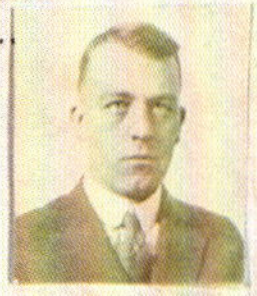

PHOTOGRAPH

Name: Beeuwkes,Henry Dr.

Born: America,August 29,1881

Home Address: Washington D.C.

Nationality: American

Notify Case Emergency: Mrs Henry Beeuwkes c/o A.R.A. London 67 Eaton Sq.

Entered Soviet Russia: September 19,1921.

No. of A. R. A. Incentity Card: 38

U. S. Passport No. 79505

REMARKS:

[Date of departure from Russia 12 June 1923 ?]

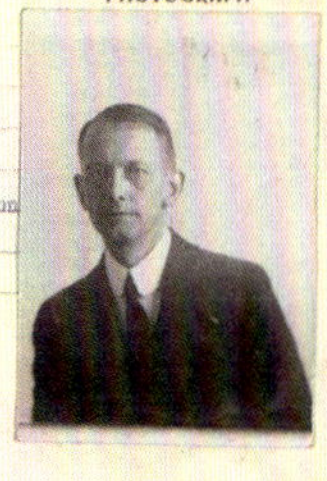

Form No. P-2, 6-50m, 8/21.

PHOTOGRAPH

Name: John B.Coffey

Born: March 30th,1895

Home Address: 312 South 12th East Salt Lake City

Nationality: American

Notify Case Emergency: Mrs.B.F.Coffey above address

Entered Soviet Russia: May 27th,1922

No. of A.R.A. Identity Card: 247

U.S. Passport No: 63421

REMARKS:

Reported May 30, 1922.

[Out June 5th 1923. Memo 395]

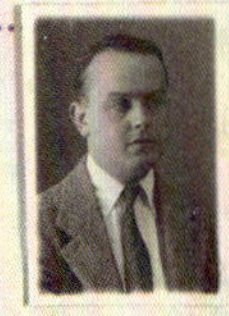

PHOTOGRAPH

Name: John E.Cox

Born: February 8th,1895

Home Address: Collierville, Tennessee

Nationality: American

Notify Case Emergency: J. R. Cox (Father)

Entered Soviet Russia: November 9th,1922

No. of A. R. A Identity Card: 351

U. S. Passport No. 225802

REMARKS:

Reported Nov. 11th 1922

[Out June 16th, 1923 Memo 407]

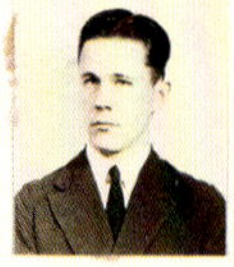

Form No. P-2, 6 50, ea, 0/21

PHOTOGRAPH

Name: Davenport Walter B.

Born: America November 14,1887.

Home Address: Washington D.C.

Nationality: American

Notify Case Emergency: John E.Davenport Holloway,Minnesota

Entered Soviet Russia: September 20th,1921.

No. of A. R. A. Incentity Card: 37

U. S. Passport No. 78897

REMARKS: Sept 21.

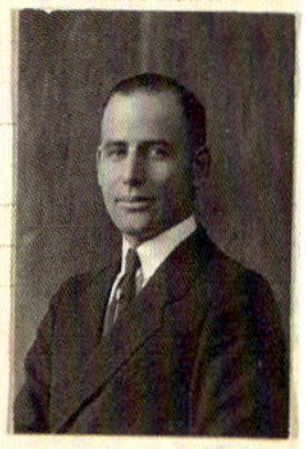

Form No. P-2, 6-50m, 8/21.

PHOTOGRAPH

Name: William Richard Doerr

Born: Hamilton-London December 7th,1893

Home Address: Coblenz Germany 10,Kaiser Friedrich Str. A.P.O. 927

Nationality: American

Notify Case Emergency: Mrs.Grete T.Doerr (wife) above address

Entered Soviet Russia: February 27th,1922

No. of A.R.A. Identity Card: 157

U.S. Passport No: 4155

REMARKS: Notify Case Emergency: Chief of Staff American Forces in Germany Coblenz Germany

[Out December 10th, 1922 Memo 313]

Arrived Moscow March 2d 1922 JM

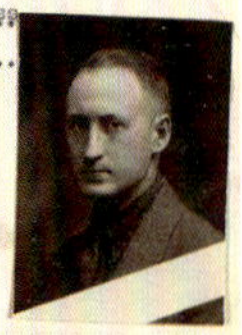

PHOTOGRAPH

Name: Frederic H. Foncar (Foucar JM)

Born: May 24th,1894 New York City U.S.A.

Home Address: 42, Broadway New York c/o A.R.A.

Nationality: American

Notify Case Emergency: Mother - Mrs. F.H.Foncar

Entered Soviet Russia: December 19th,1921.

No. of A.R.A. Identity Card: 109

U.S.Passport: 100977

REMARKS:

Arrived Dec 21st JM

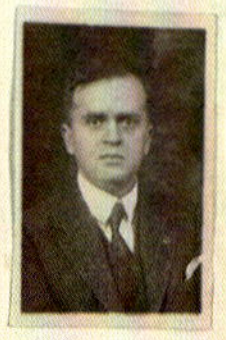

PHOTOGRAPH

Name: Dr W A H Gantt

Born: Wingina Va U S A

Home Address: Greyburn Virginia U S A

Nationality: American

Notify Case Emergency: Capt Henry P Gantt,Greyburn,Virginia U S A Greyburn Virginia U S A

Entered Soviet Russia: July 3rd, 1922

No. of A R A Incentity Card: 302

U S Passport No. 1136 Special Series

REMARKS:

[Reported July 6th]

Out June 12th 1923 Memo 399

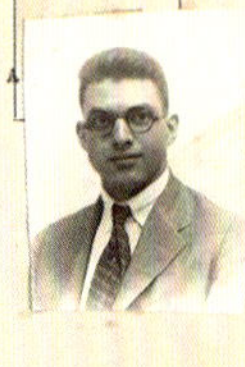

Form No. P-2, 6-50m, 8/21

PHOTOGRAPH

Name: Mark David Godfrey

Born: Ohio 1887

Home Address: Columbus Ohio

Nationality: American

Notify Case Emergency: Dr.F.Y.Johnson Waverly Ohio

Entered Soviet Russia: December 8th,1921 Rhineland Savings Co. Andernach Germany Army Bank c/o C.C.

No. of A.R.A. Identity Card: 92

U.S. Passport: 139940

REMARKS:

[Out June 12th, 1923 Memo 398]

Reported Dec 8th 1921

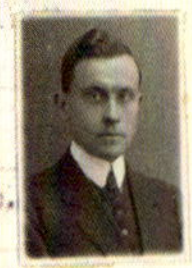

PHOTOGRAPH

Name: Ralph Herz M.D.

Born: November 24th,1889

Home Address: 56, West 35 th Str. New York

Nationality: American

Notify Case Emergency: Mrs.R.Lutyens A.R.A. London

Entered Soviet Russia: March 9th,1922

No. of A. R.A. Identity Card: 180

U.S. Passport No: 131777

REMARKS:

Arrived March 12th 1922

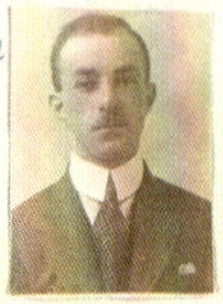

PHOTOGRAPH

Name: William E.Hurley

Born: New York March 30th,1897

Home Address: 21, Winter Ave New Brighton New York

Nationality: American

Notify Case Emergency: Mrs. Ursula Hurley above address

Entered Soviet Russia: November 9th,1922

No. of A. R. A Identity Card:

U. S. Passport No. 225711

REMARKS: [Reported Nov. 11 1922]

Out May 25th 1923 Memo 386

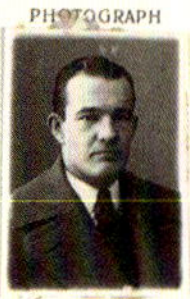

Form No. P-2, 6 50, ea, 0/21

PHOTOGRAPH

Name: Glenn I.Jones

Born: Washington November 25th,1883.

Home Address: 64, Kaiser Friedrich Str. Coblenz Germany

Nationality: American

Notify Case Emergency: Mrs.G.I.Jones above address

Entered Soviet Russia: March 13th,1922

No. of A.R.A. Identity Card: 183

U.S. Passport No:

REMARKS:

out April 1922 R.A.R. No. 16

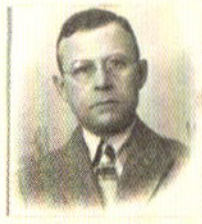

PHOTOGRAPH

Name: Raymond McK Sloan M.D.

Born: July 19th,1892b

Home Address: 519 9th Ave Huntington W.Va U.S.A.

Nationality: American

Notify Case Emergency: A.Sloan above address

Entered Soviet Russia: March 9th,1922.

No. of A.R.A. Identity Card: 181

U.S. Passport No: 118872

REMARKS:

[Out June 12th, 1923 Memo 400]

Arrived March 12th, 1922

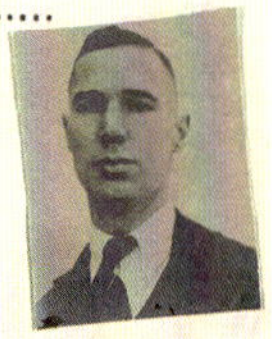

PHOTOGRAPH

Name: Frank Lynam

Born: April 14th,1866

Home Address: Duluth

Nationality: American

Notify Case Emergency: Julius Barnes New York City

Entered Soviet Russia: March 20th,1922

No.of A.R.A. Identity Card: 191

U.S. Passport No: 123082

REMARKS:

Out October 17th, 1922 Memo 256

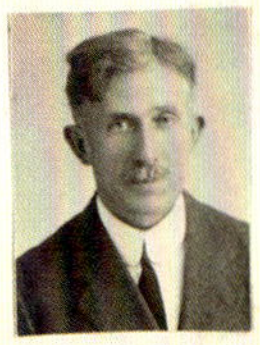

PHOTOGRAPH

Name: Jesse L.McElroy

Born: October 18th,1884 Roelsville Indiana

Home Address: Indianapolis Indiana

Nationality: American

Notify Case Emergency: Juliette McElroy Farmers Loan & Trust Co. 41 Boulevard Haussmann Paris

Entered Soviet Russia: December 5th,1921.

No. of A.R.A. Identity Card: 93

U.S. Passport: 91276

REMARKS:

Reported Dec 8th 1921

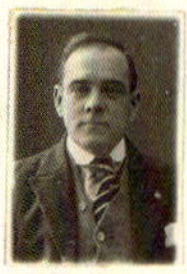

PHOTOGRAPH

Name: A.B.Muse

Born: July 16th,1888 Persia

Home Address: Webster New York U.S.A.

Nationality: American

Notify Case Emergency: Mr. K.Muse Webster N.Y.

Entered Soviet Russia: December 19th,1921. Arrived Dec 21st

No of A.R.A. Identity Card: 107

U.S. Passport No. 99648

REMARKS:

out May 1922 R.A.R. No. 19

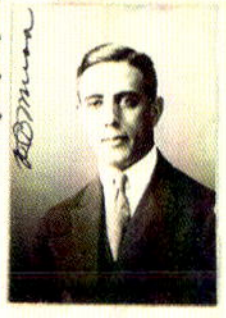

PHOTOGRAPH

Name: W.D.Nickelsen (1892)

Born: March 31st,1894

Home Address: Hood River Oregon

Nationality: American

Notify Case Emergency: John B.Nickelsen

Entered Soviet Russia: March 16th,1922

No. of A.R.A. Identity Card: 186

U.S. Passport No. S.S. 852

REMARKS:

Arrived 3/19

[Out Sept. 21st, 1922 Memo 226]

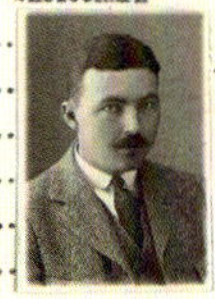

PHOTOGRAPH

Name: Dr.Francis T.Rollins

Born: Boston Mass U.S.A. December 13th,1884

Home Address: 25 Park Vale Ave Allston Mass

Nationality: American

Notify Case Emergency: Mrs H.H.Keough above address

Entered Soviet Russia: January 2nd,1922

No. of A.R.A. Identity Card: 119

U.S. Passport No: 115700

REMARKS:

[Out Apr. 21st, 22 Missing 842]

Reported Jan 5th 1922

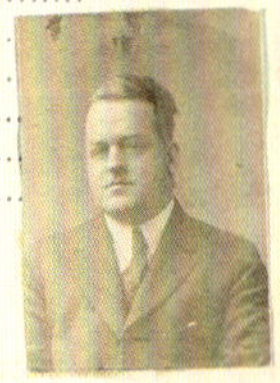

CHAPTER 5

The Plight of Physicians

"When I see what the doctors of this country have done, are doing now and are going to try to do this winter I am proud to be a doctor."

—*Dr. Henry Eversole (American Red Cross), Simbirsk, October 8, 1922*

On September 18, 1921, Carlton Bowden sent a report to ARA headquarters in London giving an account of the first two weeks of ARA operations in Petrograd. "The recruiting of the children started on Friday, September 9th, in thirty-three stations," he wrote. "Sixty-six doctors and about one hundred twenty nurses and school teachers were engaged in this work. We gave out 150,000 recruiting cards and expect to select from this number 50,000 of the most undernourished for our kitchens."

In Soviet Russia in 1921, the ARA relied heavily on local doctors in setting up and running relief operations. The ARA practice in Central Europe had been to rely on the assistance of nonpolitical "prominent citizens." In Soviet Russia such a species had become all but extinct. Some had fled or been exiled abroad; of those who stayed behind, many did not survive and most who did were in no condition to take up philanthropic work. During the revolution, refined people who had never had to perform physical labor were forced to sweep snow from the railway lines, clear forests, remove rubbish heaps—whatever it took to get a food ration and stay alive. The search for bread was everything. Now, in 1921, these people were among the first to turn to the ARA for help. Members of the former professional classes were viewed with suspicion by the Soviet authorities, and of course the Russian Orthodox clergy were anathema to them. Doctors were an exception. They knew from long residence in a community who was who, and they tended to be in good standing with the local people and regarded at least neutrally by local officials. In Simbirsk, in October 1921, when the ARA set up its local committee it consisted of two teachers, one engineer, and six doctors, in addition to a local government representative. A relief worker in Simbirsk noted that doctors were "as independently minded as any citizens of Soviet Russia can be expected to be."

Bowden expressed admiration for the Russian physicians he met during the inspections of hospitals, children's homes, and other institutions: "I have called together a committee of doctors for discussing the medical situation in Petrograd. . . . As in every other place where we have worked, I find that the doctors here are excellent people, carrying on a very fine work with practically no materials, and under the most trying conditions. If it were not for doctors and school teachers in Europe, one would almost lose faith entirely."

At the outbreak of the Great War, many physicians had been commissioned by the tsar into the army, and later many of them were mobilized into the Red

Identification records of American physicians recruited for the ARA's Soviet Russia mission in 1921 and 1922.

Army for the duration of the civil war. Throughout, they were exposed to typhus among the troops, which significantly reduced their ranks: the mortality rate from typhus was about 15 percent in the general population but nearly 50 percent among physicians. Harold Fisher, employing a military analogy, took the measure of the heroism of the doctors who remained at their posts: "Hundreds met death fighting disease, without weapons, with the same dogged courage that Russian soldiers, without ammunition, met death trying to stay the German advance."

Those doctors who survived the civil war were decommissioned and sent back into civil service only to find a dangerous lack of all medical supplies, no office space in which to practice, and a populace unable to pay for much beyond essentials. Their own pay, on average less than that for a common laborer, was used to support an entire family, all of whom were living in one or possibly two rooms. In Moscow, Dr. Samuel Ross noted that over a thousand doctors were registered at the Bureau of Unemployment, willing to assume any kind of work that would earn a living. Their degree of education made them more than eligible to be translators, clerks, and responsible warehousemen. In the meantime, they sold their household articles, clothing, and precious books; some renowned medical professors turned to making matches or even shoes.

Like members of the other dispossessed social classes, physicians engaged in the kind of manual labor entirely foreign to them before the Revolution: chopping wood, hauling water, carrying heavy packages, standing in endless lines. Some died of physical exhaustion, and others added suicide to the causes of their excess mortality, along with typhus and tuberculosis. Their surviving family members were left without any means of support and were forced to sell any remaining possessions or turn to a beggarly existence. Unlike the nobility who exited Russia for Europe when the Bolsheviks took over, physicians rarely had the financial means to leave the country and support themselves abroad.

Disregard for physicians in Russia was not a recent phenomenon. In the time of tsarist rule, civilian medicine came under the purview of the Ministry of the Interior. This nonmedical ministerial arm controlled the licensing and discipline of all physicians, considered them servants of the state to be conscripted at will to work in prisons, police stations, or the army, and subjected them to the general bureaucratic chaos and inefficiency so characteristic of tsarist rule. In other words, the state, not the physicians, governed medical practice in Russia. And it did so with great indifference to the people: while the government confirmed expenditures for the police and law enforcement as obligatory, it deemed funding for local health care and medicine optional.

In 1861, the Russian government abolished serfdom, freeing more than twenty-three million people but leaving them adrift from what little health care they may have received when in servitude. In the wake of this governmental negligence, a system of provincial councils—zemstvos—was established to meet the needs of the rural communities, including the medical needs of the peasantry, a social class that made up 80 percent of Russia's total population. Composed of local representatives, each zemstvo oversaw the town's needs with limited funding from local taxes. With no executive authority, however, the zemstvos had to apply for large-scale assistance to the Ministry of the Interior. In this way, the state retained absolute control over any local initiative.

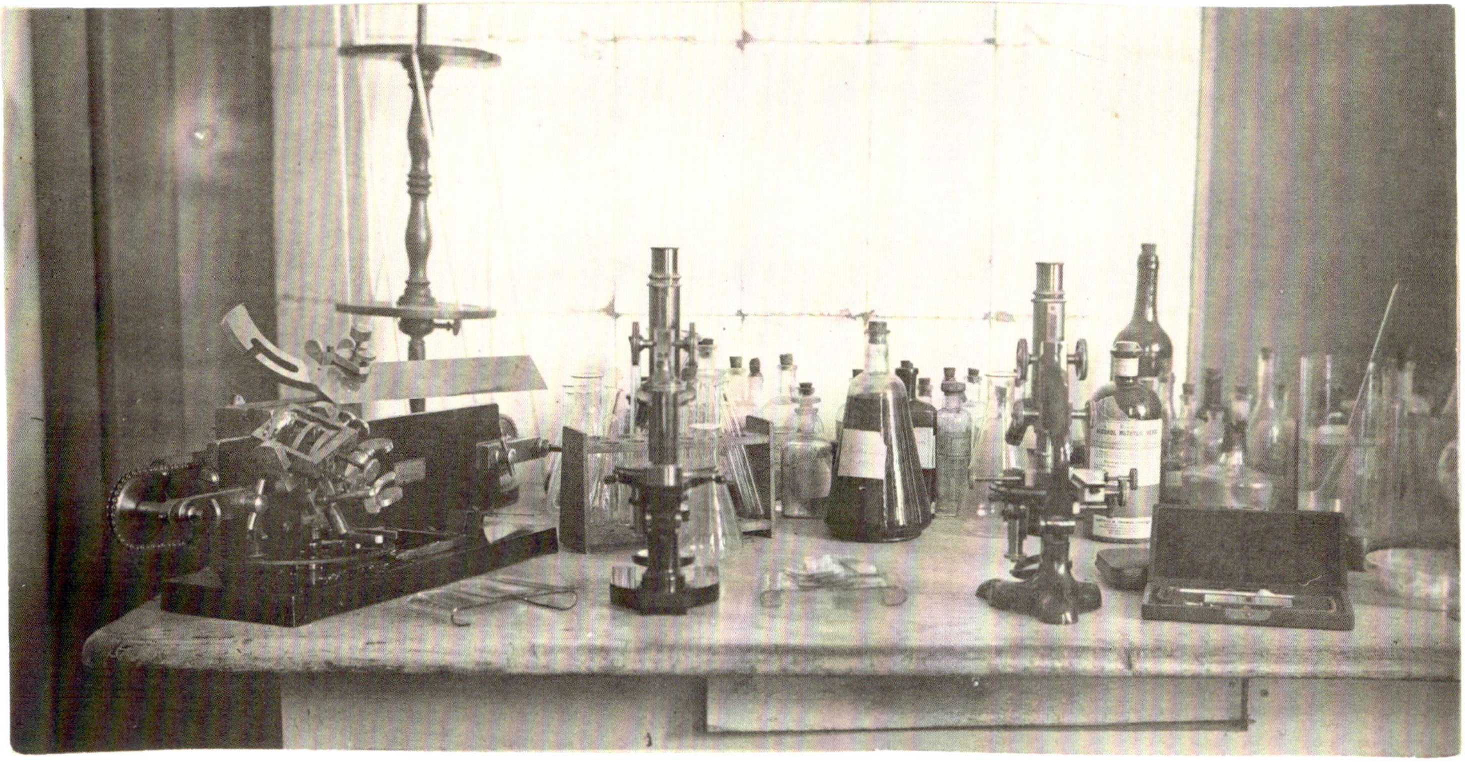

Laboratory supplies and equipment provided by the ARA, ca. 1922.

The physicians associated with the zemstvos—today we would call them community physicians—practiced at a local level, espousing high ideals and a strong social commitment. Without doubt they improved medical care in rural Russia, but given the vastness and ruggedness of the land, which made travel difficult, especially during the spring and fall when roads devolved into mud ruts, medical care by licensed physicians remained qualitatively and geographically uneven. On the eve of World War I, in 1913, the ratio of physicians to the population was 1:1,400 in the cities, similar to that found in other European cities at that time. In the rural areas of the country, however, the ratio was a staggering 1:20,300. The critical lack of health care in the countryside remained a fact of life in Russia.

In areas where there were no practicing physicians at all, a category of auxiliary medical personnel filled the gaps: feldshers. Derived from the German term for military paramedic, feldshers were armed with very limited medical training and an even smaller arsenal of medicines. Nevertheless, they provided rudimentary health care to peasants who otherwise might seek advice from local sorcerers (*znakhari*). Feldshers constituted an imperfect category of health care worker: the tsarist government decreed that feldshers could practice only under the supervision of a licensed physician; physicians, in turn, distrusted and disrespected these medics—whether they were military or civilian trained. Despite being subjected to restrictions and ridicule, feldshers persisted and practiced medicine effectively, often under no physician supervision. They were simply a necessary solution to the intractable problem of inadequate health care in rural Russia.

By the early 1900s, science, in the form of bacteriology, was beginning to influence the medical profession worldwide. The expansion of knowledge and expertise gave scientists and physicians a shared body of scientific information, making possible systematic approaches to disease, especially on a large scale. But this increasing medical expertise that gave physicians a new sense of professionalism and autonomy was perceived in Russia as a threat to autocratic control. How could a physician be at once a servant of the state and an independent-minded professional? And how could nonphysicians continue to exercise authority over medical education and research? Physicians began to insist that scientifically based knowledge and medical expertise, rather than the autocracy's privileging of age, rank, or government office, guide the direction of medical care.

When the First World War broke out in 1914, Russia discovered how medically unprepared its army and fleet were. The government wasted no time conscripting into the military the civilian physicians, whom the tsar considered to be servants of the state. At least 14,500 physicians were conscripted, almost 44 percent of the total number at that time of 33,000. As a result, civilian medical care was left in shambles, with even larger areas devoid of any practicing physicians. Those feldshers who had not been conscripted or enlisted for service filled the gaps in civilian medical personnel, attempting to deliver some measure of health care despite ever-growing shortages of all medical supplies.

The tipping point in this precarious public health situation was reached when railway trains transporting wounded soldiers—often sick with cholera, smallpox, or typhus—from the front into European Russia, started the spread of deadly infectious diseases among the civilian population. The concurrent transport of POWs and of refugees simply fleeing the fighting armies served to catalyze the widespread disease dissemination. Soon another wave of refugees took to the roads and railways expressly to outrun the epidemics. It was a mobile mass of nearly three million people, many of them carriers of cholera, dysentery, typhoid, and paratyphoid in the warmer months, or typhus and relapsing fever in winter.

This wartime medical crisis met with no practical response from the tsarist government. It might have acted, in its accustomed style, with only piecemeal measures, insisting on local rather than centralized solutions to medical care. But the war had empowered the community zemstvo physicians, who had massively bolstered the military's lean medical ranks. With newly acquired confidence and purpose, many of them participated in the newly formed Union of Zemstvos and the Union of Towns and took upon themselves larger-scale projects such as the creation of isolation hospitals and repair of sanitation systems, all done in anticipation of the arrival of disease-infected victims of war and social upheaval. In other words, preventive and sanitary needs began to receive attention equal to medical and surgical needs.

In fact, the epidemics spawned by the Great War paved the way for medical establishments everywhere to rethink their priorities. The traditional emphasis on therapeutic care as practiced in wartime in the forms of first aid, surgery, evacuation, and hospitalization now had to make room for preventive care in the form of anti-epidemic measures such as vaccinations, disinfectors, isolation hospitals, and maintenance of sanitary water supplies and of sewage disposal. This shift in emphasis stemmed directly from the developing importance of the medical fields of bacteriology, epidemiology, and hygiene. By 1915, the zemstvo physicians pressured the tsarist regime to require compulsory typhoid vaccination for the military; by 1916, this was expanded to inoculations against cholera and smallpox. And later, when the postwar demobilization of soldiers brought an epidemic of venereal disease, the response shifted from considerations based on the patient's economic class or perceived moral probity to scientific medical treatment. Physicians used the scientific advances of the very first antimicrobial drug—Salvarsan—to treat and cure the disease.

Gradually a more modern, systematic approach to medicine, based on professional expertise, scientific knowledge, and preventive planning, made the tsarist mode of piecemeal local response based on some bureaucratic minister's judgment appear obsolete and highly irresponsible.

+ + +

After the October Revolution, the new Soviet government abolished the zemstvos and zemstvo medicine altogether, without forethought as to an organized replacement. It was only the growing threat of disease that forced the Soviets out of this dangerous limbo in health care. In anticipation of a cholera epidemic that loomed large on the horizon for European Russia, on July 21, 1918, the Soviet government created a central agency, the People's Commissariat of Health (Narkomzdrav). "All hospitals, ambulatories, dispensaries, sanatoriums, sanitary apparatus, laboratories, research institutions, pharmacies, dental dispensaries and children's homes, caring for children up to the age of three were nationalized," Beeuwkes relates, "and placed under the administrative control of the People's Commissariat of Public Health, while the majority of the medical personnel including doctors, feldshers, nurses, pharmacists and hospital attendants were mobilized at the same time." Mandated to direct and coordinate medical and anti-epidemic measures, the Narkomzdrav gave Russia's physicians real hope that at long last a unified approach to medical care, the absolute antithesis of the divisive departments and competing jurisdictions of tsarist times, would serve the health needs of the people.

Despite a wariness of the Soviet government because of its hostility toward the former well-to-do classes, many physicians, even those who had organized themselves in unions during the war, welcomed the efficiency promised by the new, centralized approach to medical care and sensed that the Soviet government was likely to utilize modern technology and uphold professional expertise, both of which had been perceived as threatening by the tsarist government. For the time being, this gave them hope for progress in public health and for the increased practice of preventive sanitary measures.

The initial expectation by Russian physicians that the Bolsheviks would respect their medical training and professional experience ran up against the new regime's ideological hostility toward the former intelligentsia. Dr. Raymond McKnight Sloan attributed the disorganization in health work in the Ufa district to the fact that a veterinary feldsher served as head of the board of health in Ufa; in Chelyabinsk it was a barber; and in Ekaterinburg a laborer in a factory. Their lack of any previous training in medicine or administrative work taxed the "abilities of the trained public health man." Dr. William Dear in Kazan described a party system in the medical profession, with one group consisting of university professors who were "mostly sympathetic to the old regime and more or less passively antagonistic to the present." The second group included "men with communist sympathies who are receiving active support in their work from existing government agencies." The newest medical and scientific works by German experts were made available only to the latter group.

Apart from the disrespect shown to physicians with long-standing reputations built on experience primarily during the time of zemstvo medicine, the practice by the Soviet government of rewarding party affiliation took its toll on the trust that the peasants had formerly placed in medical care. Dr. Walter Davenport identified this attrition in a report to Beeuwkes in the autumn of 1921: "One of the doctors formerly connected with it [zemstvo] stated that the Zemstvos fifty years ago were largely responsible for introducing scientific medicine among the peasants and in so building up the faith of this class in modern medicine that they sought medical attention for the most trivial complaints." This confidence had eroded, continued Davenport, stating that "this attitude has changed now into one of untrust, primarily because there are now very few good doctors left, both on account of the severe mortality among this class due to epidemics of the last three years and the fact that many have left Russia."

The Soviets addressed the severe attrition in the ranks of physicians by introducing a fast-track educational program to create a new, loyal professional class of doctors. The numbers graduating from these medical schools grew considerably, but they came at the expense of the quality of medical training, which was generally poor. Political loyalty trumped superior medical training, recasting the original Russian problem of a dearth of physicians in rural areas into one of inferior medical care.

The Gubzdrav

The People's Commissariat of Health oversaw public health care principally through the issuance of numerous decrees to local health officials concerning the selection and salaries of personnel, and methods to combat disease, leaving little room for local initiative. These state decrees were intended to apply to even the smallest towns in Russia, but because the government agency lacked adequate resources, the decrees were not backed by funds, equipment, or personnel. The Soviet government had pledged to bring medical care to all citizens, but by nationalizing medicine it created a huge government bureaucracy that quickly destroyed what Harold Fisher called the "vital spark of private initiative and donation" characteristic of the time when zemstvo medicine and the Russian Red Cross were actively serving public health. Thus, the Narkomzdrav-initiated inoculation campaigns against infectious diseases, which made eminently good sense on paper, were impossible to achieve because of an utter lack of vaccine and syringes. Positive attempts at health care reform, in the form of preventive measures, inevitably came up against committee delays and dire economic restraint.

At first the Narkomzdrav exercised highly centralized control, but when Lenin's government introduced the New Economic Policy beginning in the spring of 1921, decentralization became the practice. Local governments swung from a situation in which central decrees had insufficient financial backing to one in which the central government withdrew all assistance, maintaining only an advisory role. The gubernias were left without resources for the purchase of food, medical supplies or equipment, fuel, or payment for personnel. Hospitals and dispensaries, already depleted of most supplies and medicines, were simply forced to close.

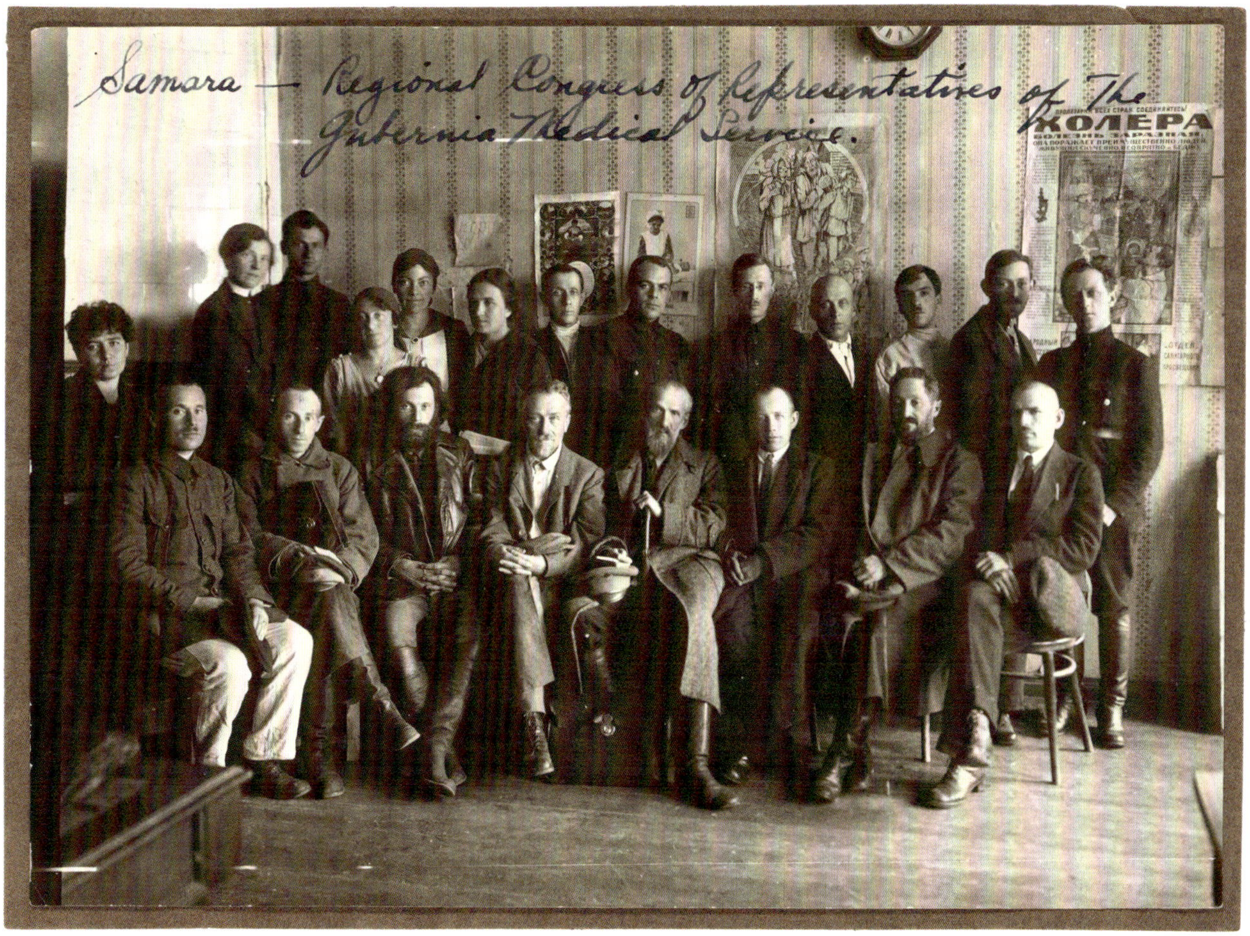

As they took up their duties in the ARA districts, American physicians became painfully aware of the shortage of physicians that continued to create staggeringly imbalanced physician-patient ratios in rural Russia. One physician in Kazan used feldshers and nurses to help him care for over 11,000 people. In Orenburg, only two doctors looked after over 1,000 children and adults gathered in thirteen collecting homes, places where orphans and refugees first landed before being assigned to other institutions. ARA special investigator James Goodrich, the former governor of Indiana, visiting a hospital north of the city of Kazan in October 1921, was informed that the hospital's best physician, "underpaid, underfed, and overworked, unable to stand the work," had committed suicide the day before Goodrich arrived. Like every other American in Russia, Goodrich was struck by the fortitude and courage of the doctors and feldshers, who carried on under what appeared to be impossible conditions.

ABOVE: Regional Congress of Representatives of the Gubernia Medical Service, Samara, 1922.

BELOW: Dr. William Dear, ca. 1921.

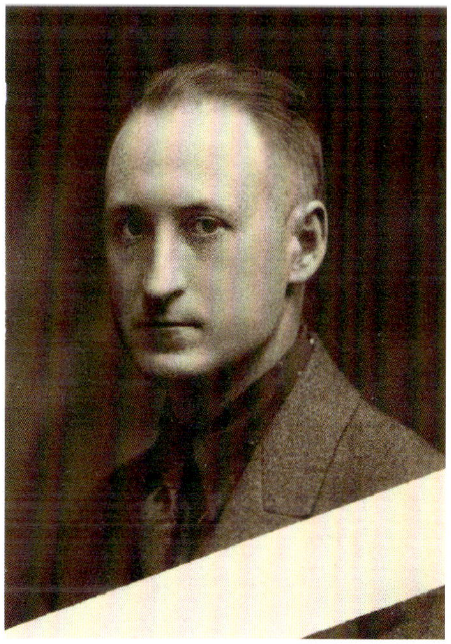

The doctors on duty in Odessa to care for 100 refugee children were "very intelligent, zealous people," observed the head of operations in Ukraine, Colonel William Grove, but they confronted a situation that was "as distressing as could be." Children huddled together, some alive but in the last stages of starvation, some too exhausted to move, and some dead. The doctors knew it was too late to save many of them even with proper nourishment. In this situation, the doctors became, in Grove's words, "only spectators of the peril of famishing and exhausted patient-prisoners."

The ARA physicians discovered an appalling shortage of hospital supplies everywhere on their initial inspections of medical institutions. Dr. George Cornick, based in Tsaritsyn, marveled at the situation in a letter to his sister:

"The hospitals . . . have absolutely no medicine, no bandages, no soap, practically no hospital garments, and the only bedding is in the form of comforts made out of rough burlap. The patients besides being sick are half starved, and cry out for food when they see you come into the wards." In Kazan, Dr. Dear was equally appalled by the conditions he found in hospitals. "What became of equipment that formerly existed in these hospitals and laboratories I am unable to say," he told Beeuwkes. "In answer to questions the reply was always that they had been 'taken.' By whom or for what purpose no one seemed to know." Trying to do the best they could with what they had forced physicians to adopt what one observer in Ufa called an "unconquerable perseverance."

+ + +

The plight of Soviet Russia's doctors was perhaps most strikingly illustrated in the country's surgical wards. Before 1914, surgical instruments and laboratory supplies had been imported from Germany, but this source was cut off at the outbreak of the Great War, and after that, hospital and surgical supplies were raided and used by the Red and White armies locked in a civil war. What did remain in 1921 was meager in quantity and nearly inoperable: rusted forceps that would flip off from where they were attached, dull knives, scissors worn at the joints, syringes with a single worn needle. Signs hung in ambulatories alerted potential patients with injuries or cuts to bring their own bandaging material. The remnants of gauze that still existed in hospitals were cleaned, sterilized, and reused. Even pharmacies and dispensaries were depleted, exhibiting on their shelves rows of mostly empty bottles and jars, and requiring customers to bring their own paper for writing a prescription.

By 1921, surgeons worldwide typically operated in an aseptic field within an operating room, with sanitized hands and surgical instruments, on patients who were made comfortable by reliable anesthesia. The surgery went quickly, and infection was rarely a complication. In contrast, the grim scene in Soviet Russia, especially in the winter, included an ice-cold operating room in a frigid hospital since there was no fuel for ambient warmth or to heat the sterilizers for the instruments. Surgeons and assistants lacked soap to wash their hands, made coarse and cracked from manual labor, or to wash the patient. One surgeon in Saratov used two pieces of gauze moistened with alcohol to disinfect his chapped hands and worried about the germs still embedded in the skin crevasses.

In such circumstances, infection became a likely outcome of surgery. Any extant hospital linens, sheets, gauze, or bandages remained a dingy color since the only water available was too cold to clean well, especially without laundry soap. Anesthesia was not always available or could be of inferior quality. When the ARA dispensed its supply of chloroform, it identified some of it as partially deteriorated due to long storage and labeled it "For External Use Only," meaning for topical use. Despite the warning, local doctors used it for inhaled anesthesia, considering it far superior to any chloroform provided by their government in recent years.

An unforgettable description of a local surgeon in action was provided by Dr. Mark Godfrey. Two weeks after arriving in Simbirsk in December 1921, he visited the government hospital and watched Dr. Vladimir Levit (also spelled Lewitt) work his magic, which he described at length for Beeuwkes.

> I inspected the instruments, sterilizer and operating room where I saw Dr. Lewitt in action and believe me he is a clever operator: positively among the best I have ever seen. Cool headed, quick, cautious and steady as a Packard, he made no false moves nor was he hindered by bungling assistants or nurses or a bum anaesthetist. The whole morning's performance was a real revelation to me as I never dreamed that these ghosts were so clever. If I had to be cut I would have no fear to let Lewitt go the limit on me.

Levit was born outside Kiev (Kyiv) in 1883 and graduated from Kharkov (today Kharkiv) University Medical School in 1906. He began his medical career in the Ardatovsk Zemstvo in Simbirsk province, first as a general practitioner and then, beginning in 1914, as a surgeon in the Ardatov hospital. By the time the ARA arrived on the scene, Levit was well known throughout Soviet Russia. The ARA named him chairman of its local committee, tasked with selecting the children to be fed in American kitchens. The day Godfrey visited his hospital, just like any other day, Levit was operating only with chloroform, and of poor quality, Godfrey noted.

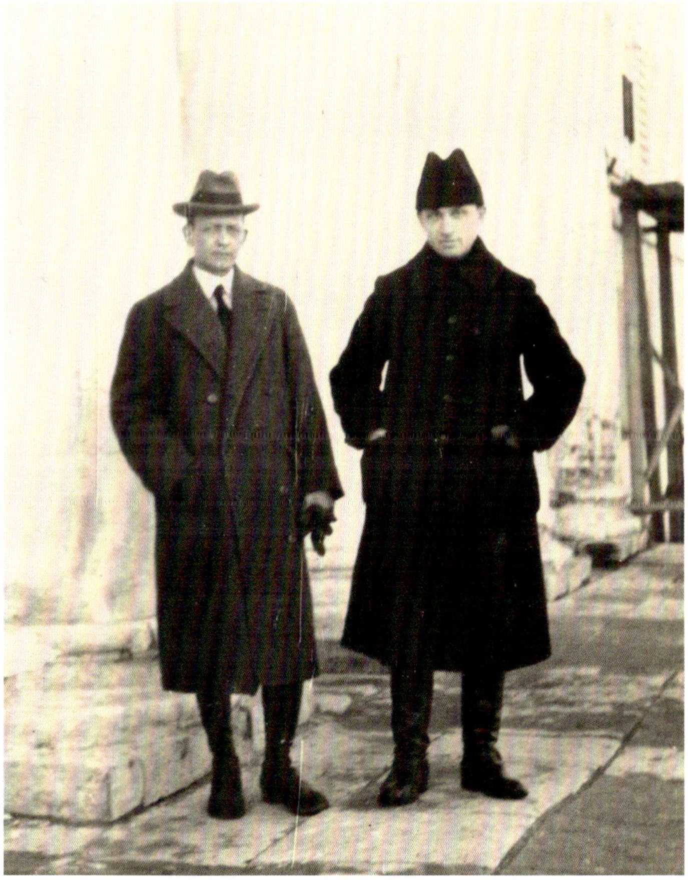

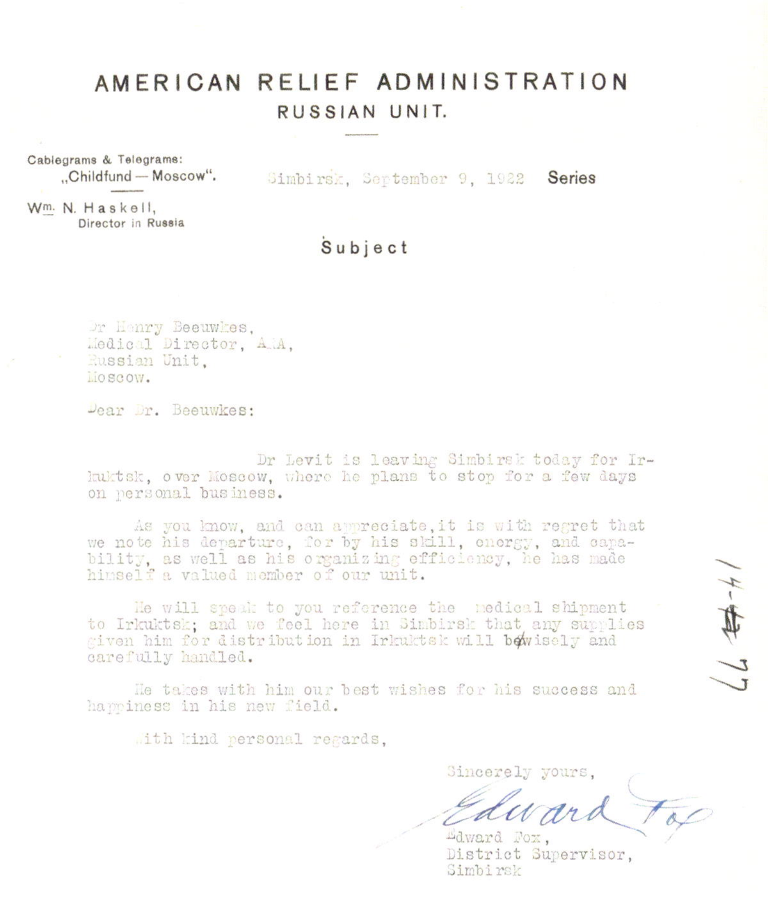

AMERICAN RELIEF ADMINISTRATION
RUSSIAN UNIT.

Cablegrams & Telegrams:
„Childfund — Moscow".

Wm. N. Haskell,
Director in Russia

Simbirsk, September 9, 1922 Series

Subject

Dr Henry Beeuwkes,
Medical Director, ARA,
Russian Unit,
Moscow.

Dear Dr. Beeuwkes:

Dr Levit is leaving Simbirsk today for Irkuktsk, over Moscow, where he plans to stop for a few days on personal business.

As you know, and can appreciate, it is with regret that we note his departure, for by his skill, energy, and capability, as well as his organizing efficiency, he has made himself a valued member of our unit.

He will speak to you reference the medical shipment to Irkuktsk; and we feel here in Simbirsk that any supplies given him for distribution in Irkuktsk will be wisely and carefully handled.

He takes with him our best wishes for his success and happiness in his new field.

With kind personal regards,

Sincerely yours,

Edward Fox

Edward Fox,
District Supervisor,
Simbirsk

14-77

ABOVE: Dr. Henry Beeuwkes and Dr. Vladimir Levit, Simbirsk, winter 1922.

RIGHT: Letter from Edward Fox, ARA district supervisor in Simbirsk, to Colonel Henry Beeuwkes in Moscow, September 9, 1922.

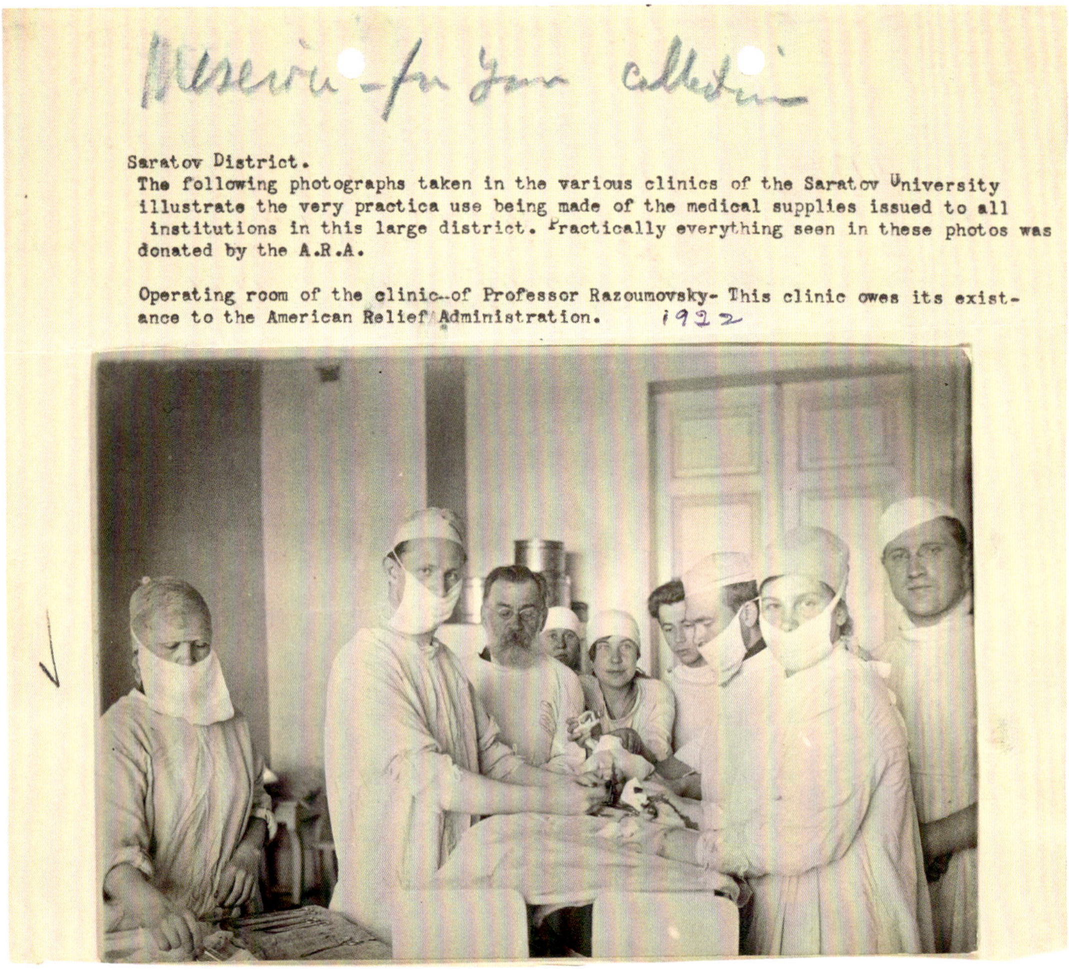
Saratov District.
The following photographs taken in the various clinics of the Saratov University illustrate the very practica use being made of the medical supplies issued to all institutions in this large district. Practically everything seen in these photos was donated by the A.R.A.

Operating room of the clinic--of Professor Razoumovsky- This clinic owes its existance to the American Relief Administration. 1922

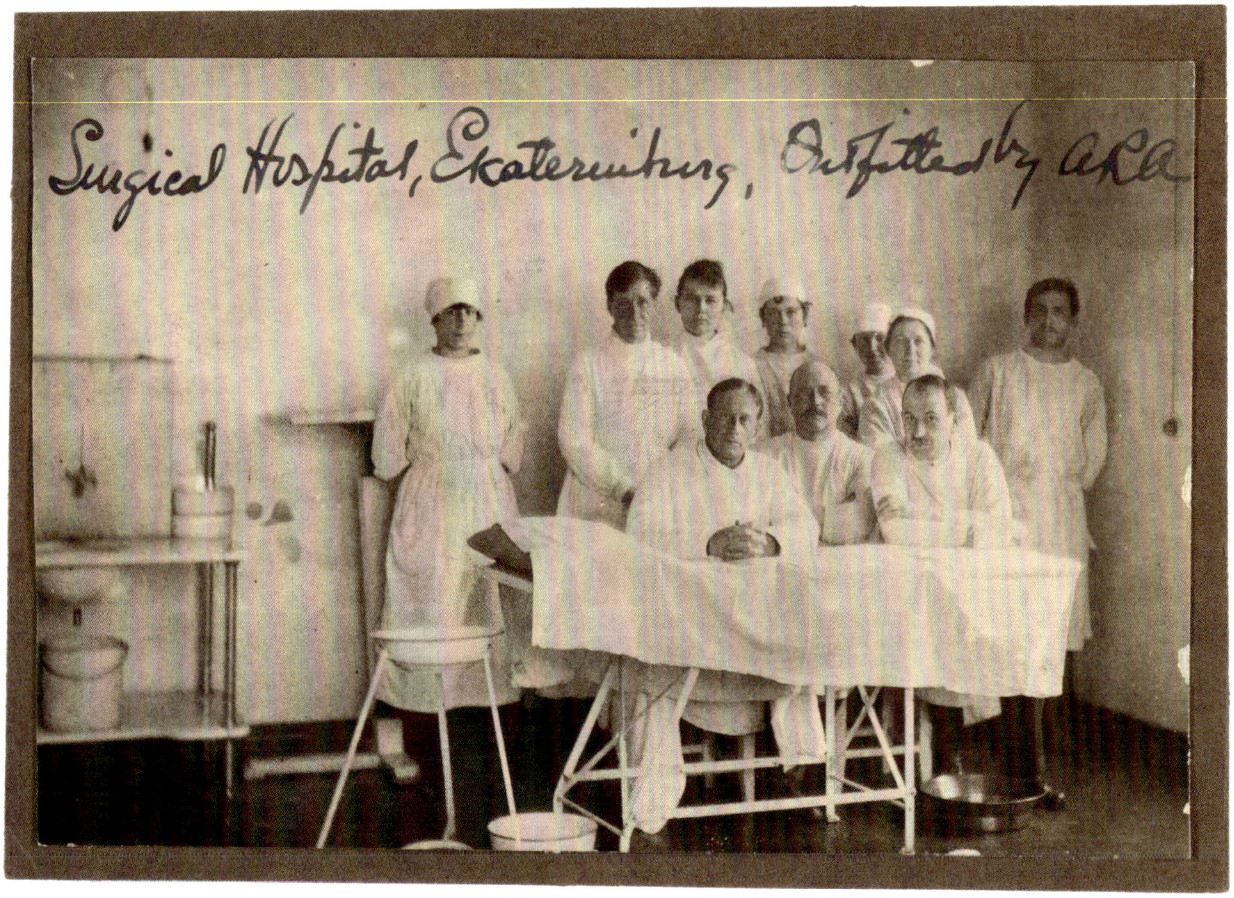

LEFT: Dr. B. Razoumovsky performing surgery at a clinic of Saratov University, with instruments supplied by the ARA, 1922.

BELOW: Surgical hospital in Ekaterinburg, in the Ufa district, outfitted by the ARA, ca. 1922.

> One patient on which a gastro-enterostomy was being performed went bad about ten minutes after the incision was made and I thought I was going to see a fatality and quite naturally turned my attention to the anaesthetist who was a woman. The patient who was an old man was blue as a Jay bird but the anaesthetist was as cool as a cucumber and very quickly gave him a big shot of camphorated oil and he came through in good shape. By that time Dr. Lewitt was washing up for the next case and when I asked him if he were not alarmed he replied that over a period of seven years of practically straight chloroform that he had only one death and that in that case it occurred an hour after the operation. He further stated that he only used this one anaesthetist and that she was a "Felcherine"—not even a nurse, mind you.

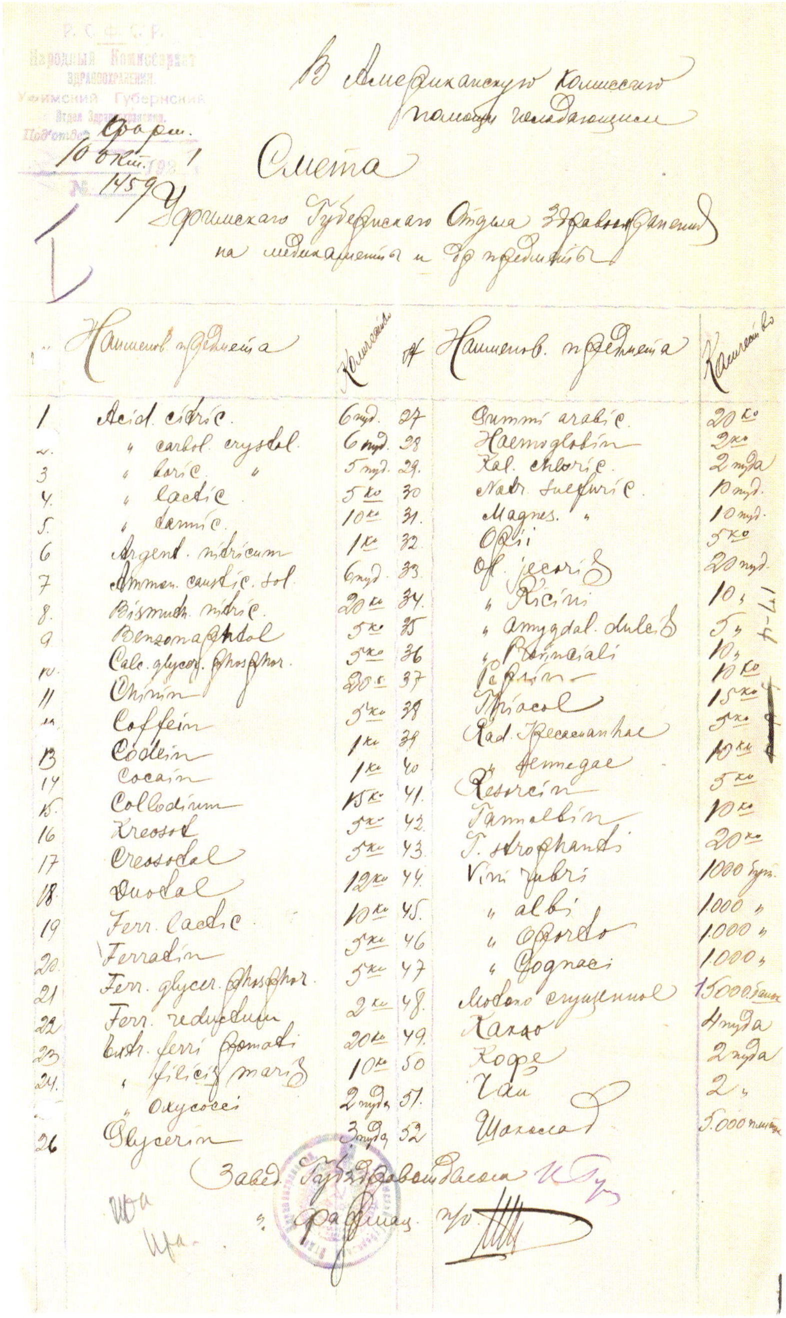

Смета Уфимского Губернского Отдела Здравоотвранения на медикаменты и др. предметы [Estimate by the Ufa Province Department of Health of required medicines and other items], list presented to the ARA on October 10, 1921.

Godfrey remarked on the freezing temperature in the operating room. "The operators and assistants' hands were blue with cold and I had to kick around a bit to keep up my circulation, even though I had on heavy clothing." When the weather was cold, physicians and scientists often worked fully clothed in overcoats, caps, and snow boots worn over their usually patched trousers and seedy coats. Dr. W. Horsley Gantt described an operating room in Petrograd in which the huge windows were covered with ice stalactites. In time, these icicles thawed, softening and cracking the putty and stucco walls until they became black and moldy, and then the ice water flooded the floors. Ingenious surgeons used moss in place of cotton or wool for pads, tongue depressors whittled from wood, and threads taken from clothing or violin strings for the missing catgut they needed to sew up an incision. Others resorted to equally unsanitary alternatives, dressing large, draining wounds with old newspapers.

The deplorable conditions of operating rooms in surgical hospitals and scant supplies forced most surgeons to perform only emergency surgeries and postpone all others. Even so, most everywhere patients were required to bring their own dressing material, gasoline for sterilization, and wood for fuel, perhaps to prevent freezing to death in a recovery bed, as happened to two patients in the city of Alexandrovsk in Ukraine.

In the town of Kishtim, located between Ekaterinburg and Chelyabinsk in the Urals, the American relief workers met a physician serving nearly 30,000 people for almost no pay. Dr. Sloan reported that despite this and his ragged clothes and worn-out shoes, the doctor worked with energy and much enthusiasm in his spotlessly clean and orderly hospital. He was but one example of a group that inspired Beeuwkes to write: "I know of no class in Russia more deserving of our admiration and assistance than the medical profession, doctors, nurses, feldshers, and assistants."

+ + +

The ARA Medical Division planned to provide local medical institutions—hospitals, ambulatories, dispensaries, laboratories—with all manner of much-needed supplies, both expendable articles and permanent equipment. These supplies gradually reached the warehouses of the Moscow ARA headquarters, and from there made the journey out to the various districts. They began to arrive in significant quantities in March 1922 and included items so basic to medical care that the lack thereof had forced Russian doctors to postpone surgeries and otherwise fail to care for their patients. Among the supplies were one thousand meters of gauze and several thousand meters of bandage; 86,000 bottles of Collodion, that syrupy surgical solution used to hold dressings in place; Albee bone sets, Hudson trephines, and radiographic tubes and plates for repaired X-ray machines; microscopes; operating tables; enamelware; ophthalmoscopes; and general operating sets. The reactions of the recipients were usually a mixture of surprise, delight, and gratitude, and also amazement that such abundant and precious supplies were a gift of the American people.

Dr. Godfrey received a letter from a rural physician in Simbirsk, thanking him for the "new style operating gowns." Perplexed, Godfrey went back to the invoice and discovered that the grateful doctor had likely mistaken the five pairs of pajamas he received for his new scrubs. ARA supplies were displayed by a physician in the small village of Promzino, in Simbirsk, "as proudly as would a small boy display his Christmas presents." Numerous physicians told their benefactors that a single ARA allotment of supplies, intended to serve for two to three months, was more than "all issues received from the government during the last two years."

The Medical Division afforded the district personnel the freedom to improvise. The Kazan district opened a free venereal disease clinic and, on the banks of the Volga, a large sanatorium for tubercular children. ARA dispensaries of many

RIGHT: ARA warehouse in Ufa, ca. 1922.

FACING TOP: ARA medical supply depot, Moscow, 1922.

FACING BOTTOM: Personnel assembled in front of the ARA medical supply depot in Moscow, ca. 1922.

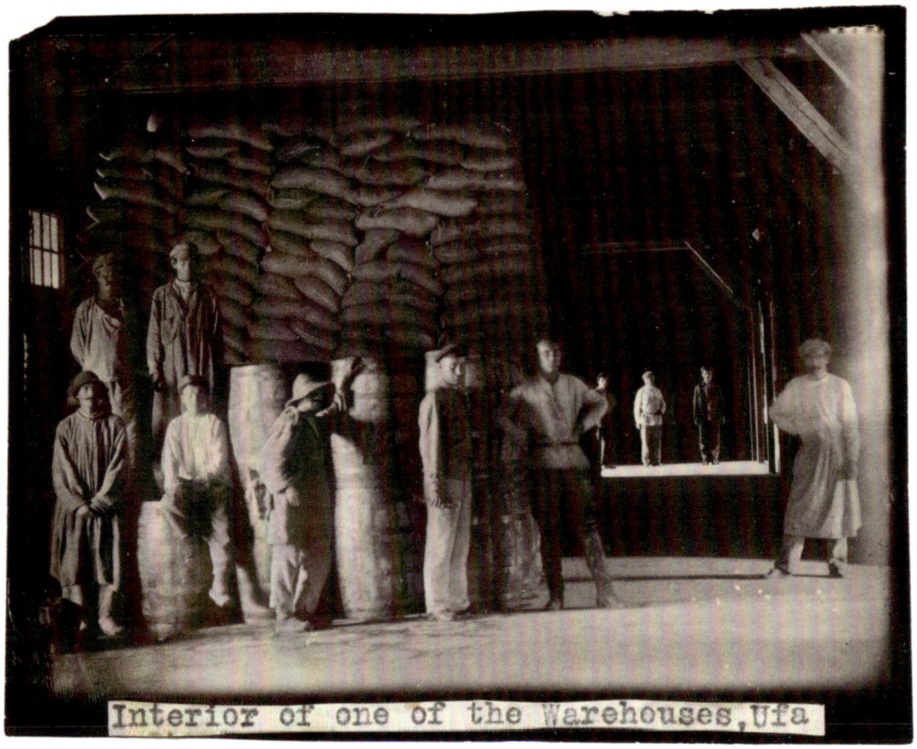

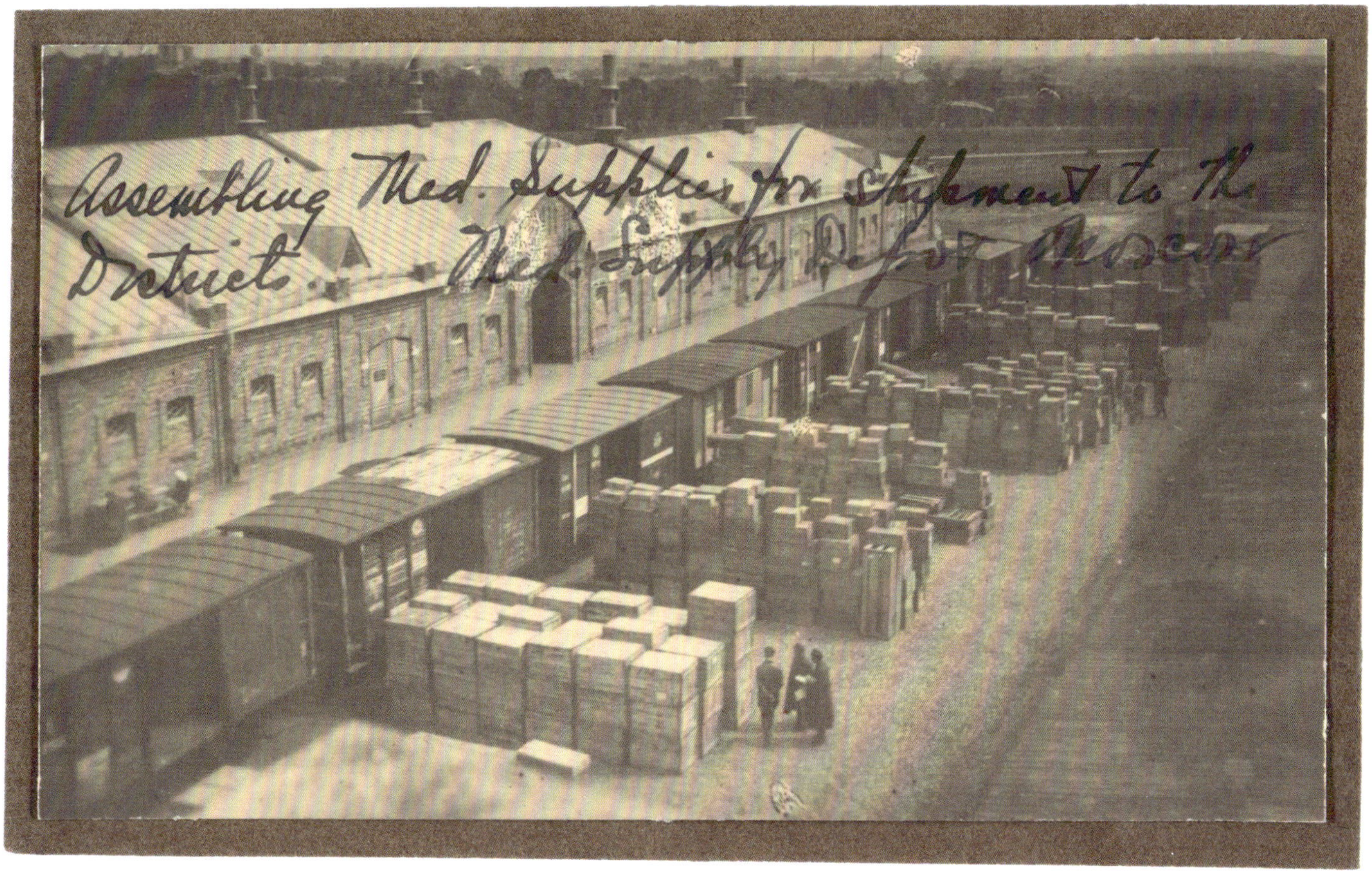

Assembling Med. Supplies for shipment to the Districts. Med. Supply Depot Moscow

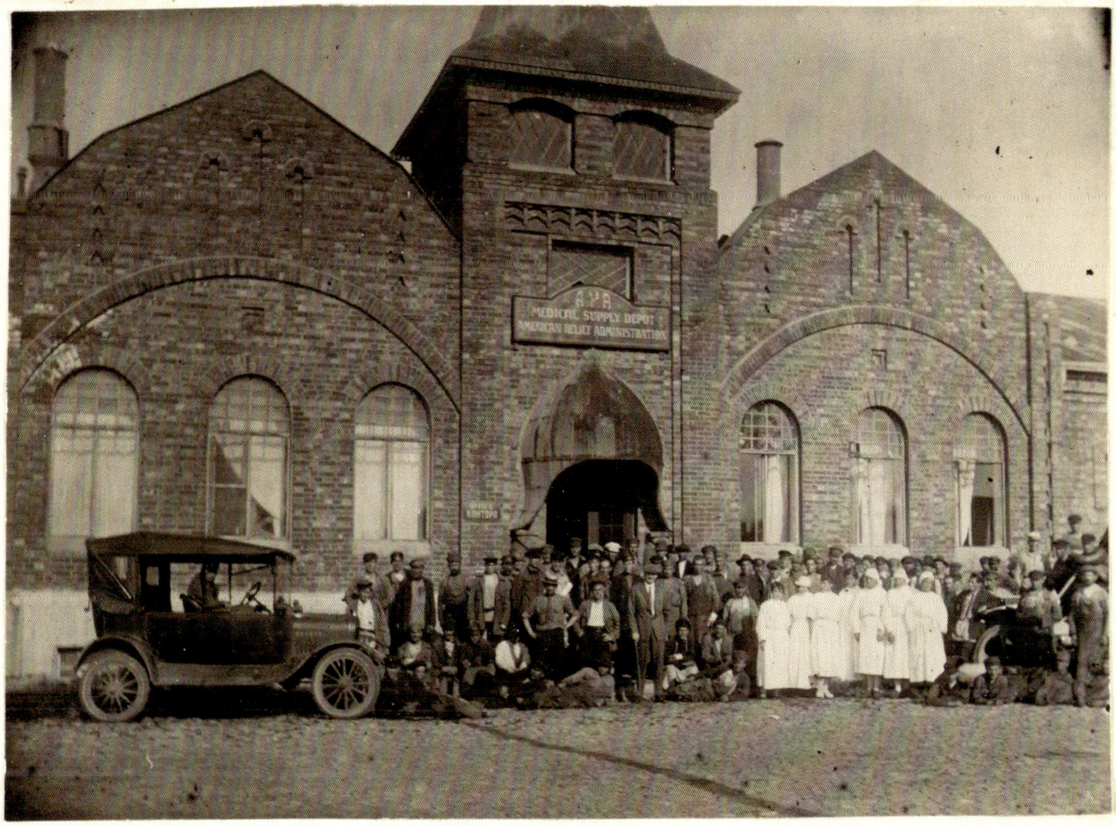

Medical Supply Depot. Moscow. and personnel.

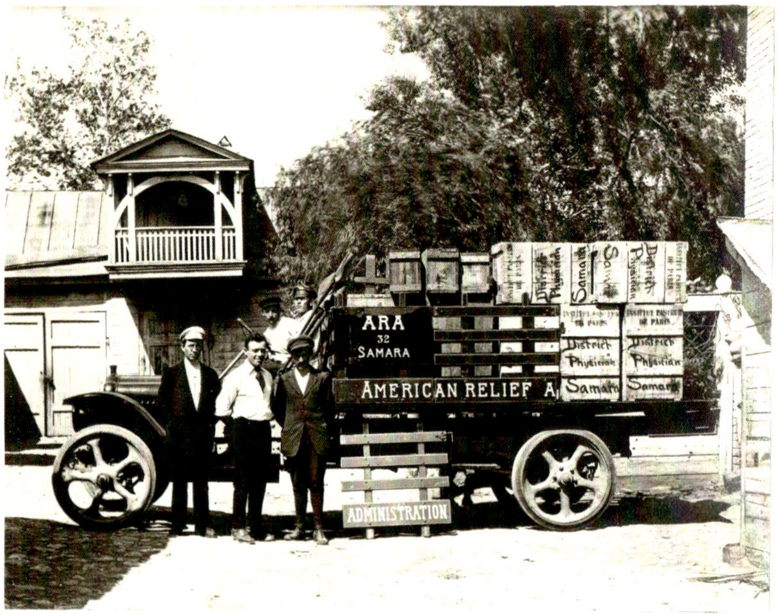

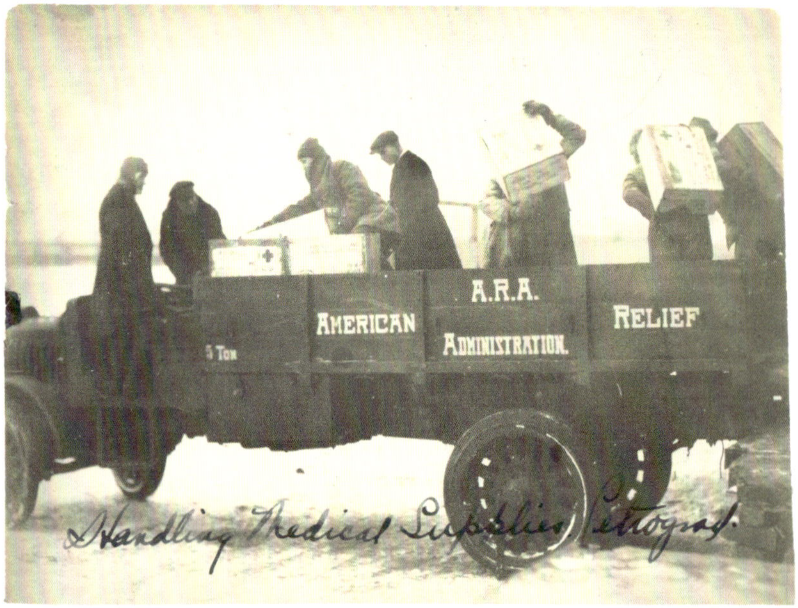

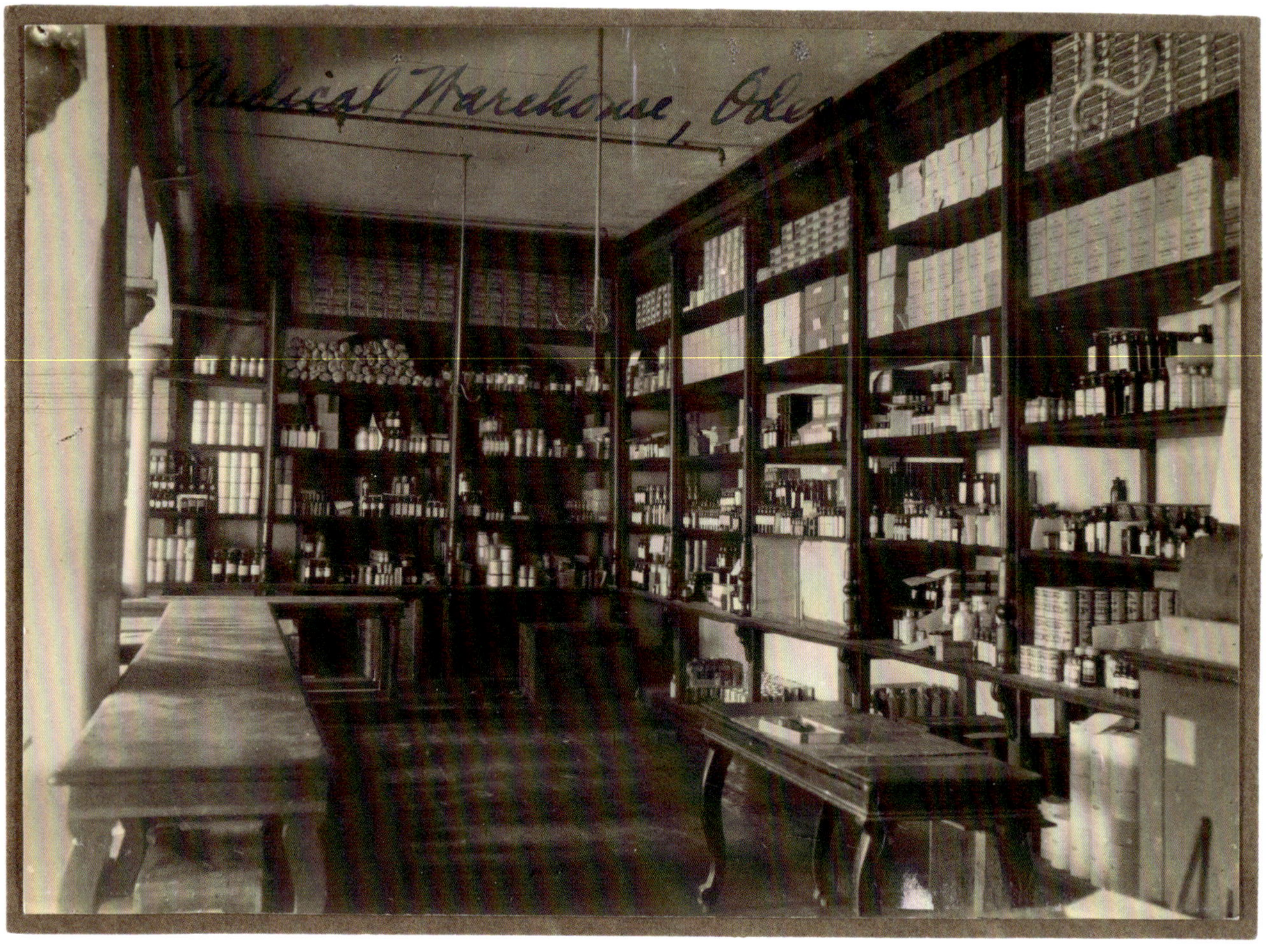

ABOVE LEFT: Delivery of medical supplies, Samara, 1922.
Courtesy of the Herbert Hoover Presidential Library and Museum

ABOVE RIGHT: Loading medical supplies, Petrograd, January 11, 1922.

LEFT: ARA medical warehouse, Odessa, ca. 1922.

FACING: ARA Odessa, Medical Division organizational chart, ca. 1922.

Chart showing organisation and management of Medical Department A.R.A. Odessa

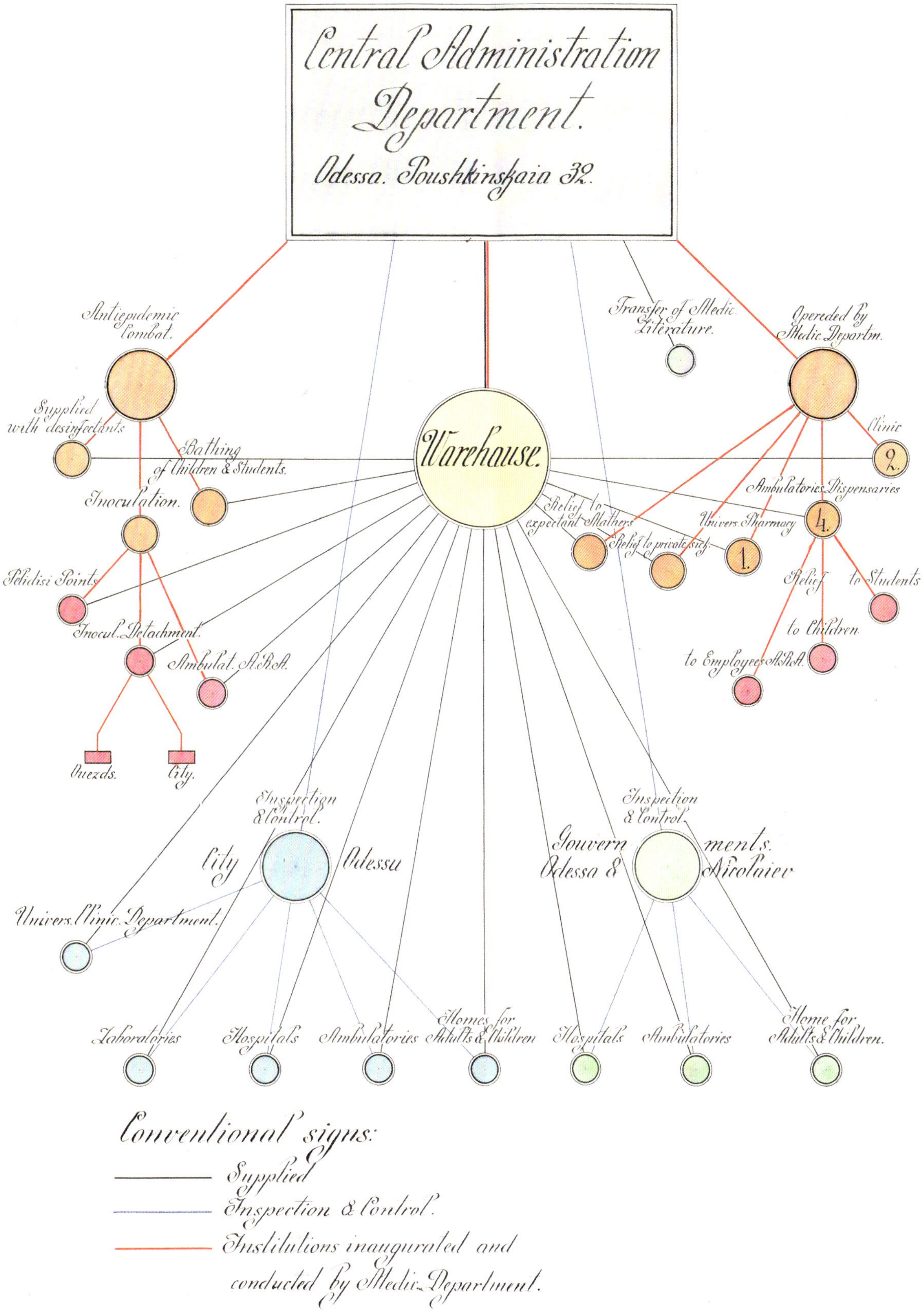

varieties became a fixture of—and a source of wonder in—major cities and towns. In Orenburg in March 1922, the ARA opened what it called a drugstore, where the needy could obtain medicines free of charge. This establishment turned out to be terrifically popular, the crush of overzealous customers sometimes making it impossible to get in the door. In August, when it was operating seven days a week, the Orenburg drugstore served some 320 customers a day.

Bolstering hospitals with medical supplies was futile if those administering the supplies were weak or sick from undernourishment and overwork. The arrival of the American corn beginning in March 1922 made it possible for the ARA to increase the feeding of hospital patients and to provide hospital personnel with corn rations. The ARA's Food Remittance program offered another avenue to assist medical personnel. The program worked as follows: Relatives, friends, and

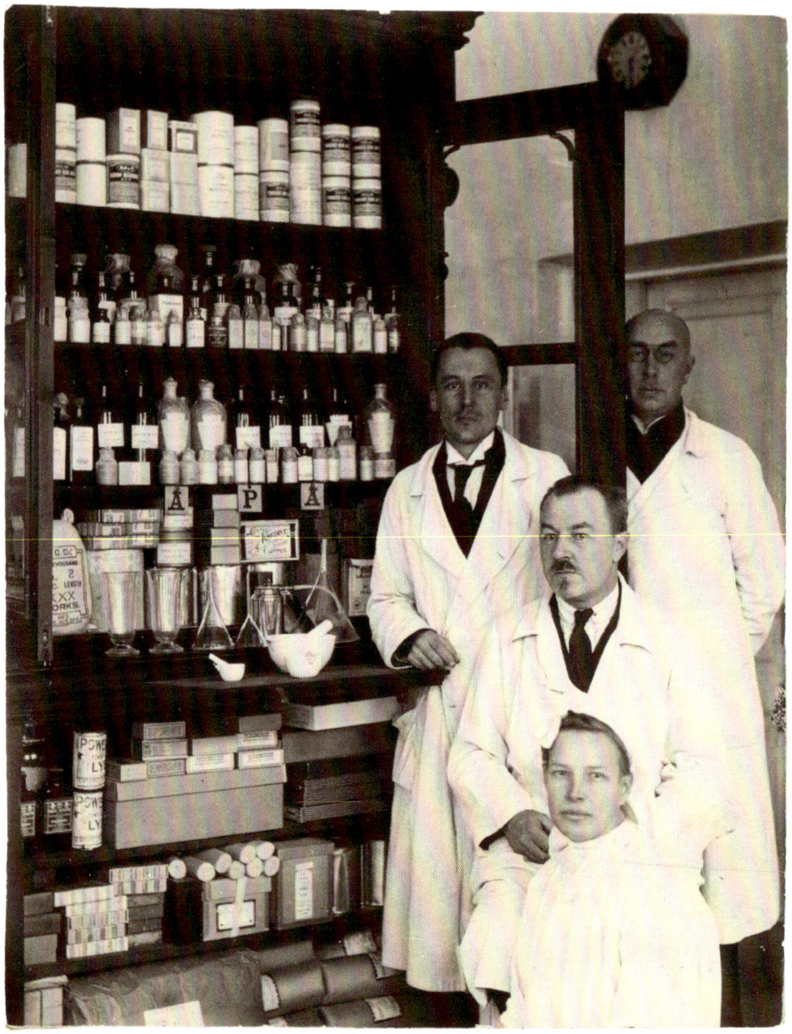

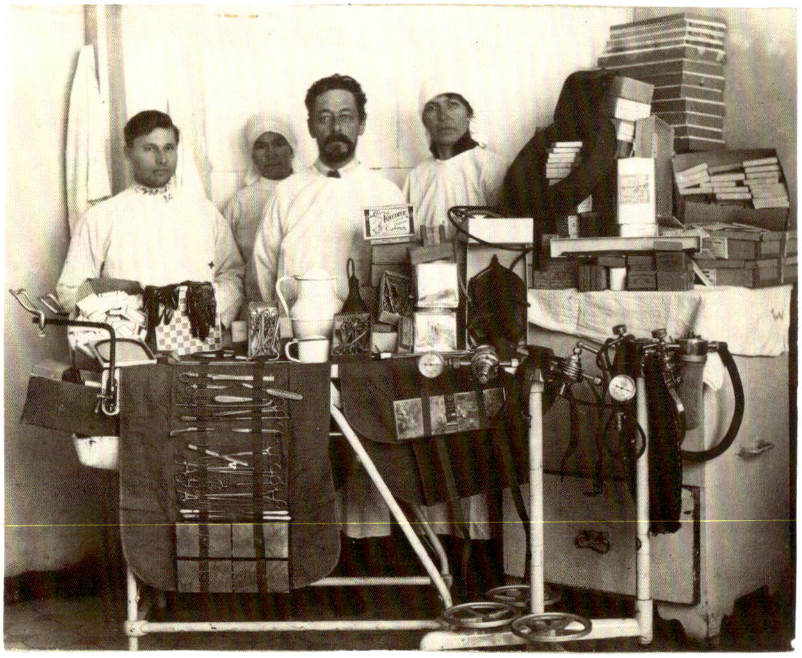

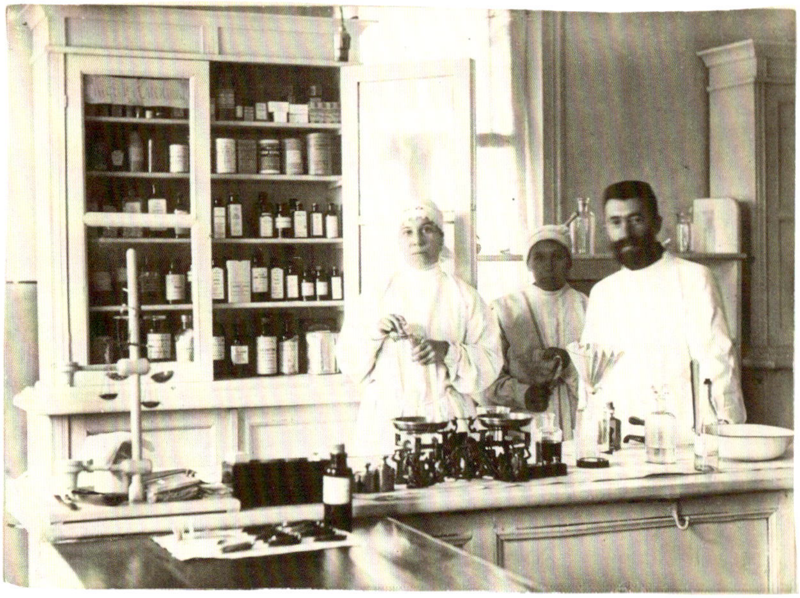

ABOVE: ARA pharmacy, ca. 1922.

ABOVE RIGHT: Hospital instruments supplied by the ARA to Samara Gubernia Hospital, ca. 1922.

RIGHT: Dispensary supply section of a hospital, ca. 1922.

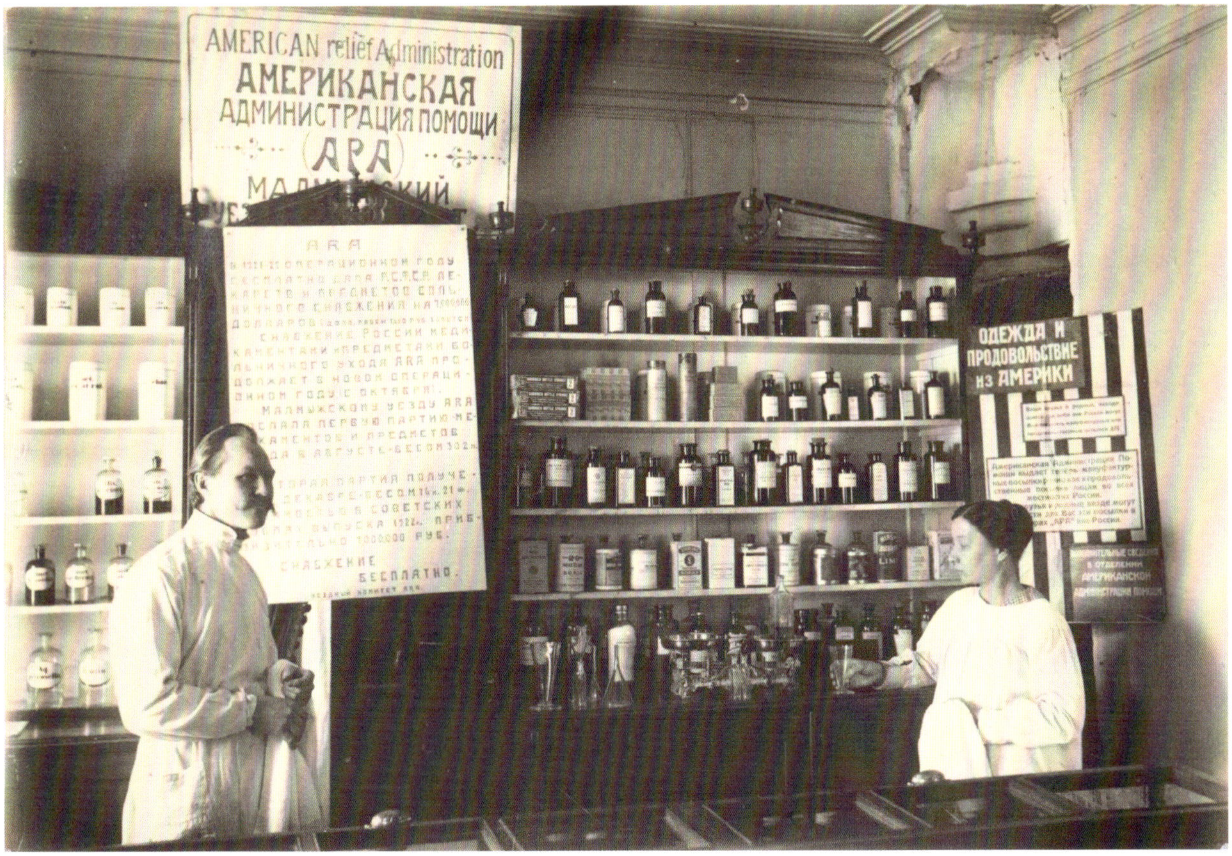

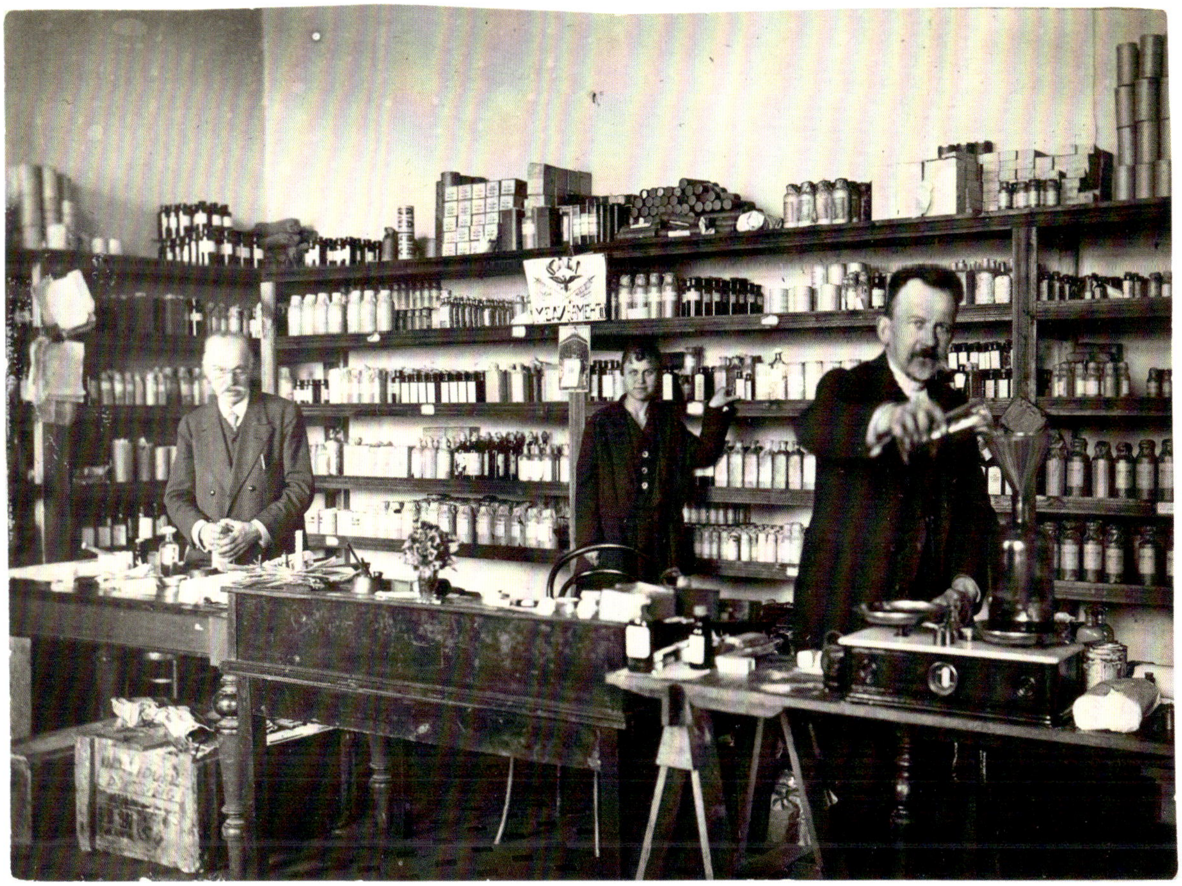

ABOVE: ARA hospital pharmacy, Malmish, Kazan province, ca. 1922. The sign at left explains that the medicine is a free gift of the American people.

RIGHT: ARA pharmacy, Saratov, ca. 1922.

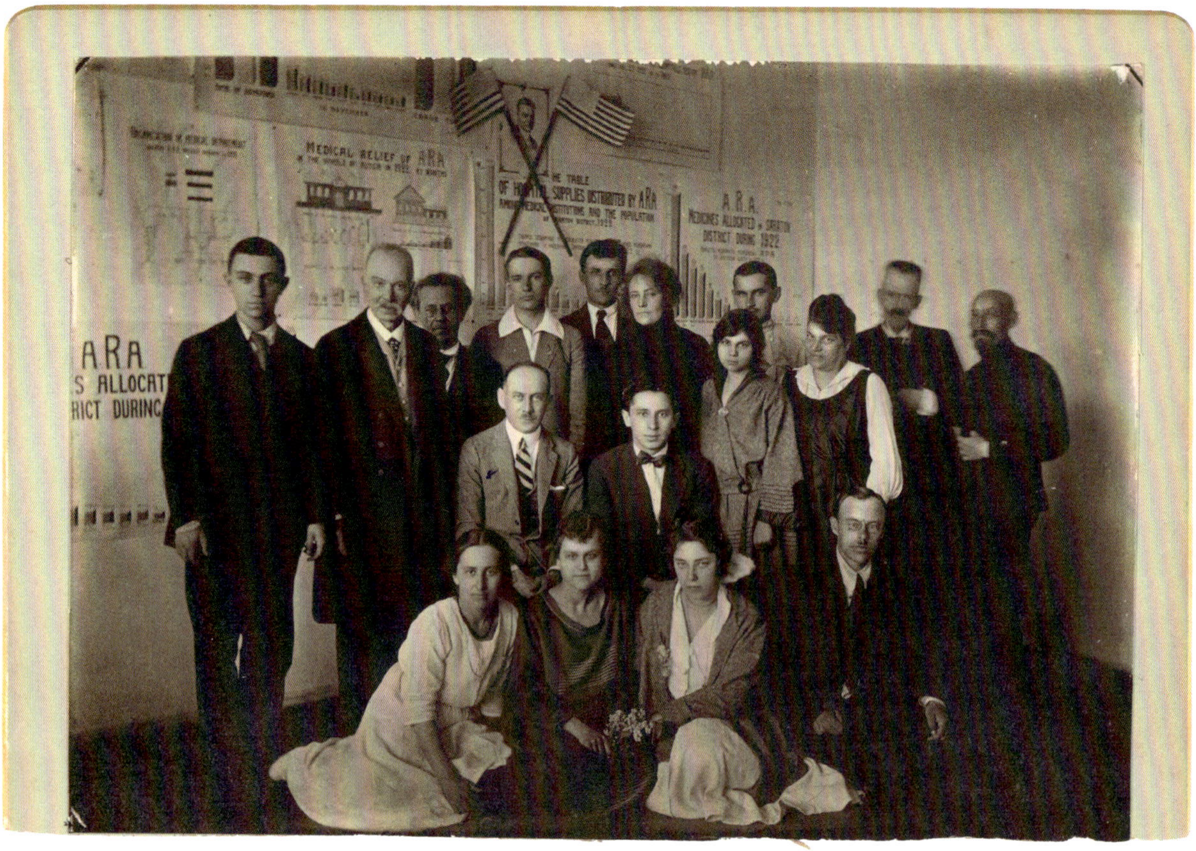

Dr. John Stack (seated at center, in striped tie) and ARA Saratov medical staff, ca. 1922. A photograph of Herbert Hoover is visible on the wall above, between the two crossed American flags.

other benefactors could put money down for a package at the ARA's New York headquarters or one of its European offices. A statement of payment would then be sent by ARA courier to Moscow headquarters, which would in turn contact the appropriate provincial ARA office, where the responsible American would send, by post or courier, a notification card to the intended beneficiary. This fortunate individual or family could collect one or more standardized food packages at one of the many ARA delivery stations spread out across the districts. By mission's end, the ARA had distributed 930,530 packages, which meant the successful delivery of 99 percent of all remittances.

The precise contents of the packages were occasionally adjusted according to the availability of certain food products and the market demand for them, but the standard ARA package during the first year of the mission consisted of the following: flour, 49 pounds; rice, 25 pounds; tea, 3 pounds; fats, 10 pounds; sugar, 10 pounds; preserved milk, 20 pounds—for a total weight of 117 pounds. The ARA also organized a smaller, though greatly appreciated, clothing package operation in Soviet Russia.

These food and clothing packages were also donated in bulk by American individuals and foundations toward relief of the Russian intelligentsia, primarily doctors and teachers, but also professors, writers, and artists. Doctors were made a priority. By December 19, 1921, Beeuwkes was able to tell district physicians in Ufa, Orenburg, Samara, and Kazan that food packages earmarked for needy doctors were on their way. The ARA encouraged individual professional groups—artists, musicians, professors, nurses, students, doctors—to make direct appeals to their professional counterparts in America. Over the course of the medical relief campaign, the ARA distributed a total of 6,900 food packages and 1,250 clothing packages to Russian medical personnel and/or their families.

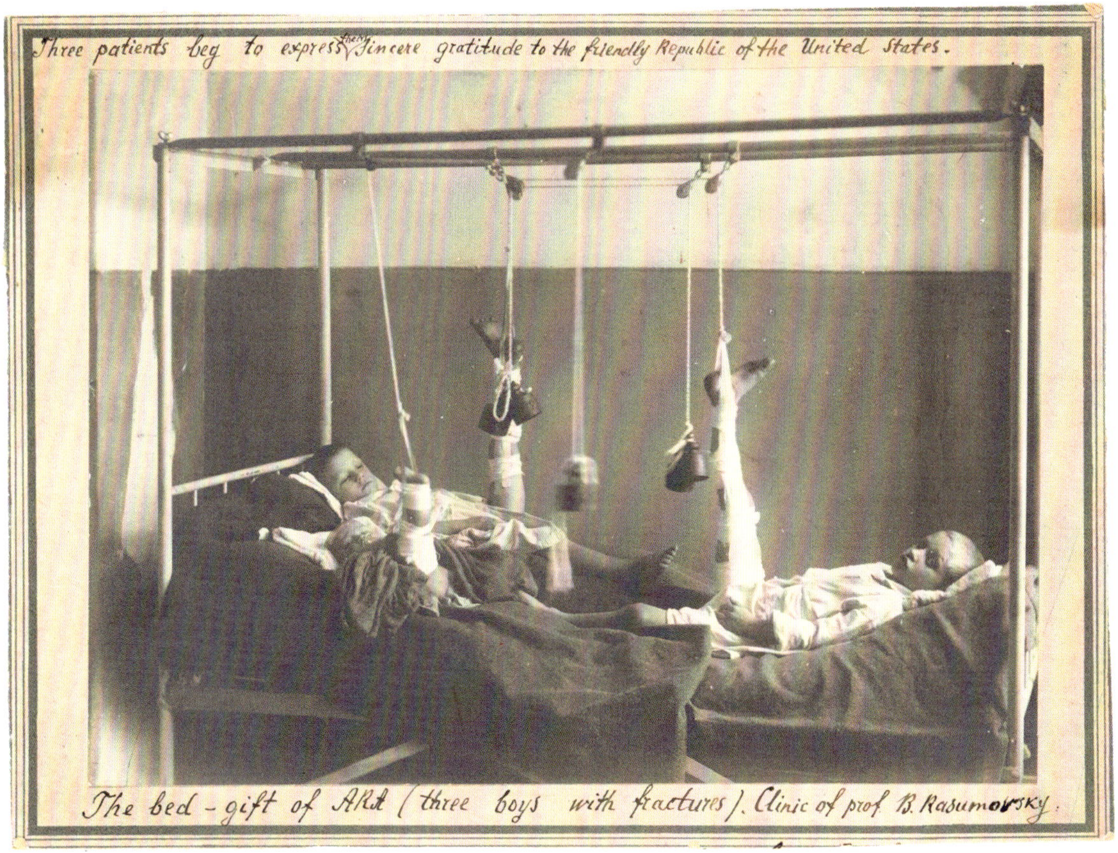

ABOVE: Three boys being treated for fractures in the clinic of Dr. B. Razoumovsky using a special bed and apparatus supplied by the ARA, 1923.

RIGHT: Letter from Colonel Henry Beeuwkes to Herbert Hoover, March 17, 1923.

AMERICAN RELIEF ADMINISTRATION.
RUSSIAN UNIT.

Cablegrams and Telegrams:
"CHILDFUND, MOSCOW."

WM. N. HASKELL,
Director in Russia.

SERIES

SUBJECT: MD 494

Moscow, Russia.
March 17th 1923

Mr. Herbert Hoover,
Secretary of Commerce,
Washington, D.C.
USA

My dear Mr. Hoover;

I have just received this rather interesting photo from Dr. Stack, district physician at Saratov. The bed and apparatus installed in the University of Saratov is from our Government Surplus supplies and you will note that the bedding, towels, bandages and practically all the supplies affording these children so much comfort are gifts of the American Relief Administration.

If, in our imagination, we multiply by a few hundred thousand, we begin to realize the amount of good that the medical division of the A.R.A. is accomplishing in Russia.

With kindest regards, I remain, as ever

Henry Beeuwkes
HENRY BEEUWKES
Chief Medical Division

HB/aer

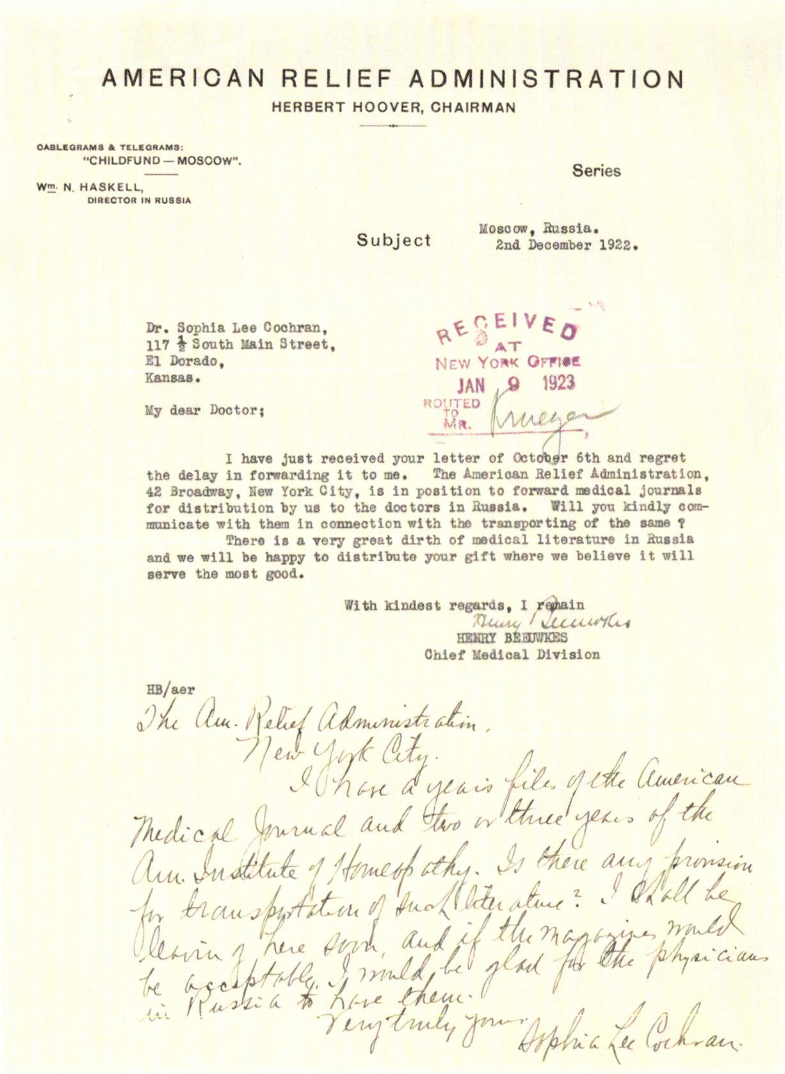

AMERICAN RELIEF ADMINISTRATION
HERBERT HOOVER, CHAIRMAN

CABLEGRAMS & TELEGRAMS:
"CHILDFUND—MOSCOW".

Wm. N. HASKELL,
DIRECTOR IN RUSSIA

Series

Subject

Moscow, Russia.
2nd December 1922.

RECEIVED
AT
NEW YORK OFFICE
JAN 9 1923
ROUTED TO MR. Krueger

Dr. Sophia Lee Cochran,
117 ½ South Main Street,
El Dorado,
Kansas.

My dear Doctor;

I have just received your letter of October 6th and regret the delay in forwarding it to me. The American Relief Administration, 42 Broadway, New York City, is in position to forward medical journals for distribution by us to the doctors in Russia. Will you kindly communicate with them in connection with the transporting of the same ?

There is a very great dirth of medical literature in Russia and we will be happy to distribute your gift where we believe it will serve the most good.

With kindest regards, I remain
Henry Beeuwkes
HENRY BEEUWKES
Chief Medical Division

HB/aer

The Am. Relief Administration,
New York City.
I have a year's file of the American Medical Journal and two or three years of the Am. Institute of Homeopathy. Is there any provision for transportation of such literature? I shall be leaving here soon, and if the magazines would be acceptable, I would be glad for the physicians in Russia to have them.
Very truly yours
Sophia Lee Cochran.

Letter from Colonel Henry Beeuwkes to Dr. Sophia Lee Cochran, December 2, 1922. Cochran's undated note forwarding Beeuwkes's letter to ARA headquarters in New York indicates she has back issues of the *American Medical Journal* [*The American Journal of Medicine*] and the *Journal of the American Institute of Homeopathy* to send to physicians in Soviet Russia.

The principal gifts of food and clothing packages were: William Bingham II, $95,000; the American Jewish Joint Distribution Committee, $25,000; Rochester Community Chest, $5,000; and Dr. Henry O. Eversole, $5,000. Bingham was a private philanthropist from Boston. His gift, which came in two installments, gave packages to feldshers and nurses as well as physicians. Much of his gift supported the vaccination teams spread far and wide in the massive effort to deliver prophylactic help to Russians threatened by cholera, typhoid, paratyphoid A and B, and smallpox.

Intellectual Famine

The American doctors in the famine zone took the lead in addressing another aspect of the medical famine. For years unable to inform themselves of, let alone apply, advances in scientific research in their fields of specialty, Russian doctors now appealed individually to their benefactors for the most important recent medical literature. The districts passed these requests on to Moscow headquarters and by spring 1922 the ARA began to relieve this kind of hunger as well.

Beeuwkes broached the idea of relief for the Russian "intellectual famine" with the Rockefeller Foundation in New York in a letter written on December 16, 1921. In response, the foundation promised to send journals directly to Beeuwkes for distribution at his discretion. Before long, multiple copies of twenty-seven different American and British medical journals were en route to Russia for contribution to the medical programs of ten leading universities. Included in the assortment of publications was a timely book, *The Etiology and Pathology of Typhus*, published by the League of Red Cross Societies in 1922. Dr. Frederick Foucar in Samara pointed out that the multilingual Russian doctors and scientists would happily receive publications in French, German, and Italian as well.

In the summer of 1922, when the ARA decided to remain in Soviet Russia for an additional year, the Rockefeller Foundation promised an even larger supply of recent American medical literature. As Davenport wrote to the district physicians in August, "The Rockefeller Foundation is particularly desirous of assisting institutions engaged in medical education work. It is requested that you forward us a list of the medical schools, hospitals used for teaching purposes, hospitals not used for teaching but possessing libraries, public laboratories and vaccine institutes, etc. in your district." A list of suggestions generated by the district physicians included such publications as the *Journal of the American Medical Association*; *Annals of Surgery*; *American Journal of Pediatrics*; *Archives of Internal Medicine*; *Surgery, Gynecology and Obstetrics*; and *The Lancet*.

In Kiev, the most interesting and important of such journal articles were translated and republished locally, and conferences were organized to discuss their findings. Dr. Dear in Kazan had loaned his copy of William Osler's *Principles and Practice of Medicine* to a local professor of medicine. The textbook was

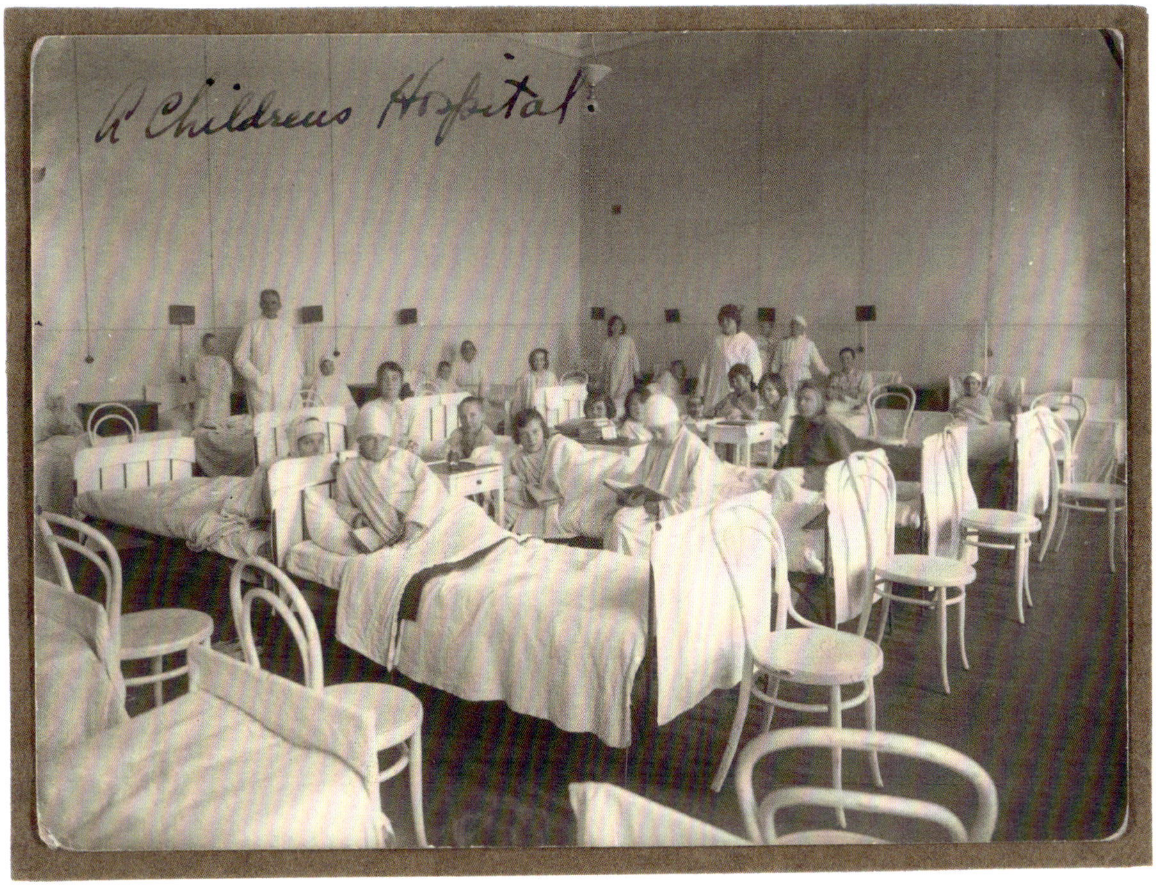

Infirmary at Obukhovskaya Hospital, Petrograd, supplied by the ARA, ca. 1922.

returned, Dear noted, "showing evidences that it had been carefully read cover to cover." Dr. Gantt in Petrograd took the initiative to have certain articles from the journals translated into Russian. He chose topics critical to Russian medical care: Nutrition and Vitamins to address deficiency diseases; and Diagnosis of Peptic Ulcers and Gall Bladder Disease considering the epidemic of ulcers largely caused by eating substitute foods.

The enthusiastic and appreciative written responses from Russian doctors and scientists and their family members were relayed from the districts to Moscow. Several hundred of them can be found in the ARA papers in the Hoover Archives. Many are addressed to William Bingham, this generous man of mystery. "We can only thank and wonder that people quite strange to us came in the most appropriated [*sic*] time to relieve us," a physician's widow wrote to him. Dr. V. Domratchew of the Perm district praised Bingham for recognizing the practical value in supporting Russian physicians: "You have understood that medical workers being the most in touch with the suffering people have to be secured so that their strengths [*sic*] should be saved for the further work of assisting their country people." Many expressions of thanks came from groups at institutions—physicians working at the Railway Hospital in Odessa, medical students at Saratov University, a conference of hospital pharmacists in Moscow—many of them trailing long lists of signatures.

In November 1922, a surgeon in Nizhni-Novgorod pointed out a display that he had arranged in his office, with photos of such scientists as Wasserman, Curie, Mechnikov, Koch, Ehrlich, all neatly placed in a semicircle around a photo of Herbert Hoover. The surgeon explained to an inquiring American that "Mr. Hoover is at the top of the list."

СХЕМА

пунктов медицинскаго снабжения Американской Администрации Помощи на Ю.-В. России с 1/V 1922 по 1/V 1923 г.

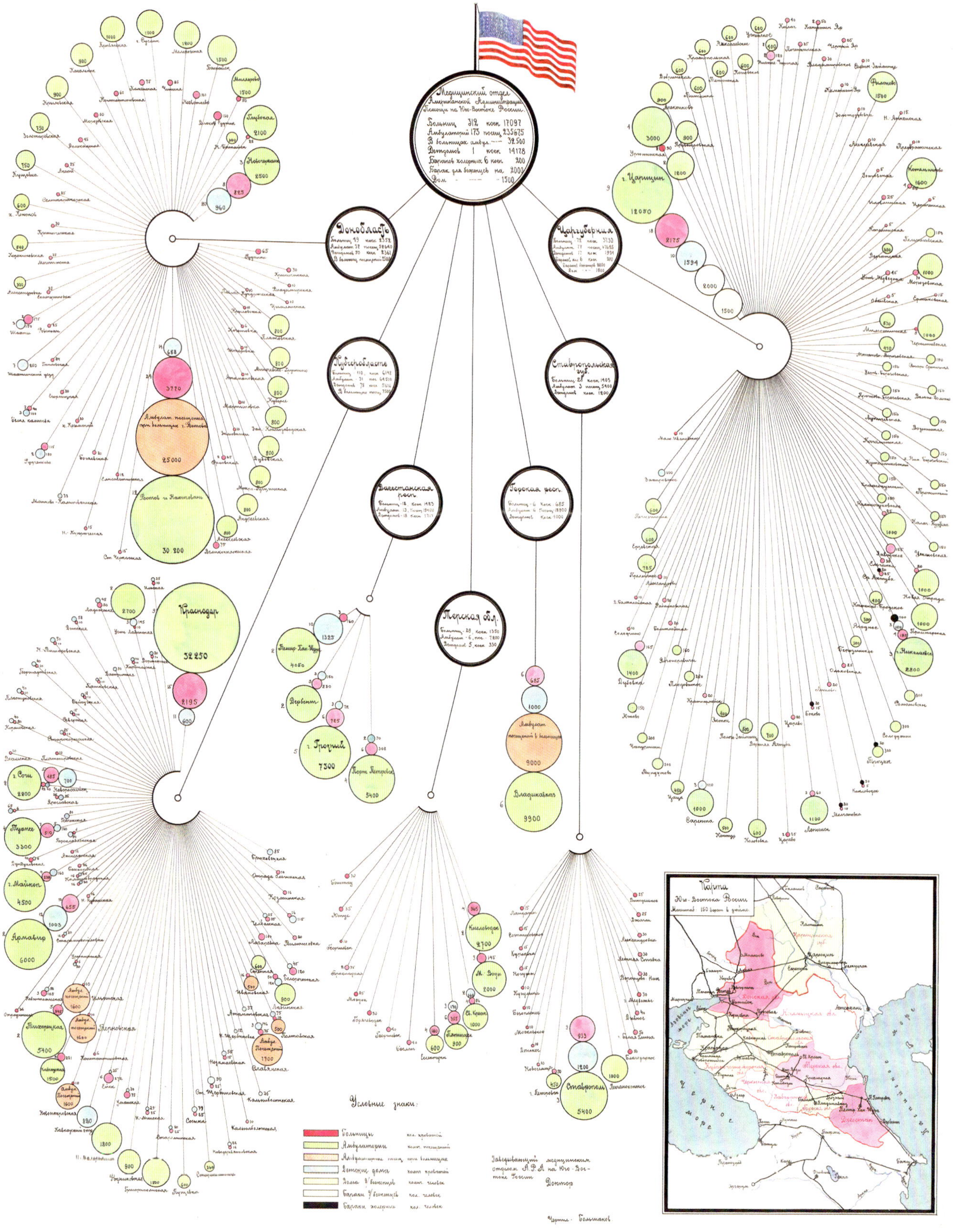

CHAPTER 6

Maladies and Remedies

"Probably the most popular drugs that we imported in large quantities were quinine, neosalvarsan and cod liver oil. Its high price made quinine practically unobtainable. Malaria was everywhere epidemic, due to the absence of this drug."

—*Henry Beeuwkes*, American Medical and Sanitary Relief in the Russian Famine, 1921–1923 *(1926)*

The story of the Medical Division of the American Relief Administration reveals what medicine in the early 1920s could do based on the understanding at that time of various diseases. The drugs the American physicians prescribed and used—bought in quantities of tons—also expose the limits of their knowledge. This was a time when arsenic, mercury, and opium were liberally used in various medicines, which by today's standards seems hair-raising. But behind every medical prescription was the effort and sincere care of a physician who faced the extreme circumstances in Soviet Russia from 1921 to 1923.

When the US government surplus medical stocks finally arrived in Russia toward June 1922, they included $1,500,000 in medicines; $1,500,000 in dressings; $500,000 in hospital supplies; and what Beeuwkes describes as "an almost unlimited amount of surgical instruments." All of it would serve to meet the "medical famine." While the Red Cross stocks were already tailored to medical relief work, Beeuwkes noted that those from the US government surplus medical supplies contained many "unrequested items or others in quantities too large." But he encouraged district physicians to "use them to advantage." Of the 230 entries in the list of medicines on the "combination invoice and receipt," at first glance only about a dozen of them would seem to be highly useful to physicians in Soviet Russia. Nevertheless, others would prove their worth as the Americans confronted diseases they no longer encountered in America or Europe because of adopted modern practices in hygiene, sanitation, and medicine.

Quackery and Cures

In the 1920s, the category of drugs called "medicine" still included botanical remedies and spurious cures in the way of elixirs and tonics, which often contained the harmful substances of strychnine, belladonna, arsenic, mercury, and cocaine. Not until 1938, when President Franklin Delano Roosevelt signed into law the Food, Drug, and Cosmetic Act, was there any regulation of the ingredients included in "medicine." Arsenic, long the killer of kings and the treatment for syphilis (together with the other poisonous metal, mercury), is now known as a liver toxin and carcinogen to the lung, bladder, and skin. The sixteenth-century Swiss physician Paracelsus, father of the phrase "The dose makes the poison," revealed a truth that is still recognized today. In the case of the metals—arsenic, mercury,

Diagram of medical supply stations of the American Relief Administration in S[outh]-E[ast] Russia from May 1, 1922, to May 1, 1923.

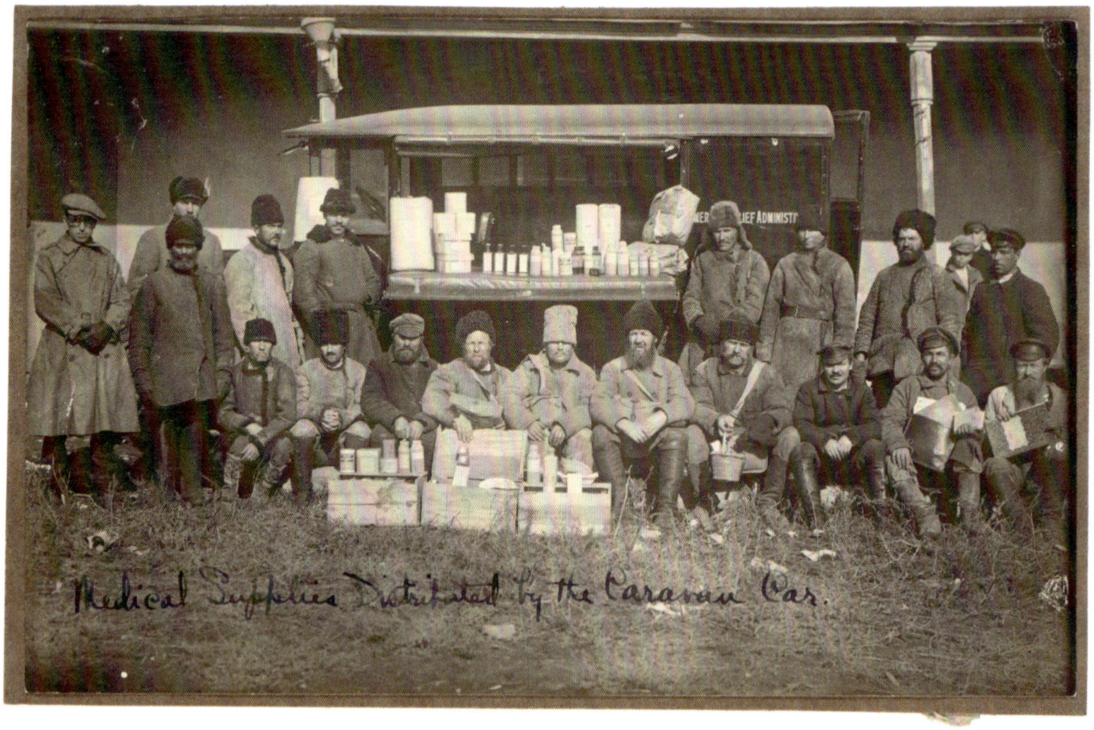

ARA caravan car, Samara province, 1923. The caravan car was a two-ton truck that served the relief workers as a dining-sleeping-passenger vehicle for feeding and inspection trips to remote destinations. It was built by American manufacturers especially for the ARA in Soviet Russia. Major Charles Hall, of the ARA Samara medical staff, stands at far left.

lead—a large dose could kill immediately, or smaller doses could accumulate in the body in a protracted process of poisoning. Nevertheless, such harmful substances continued to find their way into many adult tonics and even into teething powder for infants.

In 1860, American physician Oliver Wendell Holmes Sr., father of the future Supreme Court justice, delivered a stern verdict on the quality of medicines in the middle of the nineteenth century: "I firmly believe that if the whole *materia medica* [medical drugs], as now used, could be sunk to the bottom of the sea, it would be all the better for mankind—and all the worse for the fishes." Such warnings remained largely unheeded, and poisons continued to turn up in the arsenal of drugs that physicians used and prescribed. In their defense, it was true that arsenic and mercury "cured" syphilis, but they also poisoned the patient in the process. It was not until 1942 that physicians would have real curatives in the form of antibiotics, and until then, they observed carefully and acted empirically, hoping to uphold their oath to "Do no harm."

Medicines donated from the US government surplus stocks did include arsenic trioxide to treat skin afflictions such as psoriasis and eczema, as well as anemia, the protozoal disease of malaria, and spirochetal diseases of syphilis and relapsing fever. Strychnine sulphate (strychnine), derived from the dried seeds of the nux vomica plant, also made the list and was used to raise blood pressure. All the other medicines on the long list had basic functions: treat fever, pain, salivation, stomach acid, cough, slow or rapid breathing, low or high blood pressure, diarrhea, constipation, vomiting, itching, and hemorrhage. Many were purgatives, with ricini oleum (castor oil) topping the list. Antiseptics and astringents cleaned; styptics stopped bleeding; analgesics and anesthetics reduced pain; stimulants increased the flow of urine, enhanced nerve sensation, or boosted heart rate. Depressants slowed, numbed, and lowered body functions. Drugs for the skin were caustic, emollient, or protective like petrolatum.

Then there were drugs for specific diseases. By 1922, quinine was favored over arsenic trioxide to treat malaria. And Salvarsan, or Neosalvarsan, became the drug of choice for syphilis and relapsing fever, a pair of spirochetal diseases rampant in Soviet Russia in the early 1920s. Synthesized in 1910, Salvarsan was lauded oxymoronically as the "arsenic that saves lives." German scientist Paul Ehrlich, famed for his work with German physician and microbiologist Robert Koch on diphtheria antitoxin, teamed up with German chemist Alfred Bertheim and Japanese bacteriologist Sahachiro Hata to find a medicine less toxic than mercury and arsenic for the treatment of syphilis, which was reaching epidemic levels in Europe, the United States, and Russia. They synthesized and tested 605 compounds until they found success in number 606, an arsphenamine (arsenic) derivative that worked efficiently but less toxically against syphilis. Compound number 606, in 1910 named "Salvarsan," was in 1912 further refined into compound number 914 and called "Neosalvarsan." The latter was water soluble and easier to administer. It was the very first antimicrobial agent invented, to be replaced decades later by penicillin. Indeed, quinine and Neosalvarsan represented the only curative drugs in the entire assortment of medicines acquired by the ARA Medical Division—in addition, of course, to the three antisera specific to treating diphtheria, tetanus, and rabies.

Relapsing Fever

Hard on the heels of the influenza pandemic that raced through Russia during the autumn and winter of 1918–1919, epidemics of typhus and relapsing fever (also called typhus recurrens) were spreading through the Russian population at a pace attaining what one Russian doctor described as a "medieval character." The undisciplined demobilization of the Russian army in 1917 and 1918 was held responsible. By 1920, cases of relapsing fever reached over one million. This number dipped slightly to just under 800,000 in 1921 but escalated in the fall of 1922, as did other diseases, in conjunction with the widespread famine and lack of working public utilities. Again, the scale of disease outstripped anything witnessed in

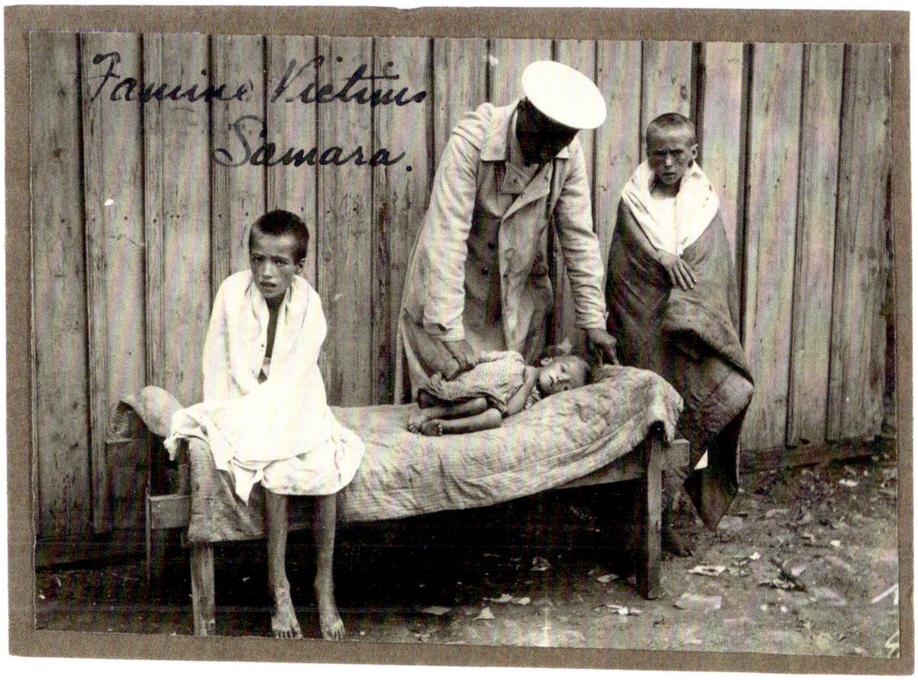

Famine victims, Samara, ca. 1921.

other European countries: in 1922, Lithuania registered 910 cases; Poland listed 40,245 cases; Soviet Russia had climbed back up to 1,479,627 cases. Russian epidemiologist Lev Tarassevitch estimated that between 1918 and 1922, 25 to 30 million citizens of Soviet Russia contracted typhus and relapsing fever: 17 million died of typhus and 7 million of relapsing fever.

Like typhus, relapsing fever is a disease of filth and dense living conditions. Beeuwkes warned the American physicians, in Medical Memorandum No. 5, that the disease was transmitted by bedbugs and "probably by lice." He was wrong about bedbugs but made a correct guess about lice. The human body louse, carrying the spirochetes of relapsing fever in its blood, simply released its fluids on human skin, and the human scratched them into his skin and bloodstream. The disease's symptoms—"relapses" of fever—and its course were usually milder than those of typhus and rarely required hospitalization. Fortunately, the spirochetes causing relapsing fever were vulnerable to treatment by that first antimicrobial drug, Neosalvarsan. The water-soluble arsenical powder was emulsified in sterile water and injected intravenously. The patient traded a loss of spirochete for a gain of arsenic in his body.

Syphilis

Over the duration of the medical campaign, the ARA physicians used the 700,000 tubes of powdered Neosalvarsan first to control relapsing fever and then to treat the high incidence of syphilis, which had increased worldwide during the war and in its aftermath. While accurate data on cases of syphilis had been kept in Russian hospitals and "feldsher points" or clinics in smaller cities and towns before the Great War, by 1922, Dr. Foucar noted, any such data "relative to the incidence of syphilis, the state in which it exists, or treatment received in individual cases were nonexistent." And serological diagnosis of the disease, previously done in the laboratories of bacteriological institutes, was rarely possible at that time because so few people were trained to conduct the test. This dearth extended as well to the expertise of physicians and specialists, those who were able to identify the disease and treat it.

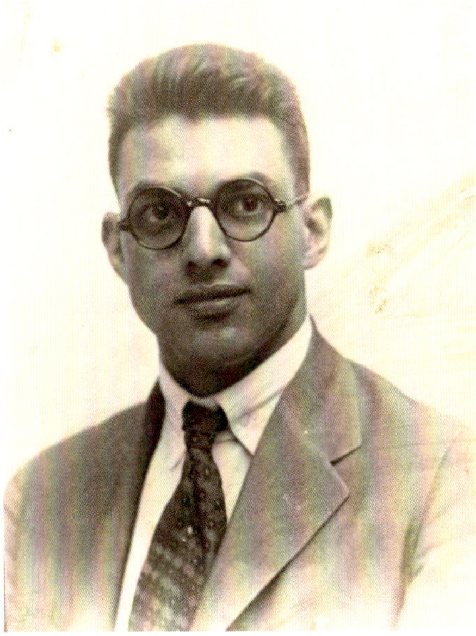

Dr. W. Horsley Gantt, ca. 1921.

American physician W. Horsley Gantt recognized the sexual transmission of syphilis, but also understood that many Russian children had acquired the disease congenitally at birth, through contact with a lesion in the birth canal. Transmission could also occur simply by contact with an open lesion on some family member, which was a direct consequence of living in such dense and filthy conditions. The telltale signs of disease in a child included a rash on the palms of the hands and soles of the feet, and presence of rhagades, cracks and fissures occurring around the mouth and nose. Dr. Gantt observed the horror of entire families infected with syphilis, a fact that made him more receptive to a claim by the People's Commissar of Health, Dr. N. A. Semashko, in 1922, that in some parts of the country 80 percent of the population was infected with the disease. Above all, a four-year lack of arsenicals, drugs to treat the disease, especially 606 and 914, or Salvarsan and Neosalvarsan, contributed most to the unchecked spread of syphilis in Soviet Russia.

In March 1923, when Dr. Foucar had completed the various medical and sanitary campaigns in his district of Samara, he launched yet another against syphilis. He formed "companies" of Russian physicians and feldshers, equipped them

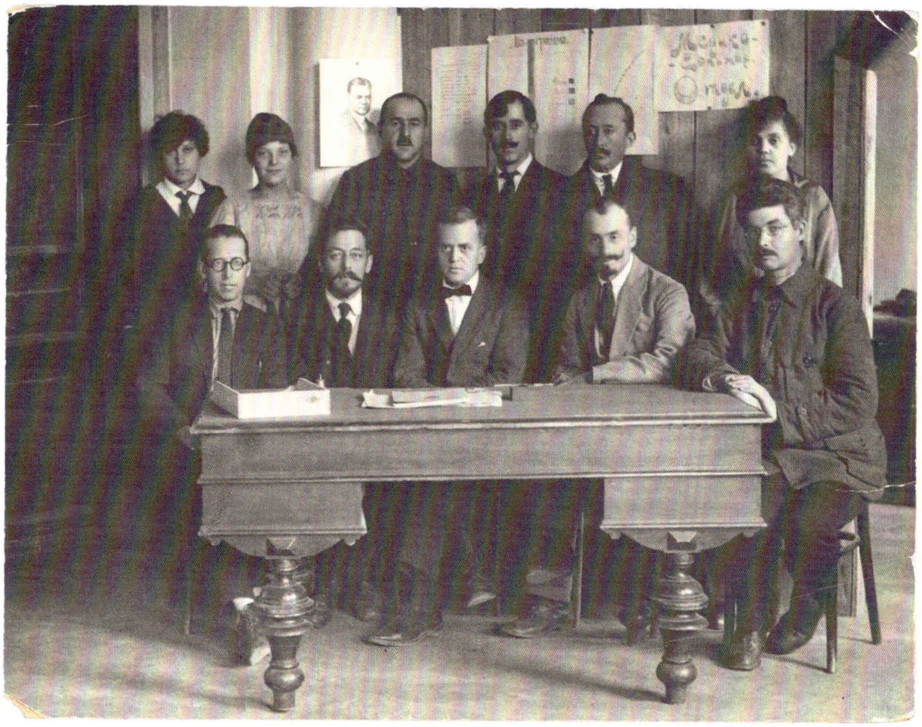

ABOVE: Dr. Frederick Foucar and his medical staff in Samara, including Major Charles Hall (seated at far left), ca. 1923. A photograph of Herbert Hoover is visible on the back wall, left of center.

with tubes of Neosalvarsan, disinfectants, syringes, and instructions for injecting the drug, and sent them out to the rural towns and villages in a dedicated anti-syphilis campaign. He assigned an additional company the job of educating people as to the critical need of medical treatment for the disease. All the workers in the companies received the food and clothing packages in exchange for their service.

Trachoma

Dr. Foucar made use of the very same system of medical companies to address the equally pressing need for treatment of the infectious eye disease trachoma, which was prevalent in the geographical area between the Volga River and the Ural Mountains, home to Tatars, Chuvashes, Votyaks, and Mordvins in the northern part and Bashkirs, Kirghizes, and Kalmucks to the south. Primitive standards of living and sanitation explained the prevalence of the highly contagious disease. A survey taken in 1913 showed that 20 out of every 10,000 people in Russia went blind from trachoma; but 95 out of every 10,000 people in the Tatar Republic suffered the same fate. The very low standards of hygiene observed throughout much of the country, and ascribed by the Americans to the general disintegration of living standards and public health in Soviet Russia, had already been the norm for many years in the areas where Dr. Foucar sent the medical companies in 1923. There would be much ignorance, superstition, and cultural resistance to overcome among the inhabitants of the villages of Chuvash and Mordova, nearly 85 percent of whom were infected with the contagious eye disease.

In the district of Kazan, Dr. John Cox confirmed that trachoma was known as the "scourge of the Tartar [*sic*] Republic inhabitants" and formed his own teams of local physicians and feldshers to travel across the district and care for victims of the disease. It was not uncommon for them to discover entire villages with untreated trachoma. In Simbirsk, Dr. Mark Godfrey also joined the medical

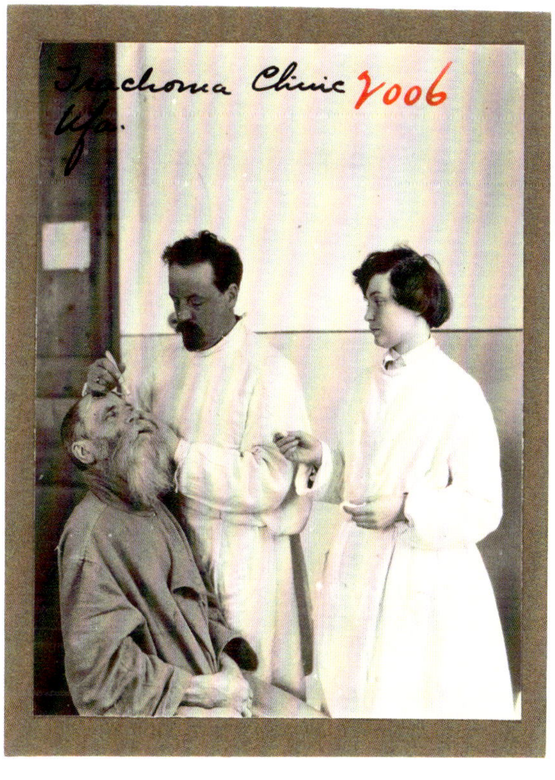

BELOW: Trachoma clinic established by the ARA in Ufa, ca. 1922.

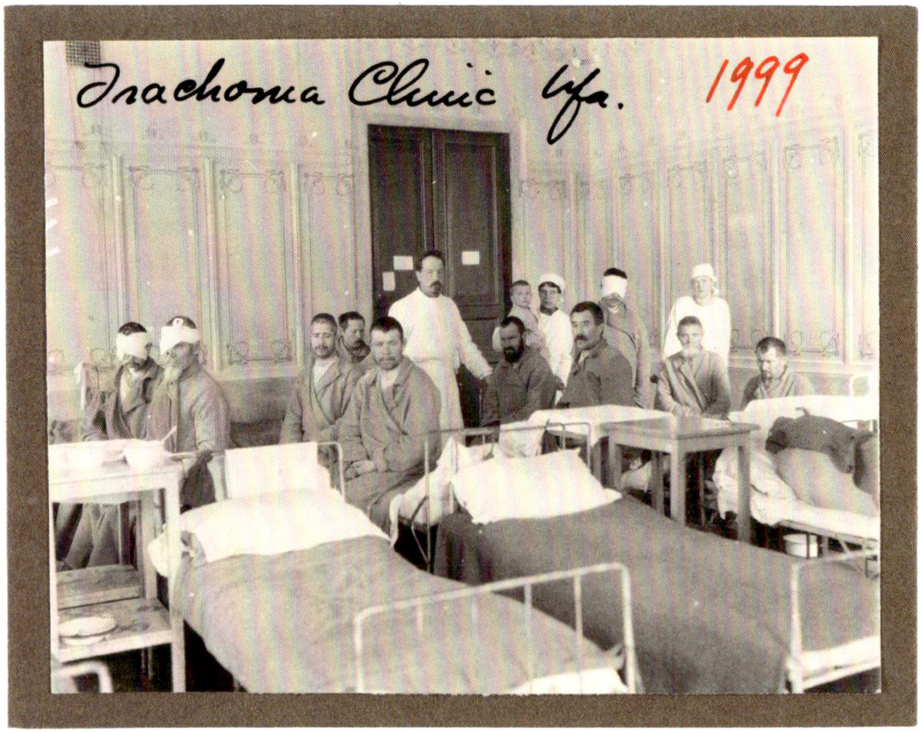

Trachoma clinic established by the ARA in Ufa, ca. 1922.

campaign to fight the eye disease when he received notice of 20,000 cases of trachoma in the county of Gorodischy, located between Simbirsk and Saratov. Once again, these victims had gone years without any medical care, or any information about the prevention and treatment of the disease.

Caused by the contagious bacterium *Chlamydia trachomatis*, and associated with poverty, poor hygiene, and dense living conditions, trachoma is spread easily from one infected person to another through secretions from the eye, nose, or throat. Flies also transmit the disease. The infection initially causes mild itching and irritation, along with discharge from the eye. Repeated infections, however, lead to scarring, and this, in turn, forces the eyelashes to turn inward and scratch the cornea. Over time the resulting corneal ulcers cloud vision to the point of blindness. Wherever cases of trachoma concentrated, the ARA dispensed the many eye antiseptics and medicines—boric acid, argyrol (silver nitrate), copper sulphate, physostigmine—along with the surgical eye instruments and binding material found in the Army surplus medical supplies.

The Physiology of Famine

By the spring of 1922, several months after the ARA had begun its relief work, there were 32.5 million people living in the Volga provinces; just over 20 million of them were threatened by starvation. In the famine districts of southern Ukraine, 3.5 million people, out of a population of 9.5 million, were also starving.

Beginning in 1914, the food shortage in Russia largely menaced the urban populations in Petrograd and Moscow, culminating in famine conditions in 1918–1919. Those living in rural, agricultural areas continued to benefit from food reserves up until 1918, at which point the Red and White armies, engaged in a civil war, confiscated everything edible in the villages they occupied or marauded. With crop failures two years in a row, in 1920 and 1921, famine came to the countryside.

THE PELIDISI SYSTEM

In conducting its feeding operations in Central Europe, the American Relief Administration had found it helpful to use an objective system to measure the level of undernourishment in order to determine eligibility for admission to its kitchens. This was the so-called Pelidisi system, the creation of Professor Clemens Pirquet, a Viennese medical doctor. Pirquet devised a formula for determining the degree of undernourishment in children up to the age of fifteen. The measurement was the cubic root of the tenfold weight of the body divided by that body's sitting height. For adults the average would be 100, for children 94.5—anything below that signified undernourishment. In Austria, the cutoff figure used was 94; in Soviet Russia, where there were tens of millions of hungry people, the standard had to be lowered to 92, and in some places less.

Here was another application of previous ARA practice that did not translate well to the Soviet Russian setting. This may have been partly due to the difference between hunger and starvation, because whereas Pirquet's system seems to have worked reasonably well in Central Europe, the relief workers in the Volga cities complained that it proved accurate only half the time. The condition of dropsy, or hunger edema—evident in the swollen bellies of many children—was a major factor. Abnormal and very reduced diets caused water to leak out of the bloodstream and into the tissues, only to be replenished by the body in the blood circulation. The result is added weight, not in any nutritional sense, but only in water. Perversely, this additional weight resulted in a high Pelidisi score that disqualified the child from eating at an ARA kitchen.

In any case, relief workers objected that the Pelidisi system was too impersonal a method for dealing with starving children, even for the businesslike ARA. As it happened, the severe shortages of time, staff, and scales prohibited the widespread introduction of the Pelidisi system into Soviet Russia. In the villages, relief operations were of necessity less standardized and regulated than the ARA was used to. For one, the scarcity of decimal scales meant that the measurement of individual food portions was less than exact. Besides, in such small communities, where everyone knew each other, there was no need to calculate the cubic root of anything in order to determine who was deserving of American food.

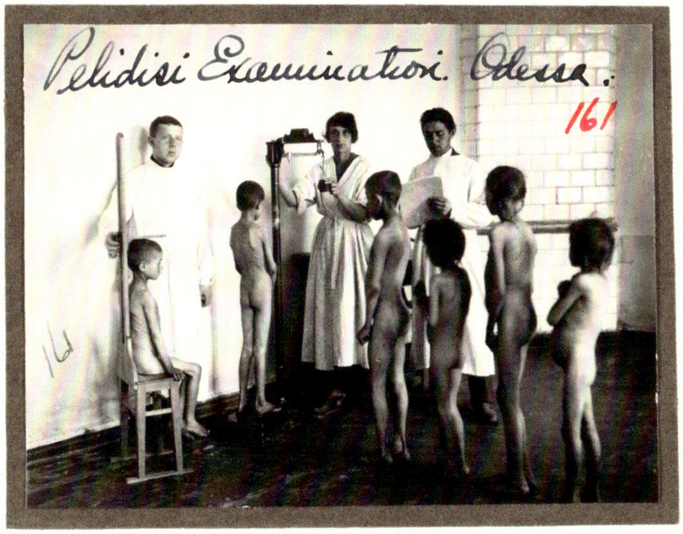

Examination of undernourished children using the Pelidisi system, Odessa, 1922.

At first, peasants collected and ate food substitutes that included the stalks of an indigestible weed known as *lebeda*, acorns, roots, tree bark, moss, camel dung, dried potato skins and pumpkin rind, rats, mice, animal bones, red clay, and sawdust. They ground these items into a "flour" for a bread that substituted for the usual black (rye) bread eaten at most peasant meals. The Soviet government even sanctioned the use of substitute foods by producing a pamphlet that listed edible plants and offered a recipe for "Bone-Dust Bread." When the ground froze and snow obscured the substitute foods, people killed and ate cats, dogs, cattle, and horses, and even ate animals that had died. In December 1921 during an inspection in a village in Kazan, Dr. M. A. Iglitzen came upon some women sitting by a fire and trying to roast a piece of horsehide. In Odessa, an ARA inspector visited a village "where typical famine conditions were found. No dogs or birds seen and the people were lying about in their homes. They were eating dogs, cats, carcasses of horses, leather, wood and at one house they had eaten half of a table." Food substitutes may have provided some sense of satiety but they contributed no nutritional value. In fact, they increased malnutrition, and the physical effects of the

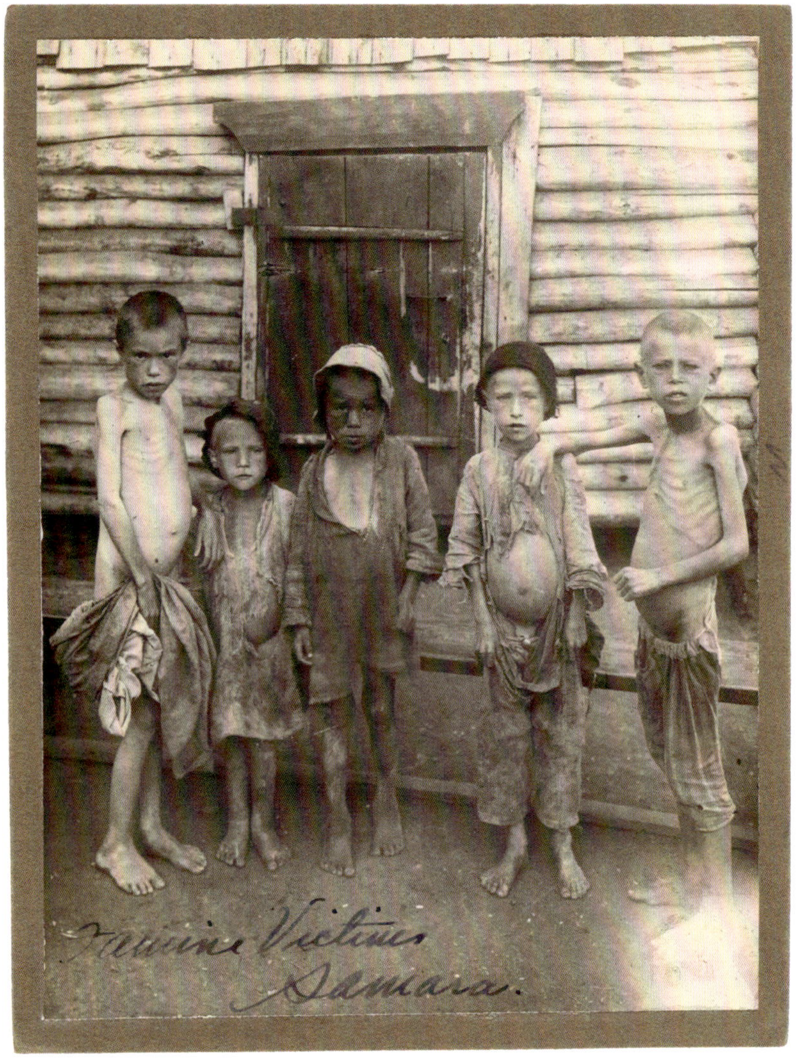

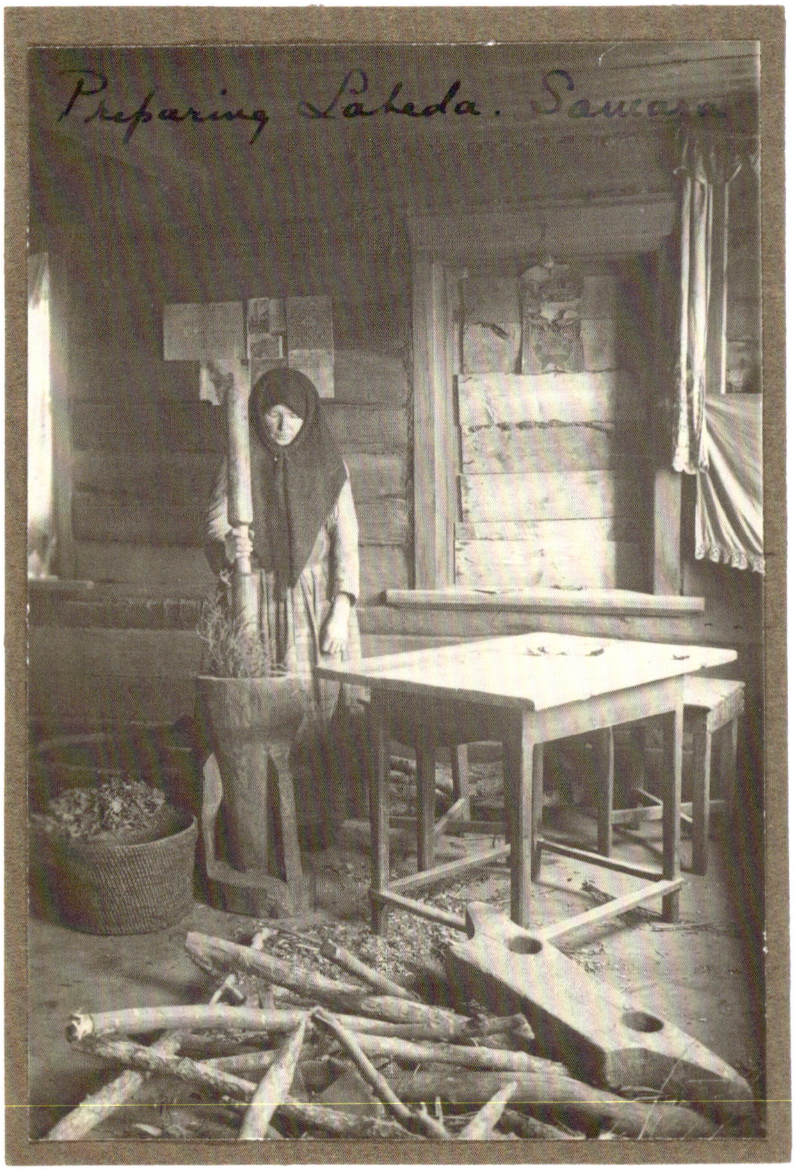

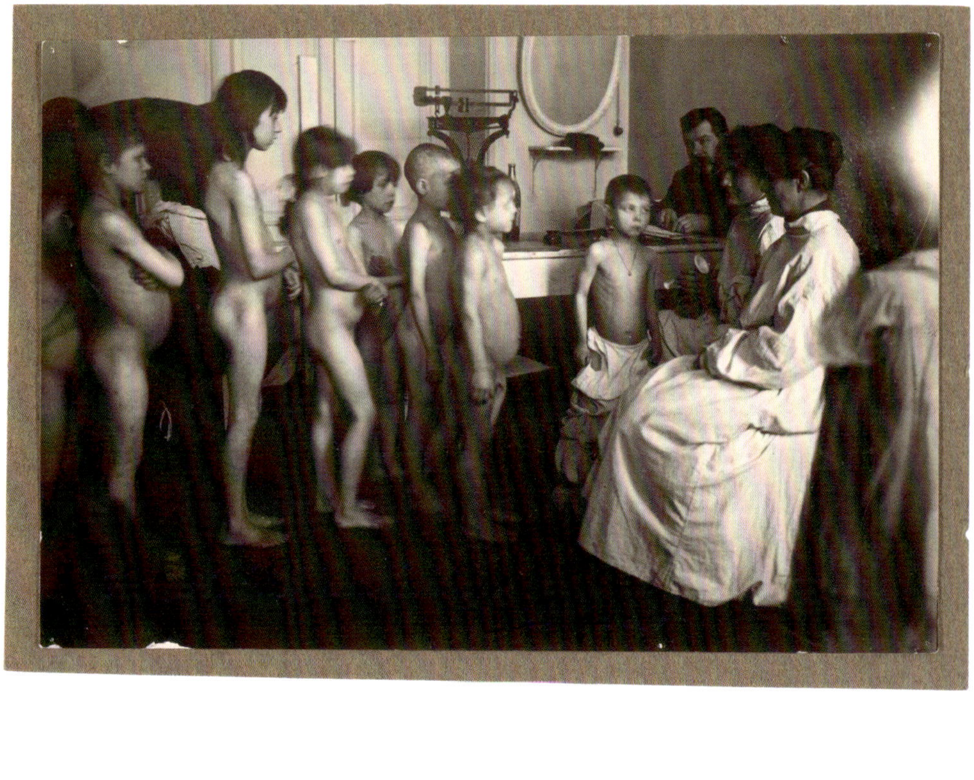

ABOVE: Famine victims, Samara, autumn 1921.

ABOVE RIGHT: Preparing labeda [lebeda], Samara, ca. 1922.

RIGHT: Children's examination, Petrograd, 1922.

abnormal diets soon became apparent, most dramatically in what one physician in Odessa described as "oedematous skeletons."

Physicians in 1922 believed that the swollen belly of a starving person was the result of a diet exclusively of carbohydrates and undigestible foods. It was an empirical diagnosis on their part. With more sophisticated technology and studies, physicians today know that the swelling or edema is caused by a diet low in or altogether missing protein; that with prolonged starvation and protein deficiency, fluid leaks out of the circulatory system and into the body's tissues, causing the abnormal swelling. The body then continues to replace the fluid in the bloodstream. Starving people with hunger edema or dropsy do weigh more, and those with anasarca, or swelling over the entire body, weigh even more. The added fluid in their tissues can impede physical movement and even reduce their visual field.

Tuberculosis

The National Russian League, an agency established in 1909 to fight tuberculosis, succumbed to the war and the social and political upheavals of the times, so that by 1921, the agency itself and any serious medical attention given to the disease had disappeared. Overcrowded living conditions, lack of sanitation, physical exhaustion, and underfeeding simply fueled the spread of the disease, and from 1914 to 1921, cases of tuberculosis steadily increased in Russia. Although diseases like typhus and cholera also existed in epidemic proportions during those years, more people died of tuberculosis in that decade, as Beeuwkes noted, than "from all other diseases combined." Famine and disease may carry off people equally, but the ones with tuberculosis are the "first to suffer."

Of the diseases directly affected by malnutrition, tuberculosis stands out. Subject to fatigue, fever, night sweats, and wasting caused by the bacterium *Mycobacterium tuberculosis*, the tubercular victim was already nutritionally challenged. The protein deficiency of starvation only increased the wasting and further reduced the body's ability to fight infection.

One Russian physician in Saratov during the famine explained the aggravation as follows: "The war and the events which followed: epidemic, lack of work,

BELOW LEFT: Tuberculosis sanitarium, women's ward, ca. 1922.

BELOW RIGHT: Children's tuberculosis sanitarium, Ekaterinburg, ca. 1922.

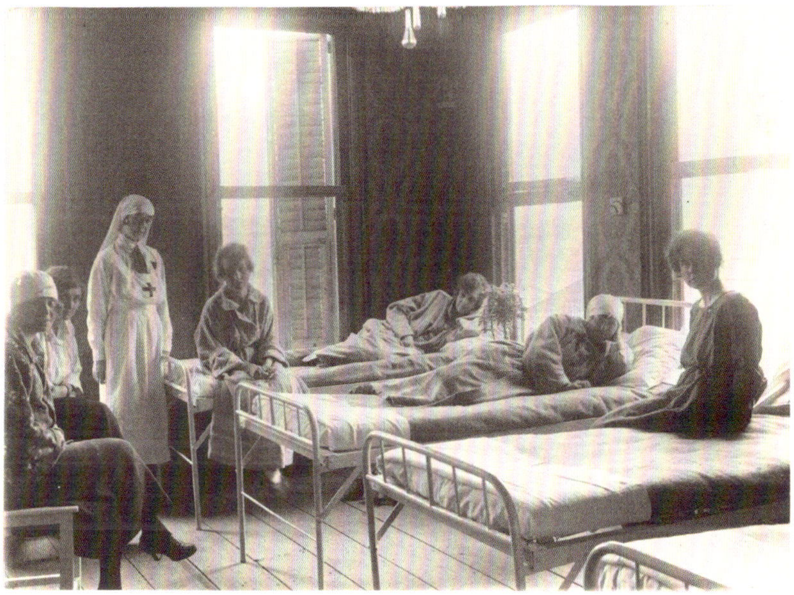

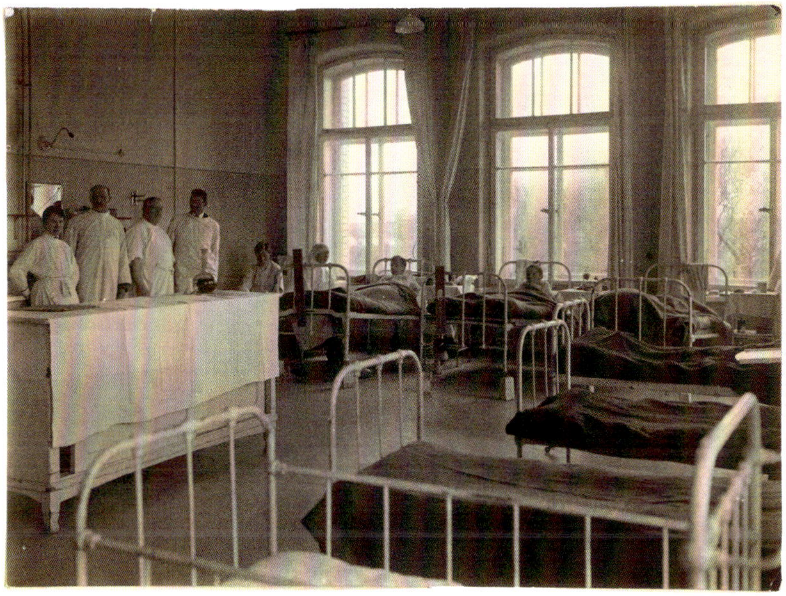

famine, fugitive movement, return of war prisoners and other abnormalities of social life both in Russia and as is stated by scientific authorities also in Western Europe have increased to a great extent the frequency of tuberculosis and made its course worse." Beeuwkes offered an interpretation on a more human scale: "The lowered resistance of the inhabitants, reduced by worry and lack of diversion, unsanitary and congested conditions, improper diet, insufficient clothing, and lack of fuel, is responsible for the increase in the incidence of tuberculosis."

This increase was especially true in children. Medical examinations in Saratov revealed that 52 percent of children between three and fourteen years of age tested positive for tuberculosis; and 43 percent of children aged fifteen to eighteen years had the disease. In one children's home in Kharkov, physicians found in December 1921 that 97 percent of the children had tuberculosis. The aerosolized transmission of the highly infectious bacterial illness combined with the density of living produced staggering numbers of children with the pulmonary form of the disease. Once in the lungs, tuberculosis could spread through the bloodstream to other parts of the body. Scrofula, tuberculosis of the lymph glands in the neck, was commonly seen among children. Unexpectedly and increasingly, it was also found among adults, who presented with large, caseous (cheesy) ulcers of the lymph glands of the neck that often erupted through the skin.

As tuberculosis spreads from the lungs to the lymph glands in the neck, it can also invade the bones (tuberculosis ossium). In March 1922, Dr. Theodore Foster reported that "30 percent of children in Kiev have bone tuberculosis," a diagnosis likely made clinically since most hospitals lacked the tubes and plates needed for X-ray machines. Physicians would have felt swellings around the long bones,

THE BEGINNINGS OF IMMUNOLOGY

In 1908, the Nobel Prize in Medicine was awarded to Russian Ilya Ilyich Mechnikov (1845–1916) and German Paul Ehrlich (1854–1915) for their individual studies in the early stages of a scientific field that would later become known as immunology. They followed on the heels of Louis Pasteur and Robert Koch, whose respective scientific experiments identified specific microbes as the source of various diseases and ushered in the revolutionary germ theory of disease. Miasmas as a suspected source of illness became a thing of the past.

Mechnikov originally worked at the Bacteriological Institute in Odessa (1886–1887) and later continued his scientific studies at the Pasteur Institute in Paris. He observed in starfish larvae that certain cells would surround and engulf foreign particles that he introduced into the larvae. Because the cells appeared to consume the foreign bodies, Mechnikov identified them as "phagocytes," from the Greek for "devouring cells." What Mechnikov discovered constituted one line of defense that a body takes against invasion or infection.

The German physician and scientist Paul Ehrlich expanded studies in immunity to diphtheria when he developed a theory to explain an immune response. He hypothesized that when a toxin—such as a vaccine—was injected into a body, it stimulated the production of a specific antitoxin, or what we now call an antibody. These antitoxins/antibodies constituted another line of defense against infection or disease.

In September 1921, when the American relief workers fanned out across the Volga region—the epicenter of the famine—they recognized immediately physical signs of starvation (cachexia, edema, anasarca, vitamin deficiencies). As they encountered the presence of several epidemic diseases in the area (typhus, relapsing fever, cholera, malaria), the men speculated as to the intersection of famine and disease and anticipated dire outcomes. That intersection, the territory of men like Mechnikov and Ehrlich and their colleagues in the young field of immunology, was in fact the human immune system. It is likely that the ARA men knew little about those lines of defense that a body mounts against infection and disease, but they reasoned rightly that when the human body is nutritionally starved and physically stressed it is more vulnerable to disease.

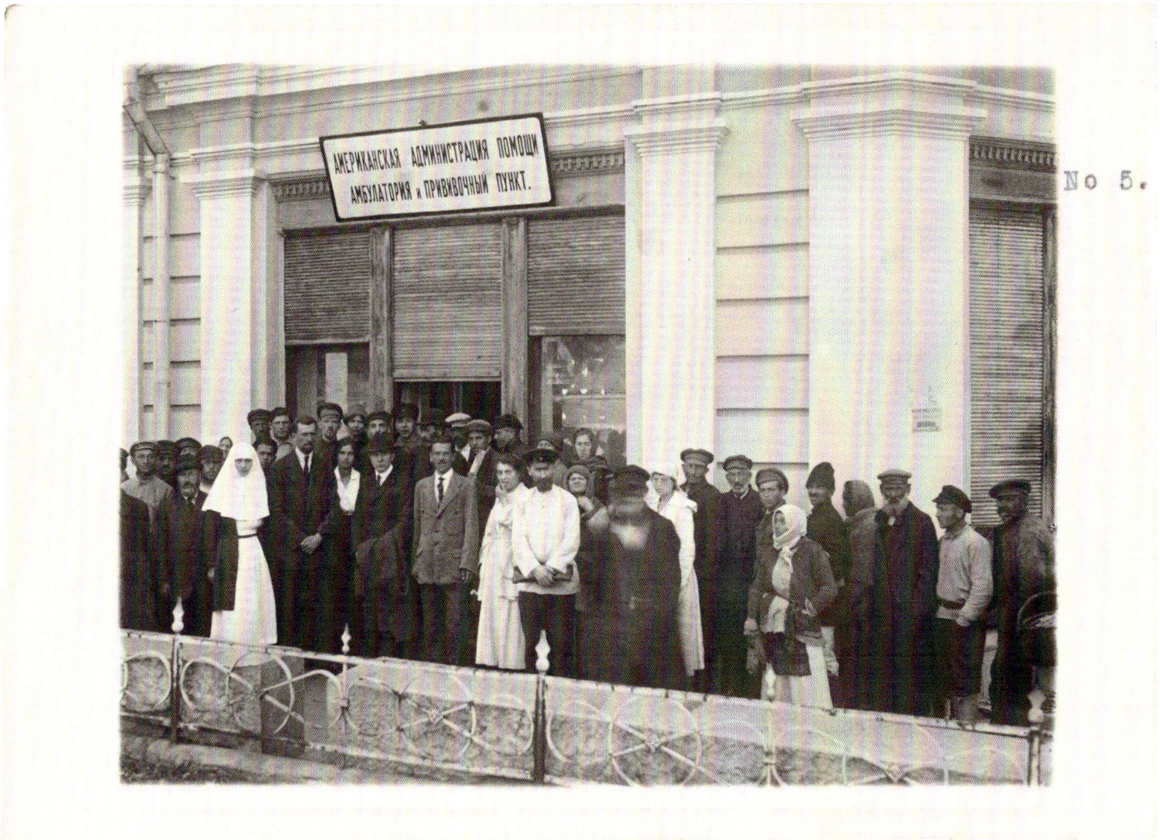

American Relief Administration dispensary and inoculation point, Kiev, May 1922. Standing near center, wearing a hat and holding his coat, is district physician Dr. Theodore Foster. American Relief Administration European operational records

knees, hips, and on the fingers of the children, which were painful to the touch. When tuberculosis spreads from the lungs to the spine (Pott's disease), a surgical procedure of the time known as Albee's operation, to relieve spinal cord compression and avoid paraplegia, was often in order. Beeuwkes knew of one surgeon in Petrograd who, "in the last few years," had performed the surgery on 250 patients with successful results. And yet the operation was far out of financial reach for most of the population.

Nearly a year after Dr. Foster reported the high percentage of bone tuberculosis in Kiev, Russian physicians in Odessa warned of an increase in tuberculosis morbidity. The disease had remained a serious public health problem. In response, the ARA fully supplied a government hospital designated as the Gubernia Red Cross Tuberculosis Hospital. It was an attempt to restore a primary "treatment": isolation of the tuberculosis carrier. The supplementary feeding program in the hospital, said Foster, was "organized after the latest most modern methods of [the] Anti-Tuberculosis League of America."

Since there was no cure for the disease until 1943, the "most modern methods" of treatment likely included the standard regimen of rest, fresh air, exercise, heliotherapy, and a balanced diet. Dr. Darkshavitch, a local physician in Orenburg, prescribed *kumis*, fermented mare or donkey milk, for his tuberculosis patients, and was grateful when the ARA sent him 251 cases of milk and rice to make the tonic. The "modern methods" of treatment also required education of the public through lectures, which in Orenburg were "made interesting and attractive by frozen and preserved pathological specimens," according to district supervisor Walter Coleman. It was one way to scare the public into practicing basic hygiene to prevent the spread of the disease.

Cod Liver Oil

In a time before antibiotics, medicine lacked many true curative therapies. Quinine treated malaria, and Neosalvarsan cured the spirochetal diseases of relapsing fever and syphilis. Lacking other cures, Beeuwkes and the American district physicians employed a single therapeutic, cod liver oil, to address an enormous array of dietary deficiencies—vitamins, minerals, essential fats—which had impaired Soviet Russia's citizens and made them highly susceptible to other diseases such as tuberculosis.

Although it was the bane of life for most American children, cod liver oil (oleum morrhuae) became the most basic and essential treatment for recovery from malnutrition. It compensated for the lack of fat in the Russian ration of food and in a diet of substitute foods, provided vitamins A and D and omega-3 essential fatty acids, and reversed anemia and many of the symptoms of starvation. Thirty grams a day of cod liver oil became a rule in the ARA kitchens. Dr. W. R. Smith in Odessa bragged that the children "lap it up like American youngsters would ice cream and yell for more." From Moscow, an ARA press release boasted that the "Russian children of this city orphanage drink cod liver oil as American children drink milk." They love the "sweet, sticky taste" and "know that a big spoonful fills the hole in their stomach and keeps them from being hungry until the next meal."

Similarly, another ARA press release likened the Russian taste for "bread with a thick coating of cod liver oil" to the way that "Johnnie Smith takes to his jam." Physicians were warned to watch for children who returned to a food line just to get a second portion of the oil. Just as quinine made the list of drugs strictly protected by the ARA warehouse staff, so too did oils have to be well guarded. "Guards furnished by the Government were not reliable, and considerable numbers were imprisoned for theft of medical supplies," Beeuwkes testified. "Their bayonets caused more loss than protection, for they used them to pierce barrels of cod liver oil for lubricant for their boots." In fact, the only complaints about

Loading cod liver oil, Petrograd, January 11, 1922.

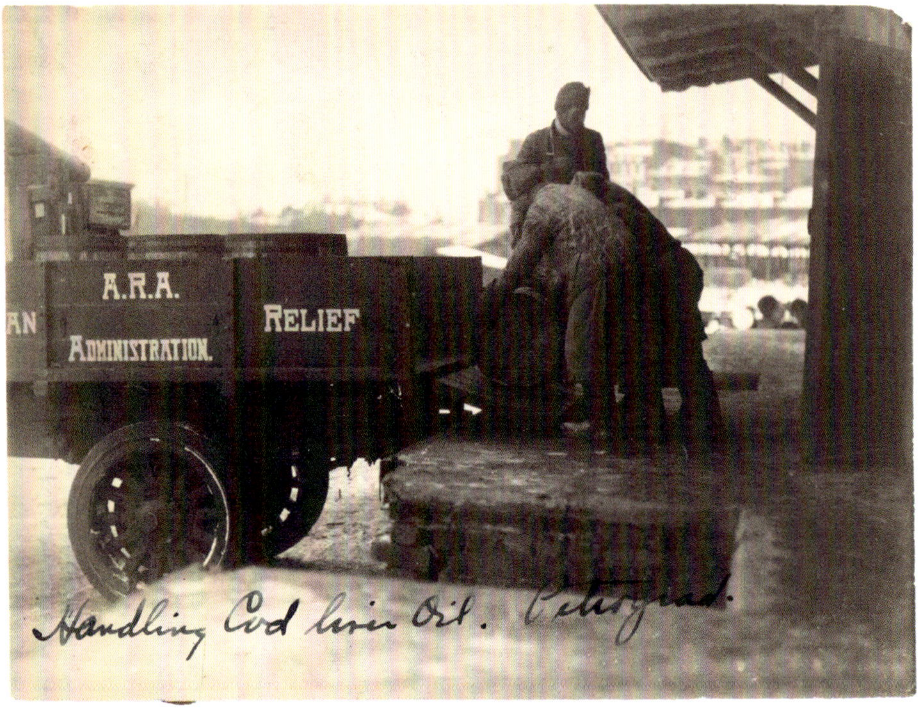

DEFICIENCY AND SKIN DISEASES

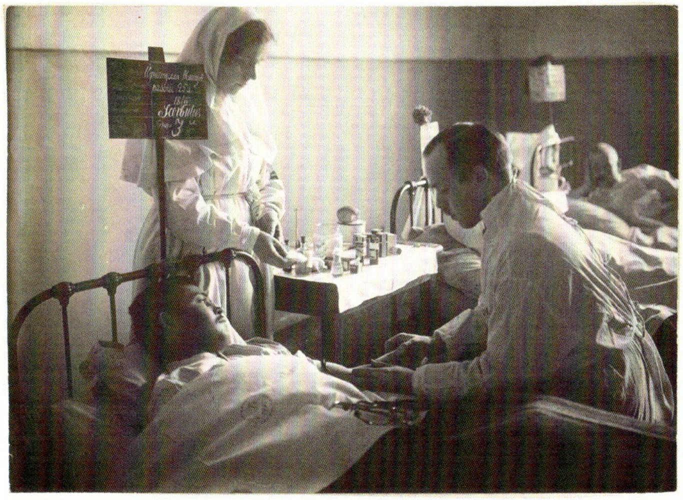

Patient being treated for scorbutus (scurvy), Kazan, ca. 1922.

On an early inspection tour in Simbirsk in December 1921, Dr. Mark Godfrey visited a children's home where he observed dirty children in rags "suffering from ricketts [*sic*], scurvy, scabies, impetigo, xerothalmia, and tuberculosis. Practically every child without exception was suffering from anemia and different degrees of malnutrition." When the starving people resorted to eating food substitutes, they condemned their bodies not only to protein deficiency but also to a host of other deficiencies in essential vitamins and minerals. Godfrey's inventory, though not nearly comprehensive, identifies several of the deficiency diseases the arriving ARA doctors found to be pervasive.

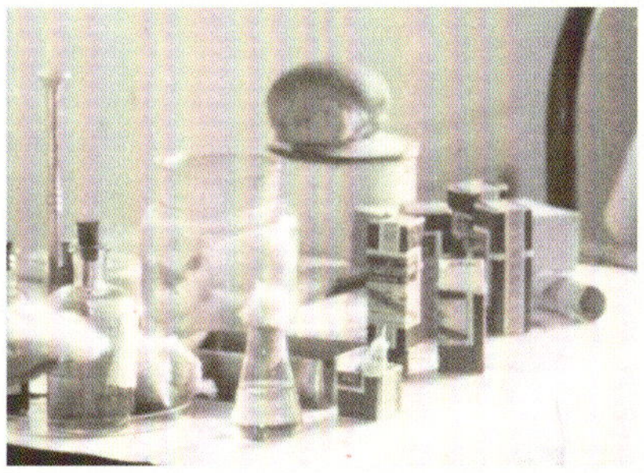

DETAIL: Close-up of bedside table reveals a white roll, a hallmark of ARA food relief, atop a container of food.

Rickets, or vitamin D deficiency, softens and weakens bones by impairing calcium absorption. Dr. W. Horsley Gantt estimated that 80 percent of the children in Soviet Russia had rickets, putting them at risk for short stature or "stunting," a condition that Dr. Theodore Foster in Kiev noted in his medical report for September 1922. Eight-year-old boys and girls, Foster observed, were now comparable in height to six-and-a-half-year-old children in prewar times. **Scurvy**, or scorbutus, caused by a lack of vitamin C, manifests itself in skin lesions, usually in the form of swollen, bleeding gums. **Xerophthalmia**, the result of vitamin A deficiency, affects the eyes and can lead to a condition in which the conjunctiva of the eyes dry out and begin to wrinkle, with the accompanying reduced vision known as night blindness. **Anemia** is brought on by a deficiency in vitamin E and iron, which also resulted in muscle weakness and coordination problems, making it difficult for some of those afflicted to walk. Children, especially those in the collecting homes, presented with the itchy skin condition known as **scabies**, caused by mites burrowing into the skin. It was known to be highly contagious, from skin-to-skin contact, but there was little opportunity to isolate children. **Impetigo**, a bacterial skin infection that manifests in red sores around the mouth and nose, was also commonly diagnosed. A lack of niacin or vitamin B3 in the diet causes the disease **pellagra**, whose symptoms include diarrhea, scaly skin sores, and dementia. Cases of "hunger belly," also known as **dropsy**, were ubiquitous in the children's homes and other institutions visited by the ARA physicians in the acute period of the famine.

the nutrient came from Dr. Beck in Orenburg in May 1922 when the large barrels holding the oil leaked in the warm weather and made a slick mess in the warehouse. Beeuwkes sent him bottles in which to store the leaked liquid. Otherwise, the 700,000 pounds of cod liver oil purchased by the ARA in Scandinavia, said to be very high quality, hit the sweet spot for the Russian children.

Malaria

Malaria had long been present in Russia, but the number of cases rose dramatically after the Revolution of 1917, the Russian Civil War, and the onset of famine. In 1922, Poland recorded 17,419 cases; Italy was beset with 234,656 cases; but Soviet Russia exceeded all other counts with 1,986,417 cases of malaria registered by the government. Russian epidemiologist Lev Tarassevitch noted several different aspects of the malarial epidemic of 1922. More commonly seen was a "more virulent tropical type"; the disease spread beyond its usual boundaries, reaching as far

ЗАБОЛЕВАЕМОСТЬ МАЛЯРИЕЙ

по Г. ЦАРИЦЫНУ

ЯНВАРЬ – АПРЕЛЬ МЕСЯЦЫ 1922–1923 ГГ.

ЗАРЕГИСТРИРОВАНО ЗАБОЛЕВАНИЙ :

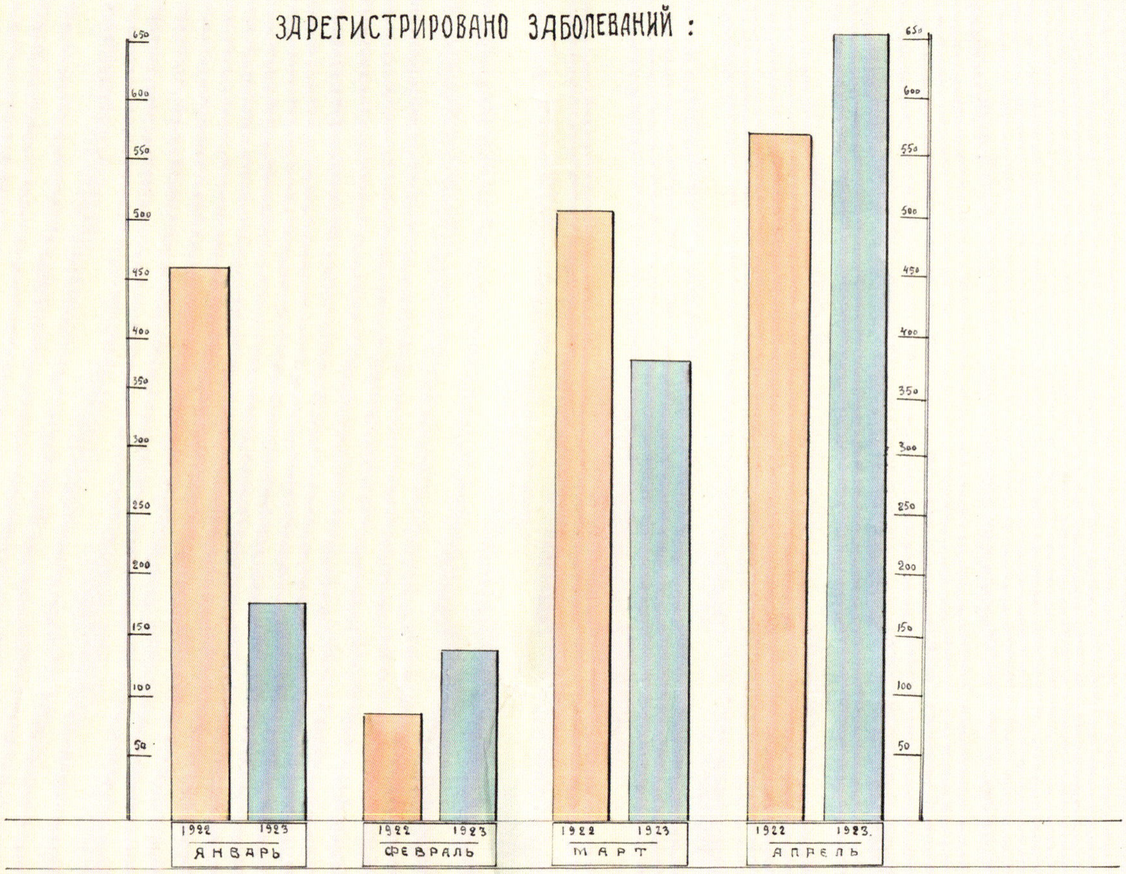

%% ОТНОШЕНИЕ МАЛЯРИЙНЫХ ЗАБОЛЕВАНИЙ К ОБЩЕЙ ИНФЕКЦИОННОЙ ЗАБОЛЕВАЕМОСТИ :

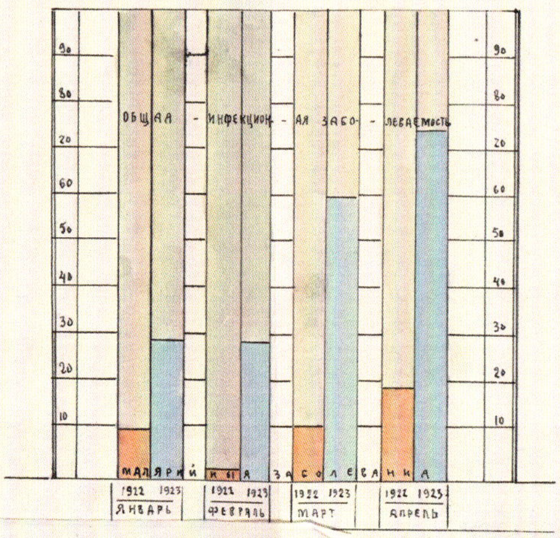

TABLE SHOWING PERCENTAGE OF MALARIA
AS COMPARED WITH FIGURES SHOWING
REGISTERED CASES OF GENERAL INFECT.
CASES IN TZARITZYN CITY.

During the months:
JANUARY, FEBRUARY AND MARCH
1922 & 1923.

000

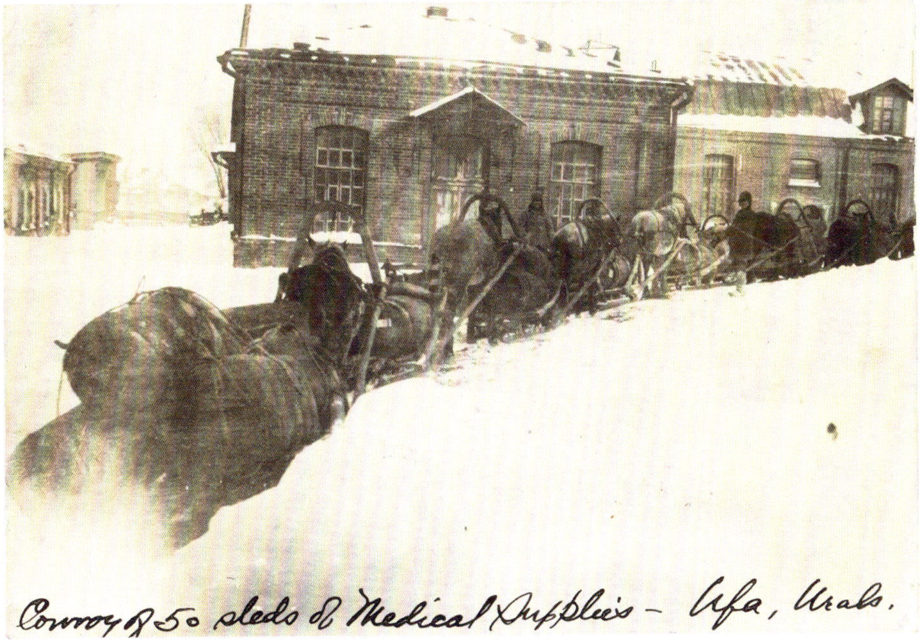

FACING: Cases of malaria as registered in the city of Tsaritsyn, on the lower Volga, in January, February, March, and April 1922 and 1923.

LEFT: Convoy of fifty sleds carrying medical supplies, Ufa, winter 1922.

north as Archangel and Murmansk on the coast of the Arctic Sea; the number of cases increased dramatically; and there was a high mortality rate. He attributed these new aspects to a change in climate, a shortage of hospitals and quinine, the mass movements of population (migration, repatriation, demobilization of troops), and a diminished resistance to disease caused by the famine.

Once again, the wartime destruction of public utilities figured into the disease prevalence, which escalated especially in the middle Volga region: the Samara, Saratov, and Simbirsk districts. The ruin of drainage systems, which had once channeled water into rivers, allowed water to pool anywhere. The inertia of the local boards of health (*gubzdravs*) and the indifference of an exhausted populace blinded all to the threat posed by the stagnant water as breeding places for the *Anopheles* mosquito, which carried malaria. In February 1922, Dr. Foucar warned that malaria, always prevalent in the Samara district, "occupies first-place among all diseases." He feared that it would surpass typhus, which at that time was epidemic. In April 1922, Dr. Godfrey in Simbirsk sent up a red flag when he wrote that "no malaria epidemic in the history of Russia has been as great as the present one." The incidence of malaria in the middle Volga region in 1922 would reach 63,200 reported cases in Simbirsk; 109,664 cases in Saratov; and 175,420 cases in Samara.

The ARA Medical Division waged a war against malaria beginning in the spring of 1922 with its cleanup campaigns. The drive to eradicate mosquitoes started with the elimination of breeding places in any body of stagnant water. Dr. Cox in Kazan wanted an all-out assault on the mosquito reminiscent of the "treatment the U.S. Government gave the Panama Canal." He was referring to the eradication campaign waged by US Army doctor Colonel William Gorgas during the construction of the Panama Canal from 1903 to 1914. Gorgas organized "mosquito brigades" to smother and suffocate mosquito larvae. Cox regretted that the local Russian government in Kazan could not initiate such a campaign, since it had no money to pay workers nor the "enterprise" to do the work. The demoralization and physical lassitude of the populace from hunger and sickness reinforced the sense of inertia.

In the spring of 1922, the promise of food from the ARA, in the form of a ration of corn, reversed this civic inertia, and soon "sanitation squads" scoured the towns looking for any empty containers holding water. The teams dug drainage ditches and oiled larger bodies of water with kerosene or oil to smother and wipe out the mosquito larvae. It was continuous work over many months due to the heavy spring rains along with two unexpected weeks of rain in July. Only the American corn rations kept the work in progress.

Like typhus and relapsing fever, malaria is a vector-borne disease, transmitted by an infected insect into the human bloodstream. But unlike those two diseases, malaria is not transmitted by human physical contact (except by blood transfusion or shared needles). Beeuwkes was thus incorrect in attributing the origin of the current wave of disease first to infected soldiers demobilized from the Turkish front and later to refugees migrating from malarial sections of Russia. Even renowned epidemiologist Tarassevitch factored population movements into his explanation for the dissemination of malaria. In fact, however, unless they transported mosquitoes and their larvae in their belongings, neither troops nor refugees could spread the disease.

The *Anopheles* mosquito, carrying the parasite known as *Plasmodium*, bites and infects a human, starting a repeated cycle of intense, shaking chills alternating with fever and sweating. Delirium can result from fevers reaching as high as 106 degrees. Physicians observing these symptoms then feel for an enlarged spleen, which indicates how the organ is working to filter and remove red blood cells infected with the parasite. Ideally, malaria is diagnosed in a laboratory by a blood smear on a glass slide that shows the presence of the parasite *Plasmodium*. But in early 1922 few laboratories or hospitals in Russia had the equipment to do any diagnostic work. Dr. Gantt observed one young intern in a hospital in Uralsk cleverly using broken pieces of glass windowpanes to prepare and analyze blood smears. He was ingenious, and also fortunate because he had a rare working microscope. When malaria is left untreated, which was often the case in Soviet Russia at that time, the cycle of chill and fever can continue for three to five days before the victim succumbs to exhaustion, coma, and possibly death.

Quinine

Exacerbating the epidemic spread of malaria in Soviet Russia in 1922 was the nearly complete absence of quinine throughout the country: in 1921, the Soviet government had only 2,000 kilos of quinine available for distribution. Large stores of the effective drug had been exhausted during the world war and civil war. In Kazan, some Russian physicians used arsenic mixed with different herbs to treat those seriously ill with malaria but reported that the results were not at all satisfactory. Apparently, the toxin—arsenic—does not deter the *Plasmodium* parasite.

"There is an incessant cry for Quinine," wrote Dr. John Toole from Saratov in August 1922. It was a notably precious commodity: "A single bottle of quinine was worth three months pay of the average laborer," Beeuwkes noted. Americans and locals working in the ARA warehouses were alert to the possible theft of drugs, especially cocaine. "The great number of cocaine addicts in Russia made traffic in this drug extremely profitable," Beeuwkes observed. Quinine was added to their list after Dr. Gantt reported the theft of a box of quinine in Saratov. The thief had cleverly covered up for the missing drug by replacing it with a discarded pair of shoes and a Russian scythe. Perhaps he thought it an even trade since shoes were also highly coveted.

TALES OF CANNIBALISM

When the famine raged, there were many reports of what was called "cannibalism." The term was applied loosely both to genuine cases of cannibalism, or anthropophagy—which implied an act of barbarous murder—and to the much more common incidences of corpse eating. In Russian, the terminology was also somewhat ambiguously used even though the language provides two neatly descriptive words: *liudoedstvo*, literally "people eating," and *trupoedstvo*, or "corpse eating." There is also *kanibal'tsvo*, which means "cannibalism" but was used indiscriminately as a label for all acts of corpse eating. "Cannibalism" is usually associated with some form of religious ritual, but there was nothing of the kind in the Russian context.

In the spring of 1922, two Russian physicians produced serious studies of the subject. One is a pamphlet by Dr. L. M. Vasilevskii, published in Ufa, whose title translates as *The Dreadful Chronicle of Famine (Suicide and Anthropophagy)*; the other a chapter in a book manuscript titled "Horrors of Famine and Cannibalism in Russia, 1921–1922," written by a doctor in Kazan enlisted by the ARA. The authors aspired to scientific analysis, and each appears to have worked carefully with the available evidence, which consisted largely of secondhand anecdotes of the most horrific kind—"surpassing all limits of the imagination," in the words of one of them.

The Ufa study examines several dozen episodes of cannibalism described in the Soviet press and speculates that in the remote countryside there were many dozens, if not hundreds, more cases left unreported. The author of the Kazan study, Dr. I. A. Violin, who supervised the ARA's vaccination campaign in the district, agrees that the incidences documented in the press were only a small number of the actual total. Based on press accounts and his own observation and investigations, Violin provides estimated totals for several famine-plagued regions. For the Tatar Republic, for example, he counts 72 cases of corpse eating and 223 incidences of cannibalism; for the Bashkir Republic the proportions are reversed, with 220 cases of corpse eating and 58 cases of cannibalism; for Samara province the respective numbers are 200 and 60.

Violin believes that the number of witnessed cases was much higher than the number reported, but that people had become so desensitized through repeated exposure to the ghastly deed—"we read [about it] with a cool indifference"—that they no longer considered it worth bringing to the attention of the authorities. This was especially true of the more common practice of corpse eating. Vasilevskii says the worst affected areas were Ufa province and two ill-fated Volga regions, Pugachev and Buzuluk. There is nothing in the ARA documentation that would contradict this assertion. Both authors advised the authorities to use discrimination in prosecuting individuals accused of cannibalism and corpse eating. Even cases involving mothers devouring children might not be what they appeared. While it seemed that the very "instinct of motherhood," this "holy feeling," has been crushed by a stronger instinctive urge, yet, "Very frequently the

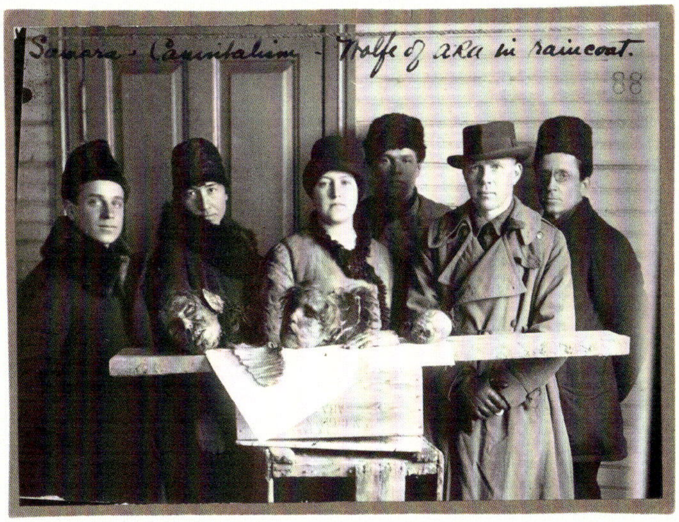

Henry Wolfe (second from right) and evidence of cannibalism, Samara, March 1922.

deed is promoted by a deep inborn feeling of motherhood. We know of a case that had been observed in the Pugachev district of Samara Province where a mother wishing to save her children from starvation, fed three of her remaining infants with the corpse of her daughter aged 13, who had died."

The photographic record of the American Relief Administration in the Hoover Archives includes numerous shocking photos of the apprehended perpetrators posed with the remains of their victims. The first such photos to reach Moscow were acquired by Dr. Iglitzen, serving as an inspector for the ARA in Kazan. He supplemented a harrowing report of conditions in Spassk canton in February 1922 with a series of gruesome photographs that seem to have struck ARA headquarters in Moscow like a thunderbolt. These photos were passed along to the chiefs in London and from there sent on to New York, though they were not given publicity.

American relief worker Henry Wolfe, of Coshocton, Ohio, spent several weeks on the trail of cannibalism as he traveled through Samara province in March 1922. Eventually he found what he was looking for, in the subdistrict of Melekes. In the ARA archive, there is a posed photograph of him standing among a row of five local citizens cultivated in appearance and dressed in Russian winter wear. Before them, set out on a wooden plank, lies the grim evidence, which appears to consist of at least two human heads and a hand.

After one has looked through dozens of ARA photographs of grotesque corpses twisted into every shape and, worse, of barely living skeletons, the Wolfe photograph fails to shock. Curiously, what attracts the eye is the figure of the lone American himself, outfitted in trench coat and brimmed hat, hands clasped before him in leather gloves. He looks as if he has walked onto the set of a horror film. His face is expressionless; his incongruous presence alone conveys the idea that something terribly significant has taken place.

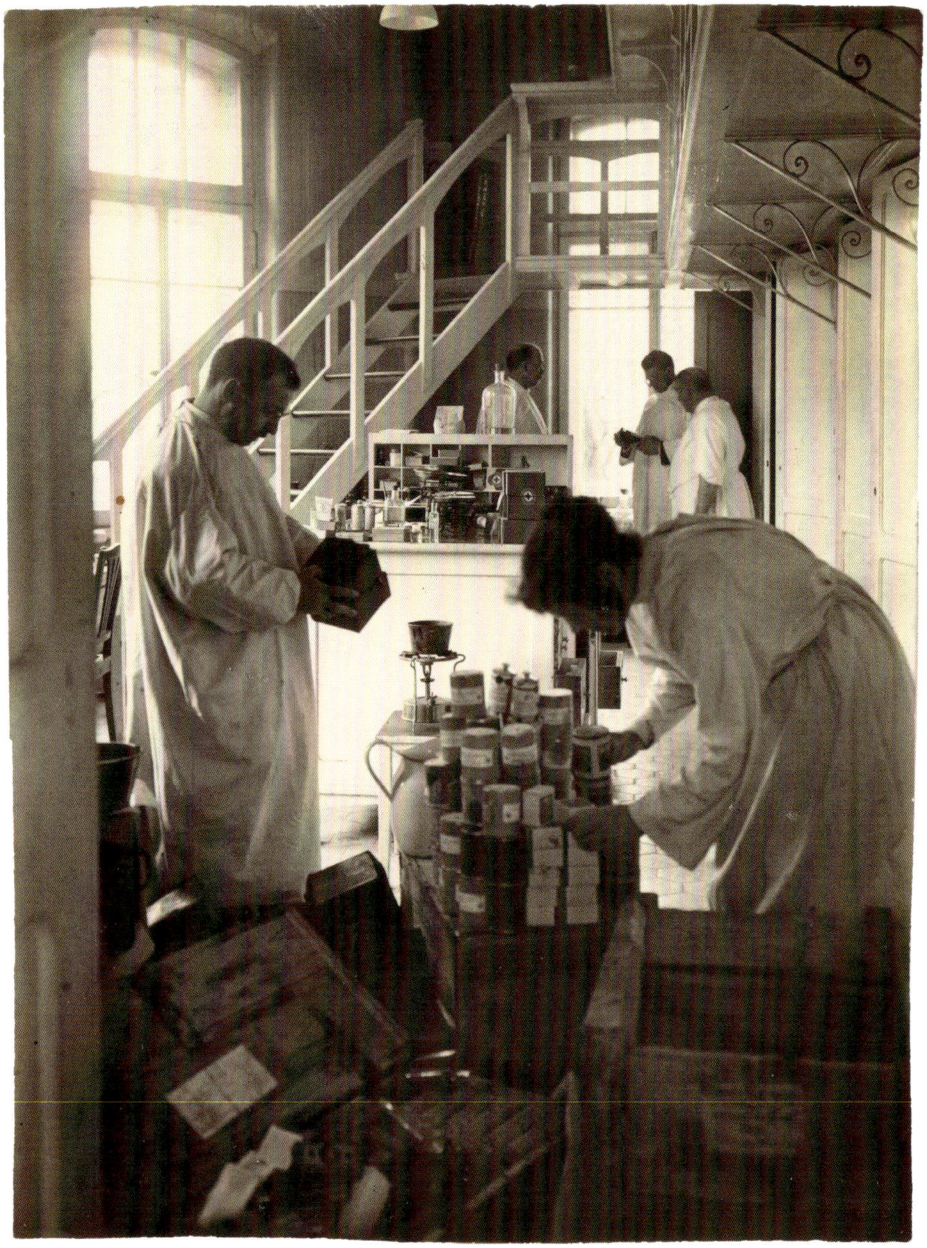

Unpacking hospital supplies and instruments, Odessa, 1922.

Quinine, taken from the bark of the Peruvian Cinchona tree, had long been known as an effective fever-reducing drug used against malaria. In fact, it is a toxin to *Plasmodium* and disrupts the growth and reproduction of the malarial parasites in the blood. It was given in the form of tablets or was injected. Additionally, quinine hydrochloride combined with urea hydrochloride produced a solution that acted as a local anesthetic at an injection site and was used often in place of cocaine. It was an important and effective drug, especially at a time when there were so few actual curatives available to physicians.

The treatment of malaria with quinine varied in drug form and regimen. Dr. Gantt prescribed "large doses of IV quinine hydrochloride, repeated in 2–3 doses on successive days." In Rostov, Dr. Patrick H. Kennedy found best results when the drug was given intravenously but accepted the Russian practice of giving an intramuscular injection in the thigh. Local Russian physicians in Samara followed several practices: an intravenous injection on the first and second days of treatment; followed by a subcutaneous injection once daily for ten days along with .5 grams of quinine sulphate by mouth three times a day. "The above therapy is complicated and difficult, in fact impossible to carry out on a large scale and in the regions," complained Dr. Foucar in his monthly medical report for July 1922. Foucar preferred the easier quinine-by-mouth therapy over the quinine-injection therapy for most cases.

Preventive measures figured prominently in Foucar's medical arsenal. He secured enough quinine tablets for all the ARA personnel to take "every night at bedtime or with the evening meal." And he prescribed a similarly simple regimen for the medical staff working in malarial clinics.

The district of Sorochinskoye in Samara opened a malarial clinic offering free care, courtesy of a supply of quinine from the ARA along with food rations supplied to the medical staff. In the first few days of the clinic, Russian physicians treated 398 patients for malaria. They prescribed 20 grains of quinine sulphate (tablets) to be taken daily for a succession of six days; stop for four days; take 20 grains for five days; stop for fourteen days; finally, take 15 grains for four days. Detailed records of each case remained on file. Even after such a laborious treatment regimen, symptoms could in fact reappear, and patients were advised to return to the clinic. Two malarial stations were set up in Rostov, and each treated over 300 cases a day. The large treatment center in Penza (Simbirsk district) saw over 250 patients a day.

Research on malaria resumed in the Bacteriological Institute in Tsaritsyn after it was supplied with equipment to analyze blood smears and confirm the diagnosis of malaria. Russian soldiers returning from Tashkent and Astrakhan were suffering from a more serious, tropical form (aestivo-autumnal type) of malaria that was not responding well enough to quinine alone. Often called pernicious malaria and caused by the *Plasmodium falciparum*, this malarial type caused attacks every forty-eight hours involving cerebral, renal, or gastrointestinal symptoms. Because it was a severe and fatal type of the disease, physicians began to experiment with an unconventional solution of Neosalvarsan added to quinine and gave it intravenously. Some even added an antipyrine to further reduce the fever.

Keenly aware that malaria threatened to derail ARA relief efforts, Dr. Foucar decided to supply prophylactic quinine to all ARA local personnel, men holding public offices in the district, and railroad personnel, to keep the ARA work and supplies steadily moving forward. In the spring of 1923, as the ARA mission was winding down, Foucar continued the anti-malarial campaign and organized seven "companies" each composed of a doctor-instructor and a feldsher. Their assignment was to fan out into villages, and their duties included safeguarding the quinine, instructing local physicians in the technique of quinine injection, educating all as to the prophylactic use of quinine, and reporting on the sanitary measures being taken to control the breeding grounds of the mosquitoes.

Foucar planned to use the ARA corn ration to pay all the workers. Dr. John Stack in Saratov also instituted similar prophylactic measures in the final months, equipping two large "malarial missions with various forms of quinine and syringes and other medicaments." The epidemic peaked in the summer of 1923 when over six million cases were registered, including several American relief workers, a figure likely representing only one-third of the actual number of cases. Right down to the final days of the medical relief effort, the sixty thousand pounds of quinine provided by the ARA was making a difference.

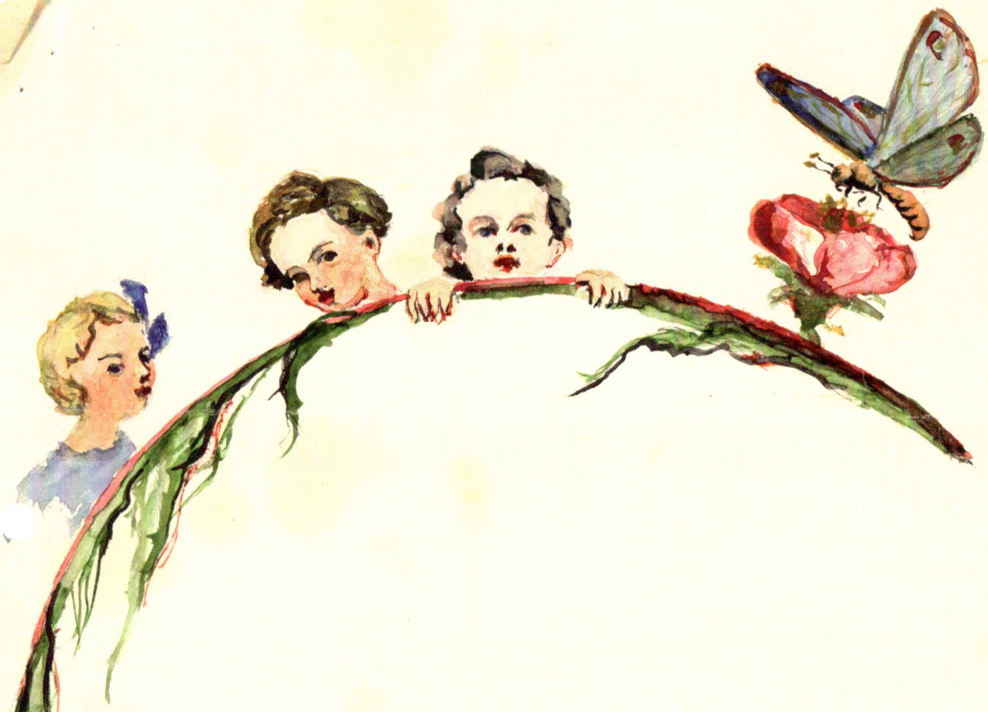

Горячее спасибо „дядям-американцам" за белый хлеб и сладкий какао и другую помощь, оказанную в 1922 году, тяжелом для всех.

Дети детских садов гор. Тетюш:

ПАША КАТЯ
ШУРА ЛЕЛЯ ГАНЯ
ПЕТЯ
ШУРА ЛЕНЯ НАСТЯ
МАНЯ ЛИЗА ЗОЯ
НЮРА КОЛЯ МИША
НЮРА
ИВАН КАТЯ СОФЬЯ
А. ЛЕКСЕЙ АНА Костя
КОЛЯ СИМА Коля
Валя
ПЕТЯ ПОЛЯ Володя
ШУРА Петя НАСТЯ
ПЕТЯ Кондратий

CHAPTER 7

More Precious Than Bread

"The need for continued assistance is great. I believe, however, that Russia should learn to bear her own burden. This should be taken into consideration when making a decision as to the time when medical relief operations shall cease."

—*Henry Beeuwkes, July 22, 1922*

The culmination of the ARA's food campaign was the great surge of American corn and wheat seed into the famine zone in the spring of 1922. The ARA's medical program experienced its own great surge a short time later. During the initial months of operations, because of the late arrival of the American Red Cross supplies that had been ordered on the eve of Beeuwkes's departure for New York, the Medical Division struggled to keep up with the demand for medicines and equipment from the districts. One advantage of this delay was that Beeuwkes and his staff had more time to secure adequate warehouse space in Moscow. The US government surplus medical stocks, authorized by the congressional appropriation in January 1922, were slow in arriving owing to the time needed to round them up and ship them from the United States, and also to the fact that the American corn and seed were given priority in the Soviet ports.

In June and July 1922, the Medical Division was inundated with arriving supplies, mostly the government surplus stocks, but also a new wave of Red Cross supplies. Anticipating the expansion of its operations into Ukraine and Belorussia in December and early January, the Medical Division had made several very large requisitions from the Red Cross. These supplies now began to arrive in Moscow. Adding to the burden, as Beeuwkes lamented, most of the Army surplus stocks were shipped from the Atlanta Medical Supply Depot, where the invoices and packing lists were so carelessly prepared—Beeuwkes said they were "like a dog's breakfast"—that it made the job of identifying the contents of the cases nearly impossible "without infinite labor," causing a considerable loss of time.

Harold Fisher, ARA historian and future director of the Hoover Institution, arriving in Soviet Russia at the beginning of June, wrote to New York headquarters on June 7:

> The Medical Div[ision] is the one which really has the biggest job on its hands right now. The stuff is coming in very fast, and as warehouse space is limited here, it has to be sorted and sent on its way about as fast as it comes in. The accounting for so many different kinds of drugs is in itself a full sized job. Just at this writing Beeuwkes is sweating blood over some 90 cars of supplies which have just arrived. He estimates that he has some

Appreciation signed by the children of the kindergartens of the city of Tetyushi, in the ARA's Kazan district. The text reads: "Warm thanks to our 'American uncles' for the white bread and the sweet cocoa and the other help shown to us in 1922, a difficult year for everyone."

40,000 different packages, the contents of which he does not know until he has located them on his invoice which is 200 pages long.

The ARA was proud of its reputation as an efficient machine, yet the success of the American medical program owes much to the talents and resourcefulness of Beeuwkes. He remained calm and resolute in the face of adversity, which included a slow-moving and at times obstructionist Soviet bureaucracy, the theft of medical supplies, transportation problems, importuning American physicians, etc., all the while maintaining his sense of humor. "Beeuwkes impresses me as being extremely able, and he is unquestionably very amusing," Fisher wrote, an assessment echoed by numerous ARA men. Dr. John Toole told his diary that Beeuwkes had become a mentor to him, offering career advice during their many late-night conversations in Moscow. George Cornick, the Texas medical doctor based in Tsaritsyn, remarked to his father in a letter of January 10, 1922, shortly after arriving in Soviet Russia: "He is only about forty years of age, and seemingly a very pleasant and capable man." Dr. Walter Davenport, the assistant director of the Medical Division, noted in his understated style: "Beeuwkes has put over a good job."

Adding to the pressure on Beeuwkes in June and July was his assumption that the clock was running down; that he had precious little time to distribute all these incoming supplies to the districts before the ARA ended its operations in Soviet Russia. It was assumed within the organization—though not revealed to the Soviet government or the American public—that with the back of the famine broken, the ARA would likely wind up operations at the harvest. Beeuwkes knew that when it came to medical supplies, the wealth would have to be carefully spread out across many local medical institutions. As he told Haskell, "Overstocked storerooms will always make for temptation on the part of the Government to requisition supplies after we have discontinued operating."

+ + +

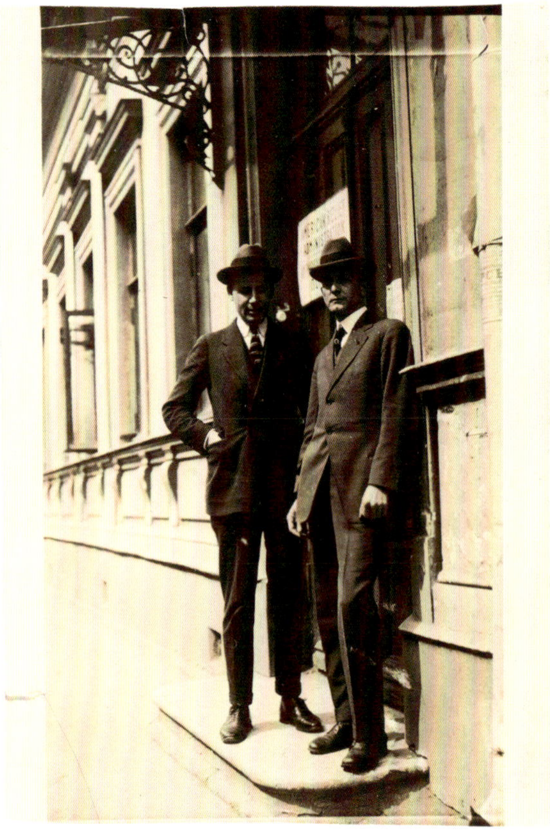

ABOVE: Dr. Walter Davenport (left) and Dr. Henry Beeuwkes, Moscow, ca. 1922.

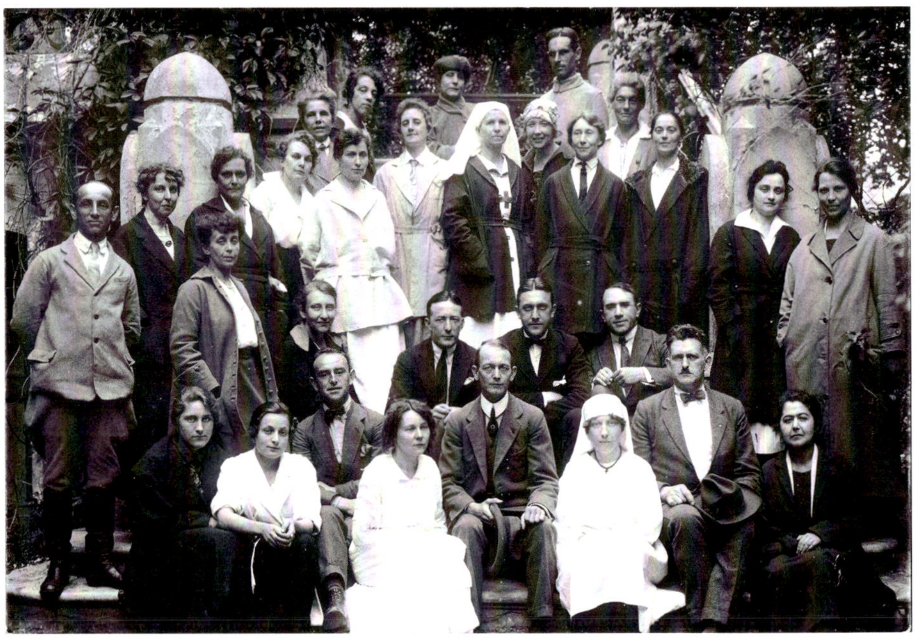

BELOW RIGHT: Moscow staff of the ARA Medical Division, ca. 1923. Colonel Henry Beeuwkes is seated at center, hat in hand. Behind him to the left (over his right shoulder) is his secretary, Arnold Rattray; over his left shoulder is Dr. John E. Toole. Courtesy of Bess Rattray

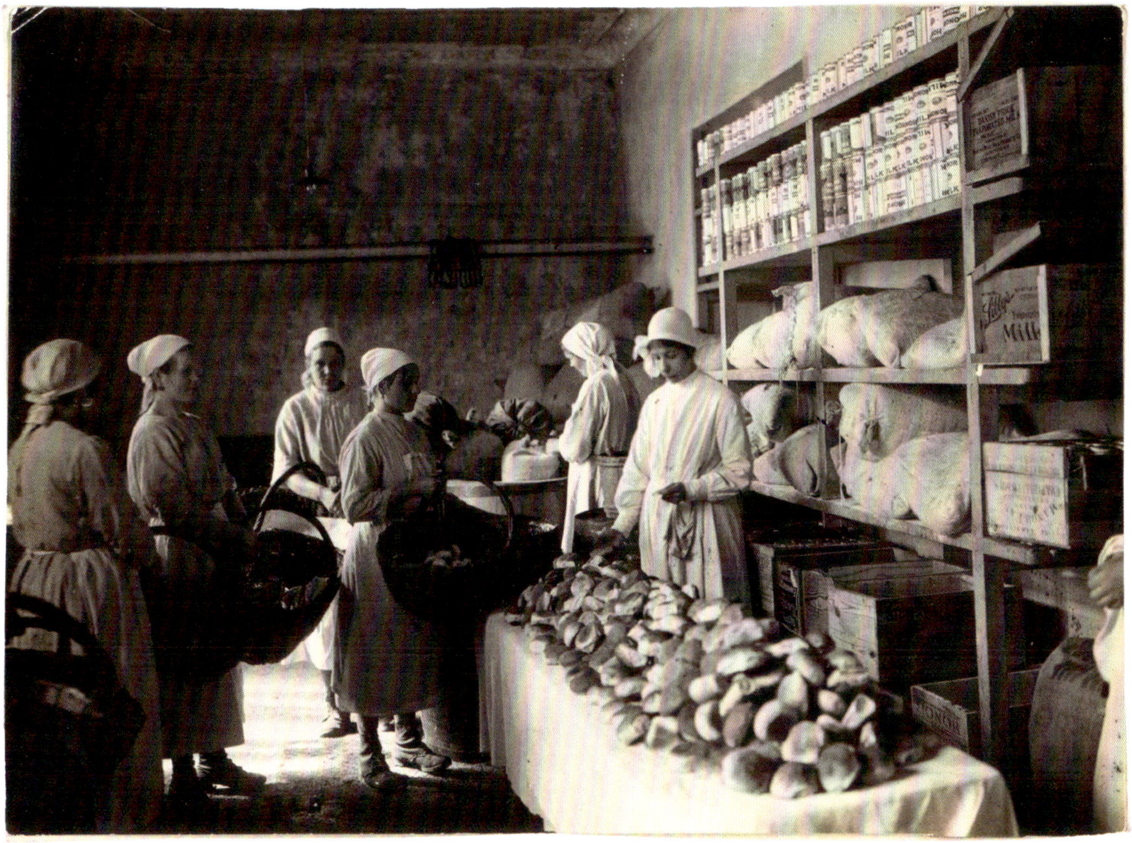

ARA kitchen at the Obukhovskaya hospital in Petrograd, ca. 1922. Two favorite menu items are visible here: freshly baked white rolls and canned milk.

Herbert Hoover convened a meeting of the ARA's executive committee and officers in New York on July 30 for the purpose of deciding the future of the Soviet Russia mission. Two days prior to the conference he wrote to Secretary of State Charles Evans Hughes to follow up on Hoover's suggestion that the American Red Cross assume responsibility for the conduct of all further "charitable activities" in Russia. Such a handoff made perfect sense, Hoover wrote. "The American Relief Administration in its whole inception, character of its organization and personnel, is a famine fighting organization. The great famine in Russia is over with the present harvest."

True, Hoover allowed, the Russian unit had been carrying on a substantial medical relief program, "not only in support of Russian hospitals but in a great campaign against the conflagrations of contagious typhoid, typhus, smallpox, and various virulent fevers. Millions of human beings have been inoculated and vaccinated and large sanitary measures have been undertaken." But medical and sanitary work was not a natural fit for the ARA, Hoover maintained; a typical Red Cross mission would be far better suited to mount the large-scale operation necessary to fight contagious disease. The Red Cross could also administer a supplemental program to provide food to the many thousands of homeless children who had survived the famine.

"In all these circumstances," Hoover told Hughes, "it appears to me that there should be a change in the organizations undertaking the Russian problem from the American Relief Administration—a food and famine organization—to the American Red Cross, a medical and sanitary relief organization." Such an arrangement would be not only reasonable but just, Hoover wrote. "The American Relief Administration being a voluntary body grown out of the war, composed of professional and business men who have given many years of voluntary service,

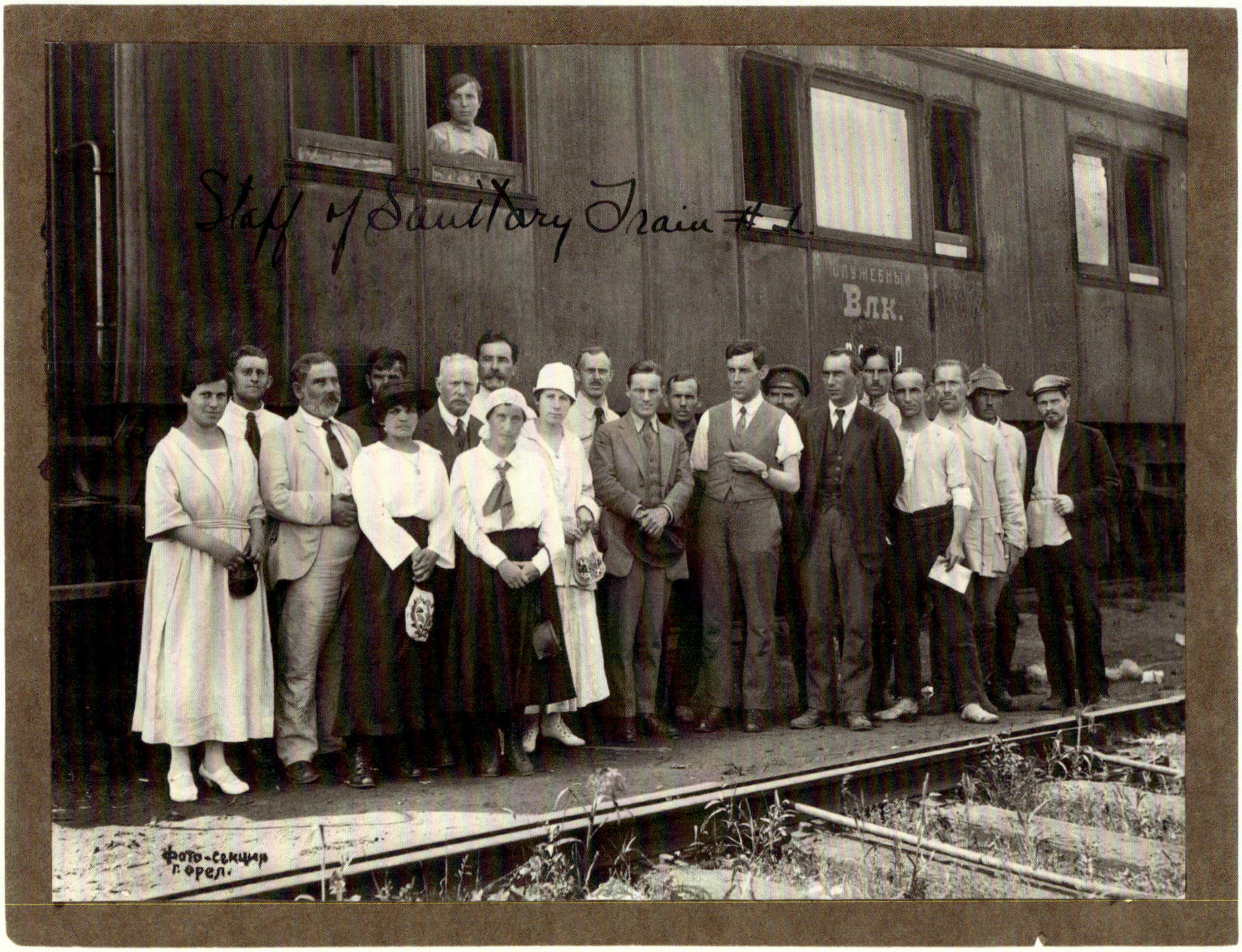

Staff of Sanitary Train No. 1, Orel, September 1922. Dr. Samuel Ross stands at center, hands clasped in front of him.

During the spring of 1922, the Medical Division expanded its activities to all the regions where ARA child feeding and food remittance operations were under way. The areas in European Russia not supplied with American food consisted of sparsely populated villages in the north and the provinces surrounding Moscow, places not stricken by famine. Yet as Colonel Beeuwkes remarked, the medical famine was not limited to the regions afflicted by "food famine." Medical stocks and equipment were severely depleted, and contagious disease took its toll, across a much larger area. Beeuwkes judged it impractical to try to supply the northern territories because they were sparsely populated and difficult to reach by river or rail. Nor would it have been feasible for the ARA to establish new medical districts in the central provinces. But with the Soviet government's assistance, Beeuwkes made arrangements to distribute medical supplies to major cities in the provinces south of Moscow—Tula, Orel, Kursk, Voronezh, Kozlov, Tambov, and Ryazan—by means of sanitary trains.

Sanitary Train No. 1, under the charge of Dr. Samuel Ross, left Moscow on August 3, 1922, with twenty-one carloads of medical supplies. Convoyed by Russian Red Cross Train No. 5, the ARA train traveled nearly two thousand miles over the course of a month, distributing supplies throughout the region, using the seven major cities as bases of operation. The supplies consisted of four thousand cases and bales of medicines—common varieties of drugs and vaccines—along with enamelware, rubber goods, hospital clothing, bed linen, and ten thousand blankets, all supplied to nearly 1,200 institutions. High on the priority list were 750 pounds (12,000 ounces) of quinine, more than 33,000 pounds of toilet soap, and nearly 35,000 pounds of common soap. Dr. Ross and Sanitary Train No. 1 returned to Moscow in early September.

In March 1923, as the ARA program in Soviet Russia was entering its final phase, Beeuwkes dispatched Sanitary Train No. 2 to seven of the largest cities north of Moscow suffering from "acute medical famine": Yaroslavl, Kostroma, Vladimir, Ivanovo, Tver, Rybinsk, and Rostov, with stops in Kaluga and Bryansk, south of Moscow, added later. Dr. John Toole took charge of the second sanitary train, adopting a new procedure: rather than form a well-stocked train to tour the cities, he first visited those cities in order to take stock of the needs of individual hospitals and institutions and then returned to Moscow to assemble specific allocations for each institution, before setting out again to deliver the supplies. "The method selected, I believe proved more efficient and economic under the circumstances which were the essential considerations of the time," Toole wrote. "Then too, the dangers of railroad travel in third class wagons of the previous years, such as typhus, relapsing fever and cholera were not to be feared at this time."

Dr. Toole traveled with an interpreter and one laborer. Doctors in each district arrived at the respective railroad warehouses well before the railroad car was to be unloaded, and Toole made a point of personally parceling out the supplies to each physician or representative. It was a touch of courtesy and, more importantly, a way to ensure that the supplies reached the intended beneficiary. Once these distributions were completed, Toole set off to the south of Moscow to check on the institutions in all the cities and towns that had been supplied six months earlier by Sanitary Train No. 1. The results were heartening: "In inspecting the hospitals, it was a pleasure to see beautiful Red Cross blankets on practically every bed," Toole wrote. "Everywhere one turned one's eyes, some articles provided by the American Relief Administration were visible: sputum cups, urinals, bed pans, sheets, blankets, nurses gowns, slippers, fracture beds, dental cabinets, eye cases, surgical instruments, towels, etc., etc."

Toole saw cabinets stocked with supplies that he estimated would not last more than a couple of months. While inspecting what he called the best surgical hospital in Tula, he noticed something unusual: practically no visual sign that it had previously been provisioned by the ARA. Old, tattered blankets covered the beds, while patients wore dingy hospital clothing. Toole learned, to his dismay, that the American medical supplies were being stored under lock and key. The chief surgeon informed him that he allowed the use of good blankets and hospital linens only on Sundays and holidays. Otherwise, he said, the supplies were strictly rationed, as he could not imagine where any replacements for these precious items would come from. Toole insisted that the supplies be used immediately, explaining that he feared such a trove could be requisitioned by the Soviet authorities. He reassured the surgeon that the ARA would return with an allotment of medicines to round out the original supply.

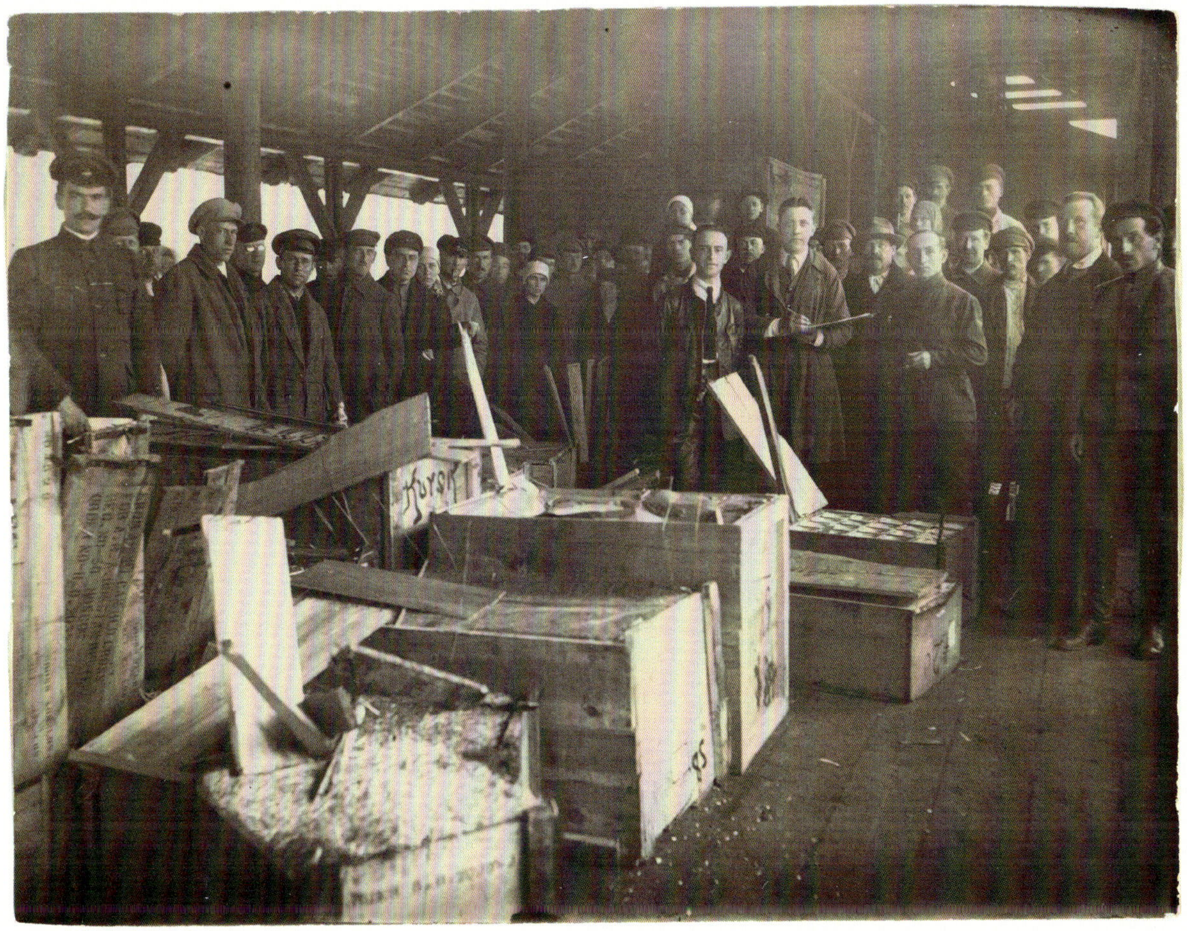

Distribution of supplies from Sanitary Train No. 2, on the station platform in Kursk, May 9, 1923. Dr. John Toole stands at center, holding pen and clipboard.

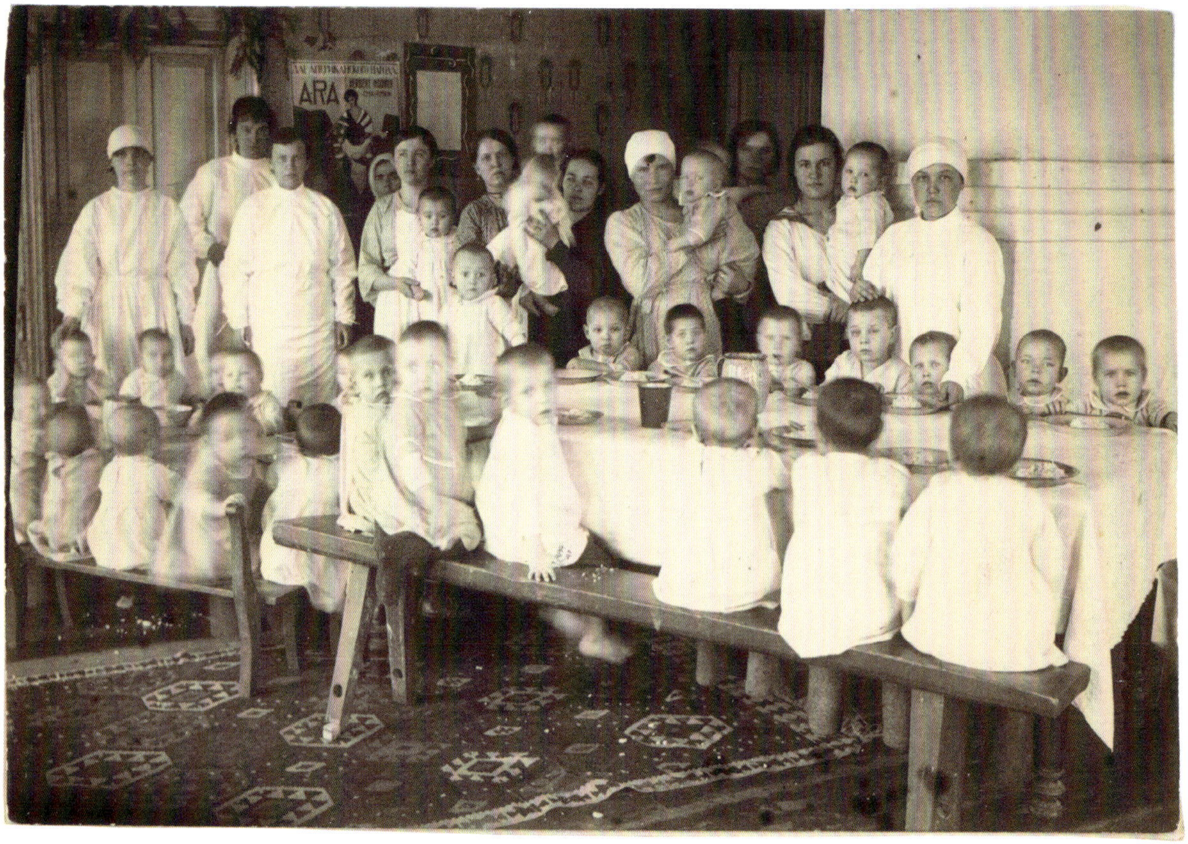

Child patients in a hospital dining room provisioned by the ARA, ca. 1922.

has a right now of laying down its burden, having dealt at one time or another with upwards of two hundred millions of people."

The proposed Red Cross solution, whatever its actual promise, was nullified two days later by the decision taken at the New York conference to commit the ARA to remain in Soviet Russia with a reduced program until the harvest of 1923. The conference report, in setting down the reasons for the decision to continue for another year, noted the persistence of hunger and the potential for the return of areas of famine. Mostly, however, the task at hand was to deal with the aftermath of the disaster. "The famine has left a heritage of numerous waifs and displaced children, who will need to be settled into public homes and for whom service must be given in the interim," the report noted. The concern of the American relief workers about the large and growing number of orphaned and abandoned children they encountered in the autumn of 1921 had been a principal motive behind the decision to expand the ARA mission to include adult feeding. During the second year of the mission, the focus of relief would shift from the villages to urban areas, with special attention to the homeless children roaming the cities in packs like wild animals, a problem so acute that it would persist throughout the 1920s.

A principal reason for the ARA's decision to remain in Soviet Russia was the fact that the campaign to contain and combat epidemic disease was far from completed, and held potential ramifications beyond Soviet Russia's borders. "Contagious disease is still prevalent in Russia," the report states, "and without the A.R.A. medical direction and imported supplies, it is likely to increase and involve the infection of not only Europe, but the entire world. The medical and sanitary necessities far outrun the problems of children's care."

"If the A.R.A. retired," the New York conference report concluded, "it would create a great shock of abandonment." There was no hint that Hoover had been determined to withdraw his organization from Soviet Russia. Instead, the tone was that the time had come to move on to the next logical phase of the work: "It is proposed that, as the great famine battle is over and the problem is now one of re-adjustment of the aftermath of famine, the time-honored policy of the A.R.A. of building up local institutions to take the responsibility for hospitalization, orphan asylums and other public institutions on the charge of the community, should be undertaken."

+ + +

Back in Soviet Russia, the late summer reversal caught the American physicians by surprise. Beeuwkes's office had been pressuring them to distribute their supplies expeditiously. Now they were instructed to "husband" their stockpiles and to enforce their usual standards of inspection and control over the beneficiary institutions. The word took some time getting out to the districts. Cornick wrote to his father, August 27, 1922, from Tsaritsyn:

> I received a very interesting and significant letter from Dr. Beeuwkes yesterday. Only about six weeks ago I received a letter from him practically telling me to 'Dump' my supplies as quickly as possible as a move was imminent. In yesterday's letter, however, he stated that the Medical department

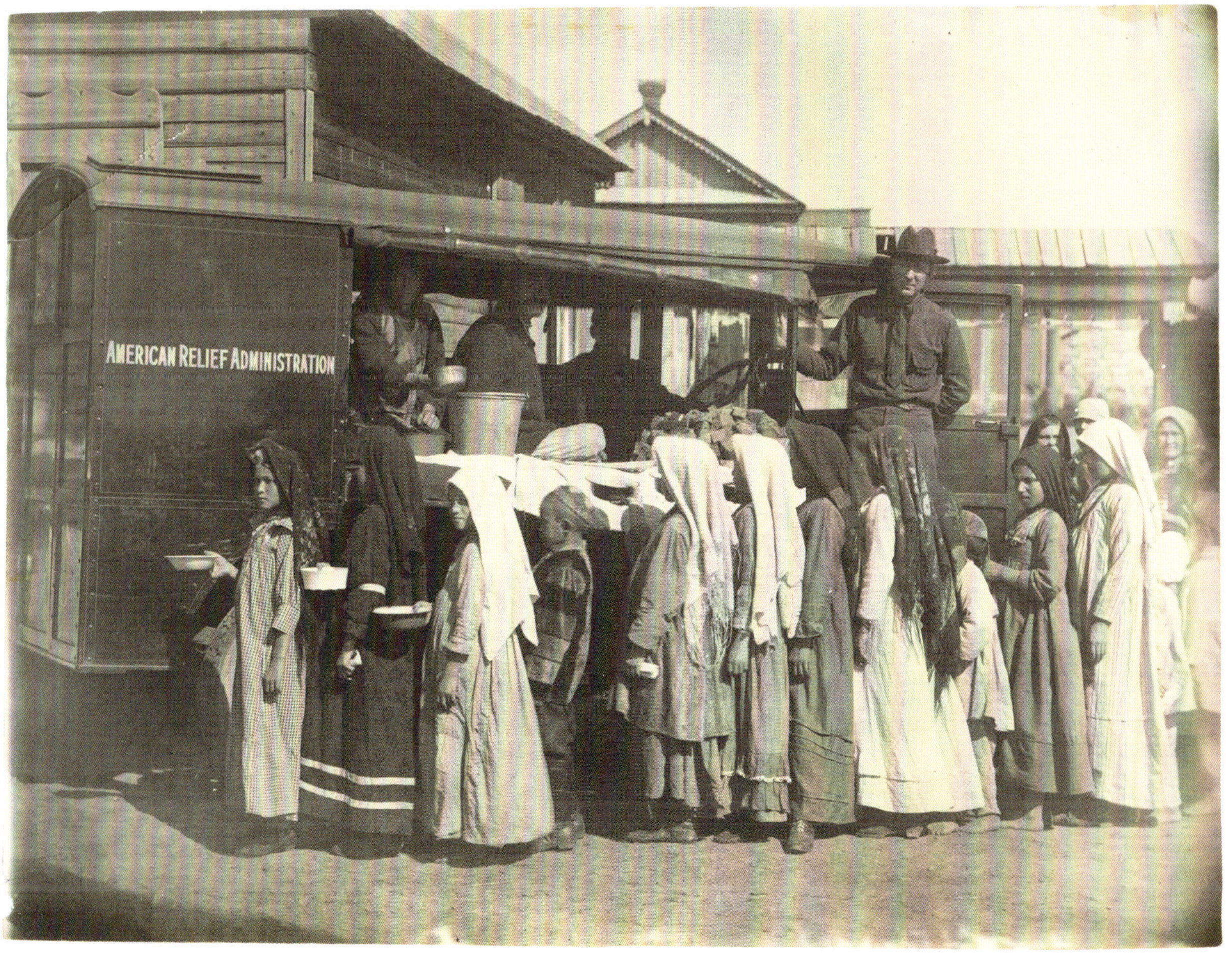

American relief worker Charles Willoughby serves meals from the ARA's caravan car to Bashkir children in Pugachev, Samara province, September 1922. The Bashkirs are a predominantly Muslim Turkic ethnic group.

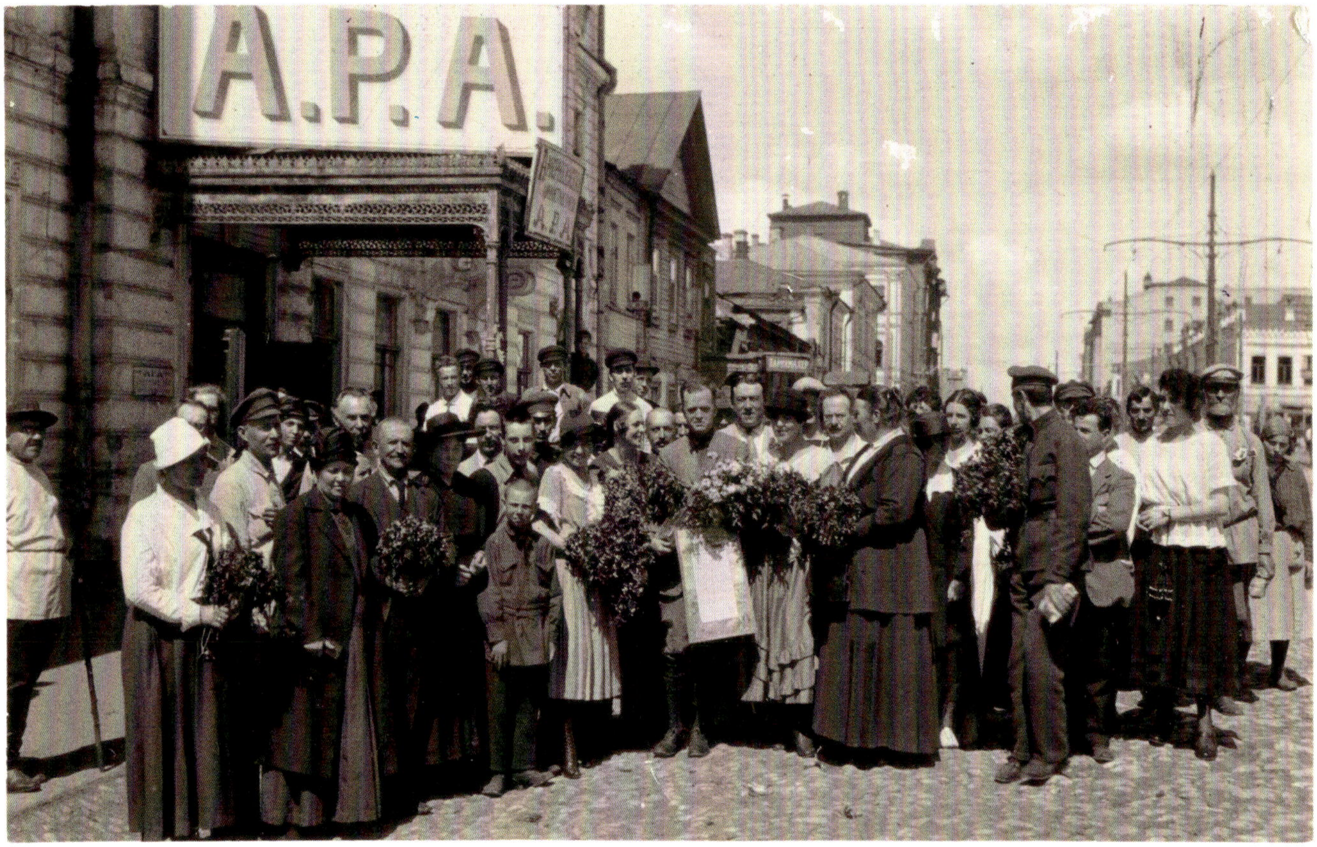

Dr. Frederick Foucar's send-off in Samara, June 1923.

> would function for at least eight months longer and that I should guard my stock carefully as I would probably receive only about six more cars for that time. This really suits me quite well as I do not like the idea of giving things away too promiscuously, when I know that they will not be properly used without some sort of inspection once in awhile to see that supplies are left in the hospitals to which they have been issued, rather than being moved to Red Army hospitals which we of course do not help.

The additional ten months of operations were crucial to the mission's success, as Beeuwkes noted in his history of the medical program: "Only continued assistance of the American Relief Administration prevented the wholesale elimination of medical institutions." And yet, in spring 1923, as the ARA prepared to depart Soviet Russia, the American physicians heard local health care workers express concern, if not outright certainty, that their institutions would not be able to survive if they were taken off American life support. "The doctors even dread the departure of the A.R.A. saying that when it leaves they will have to close," Dr. Raymond McKnight Sloan in Ufa wrote in his final report.

In April 1923, as the district headquarters began to send their office files on to Moscow for archiving and the relief workers made preparations to depart, an ARA press release observed that "American charity has done much for Russia in the zone of famine but it has given Russia something more precious than bread, from the standpoint of hygiene and disease prevention." More precious than bread—and yet, every American doctor on the scene, starting with Davenport during his scouting expedition to Samara in the fall of 1921, testified to the indispensability of American food to the success of the American medical campaign. In September 1922, as the ARA mission was scaling back its food relief operations,

Charles Willoughby, fresh from a trip to Pugachev, in Samara province, to distribute medical supplies, stated emphatically: "It is useless to try to keep these people out of the grave by furnishing them with medicine alone. They must be fed. Without food, the medicine will tend to merely counteract the diseases from which they are suffering, and save them for an even more horrible death by starvation." Sloan, writing in spring 1923, underscored the vital role played by food: "In addition to medical equipment the A.R.A. in this district has at all times fed hospitals 100 percent. Had it not, its medicines would have done little good, for the hospitals had no other food sources." He echoed the point at the close of operations: "The common chorus of medical institutions throughout the district is that they would have had to close had it not been for A.R.A. medicines and food."

As the ARA mission came to a close in the summer of 1923, tributes poured in from beneficiaries, including many doctors, medical institutions, and medical students. These conveyed gratitude to the relief workers, the American people, and Herbert Hoover for coming to Soviet Russia's aid at a time of extreme need—like an answer to a prayer, in an oft-repeated phrase. Many expressed great sadness that the ARA's departure meant the end of their magical connection to that fairy-tale land: *Amerika*. "At this nightmarish time, destiny saw fit to send us a bright warm sun," wrote Grigorii Sobolev of Simbirsk on May 27, 1923. "And now our sun is sinking once more. You are going away to your dear America." These accolades often contain long lists of signatures, and many are adorned with artwork. The most affecting were composed by children from the homes, hospitals, and schools nurtured by American relief. Those paying tribute assured their saviors that the memory of America's errand of mercy in Russia's darkest hour would never be extinguished. "A.R.A." a Kiev intellectual observed. "Those three letters will never be forgotten."

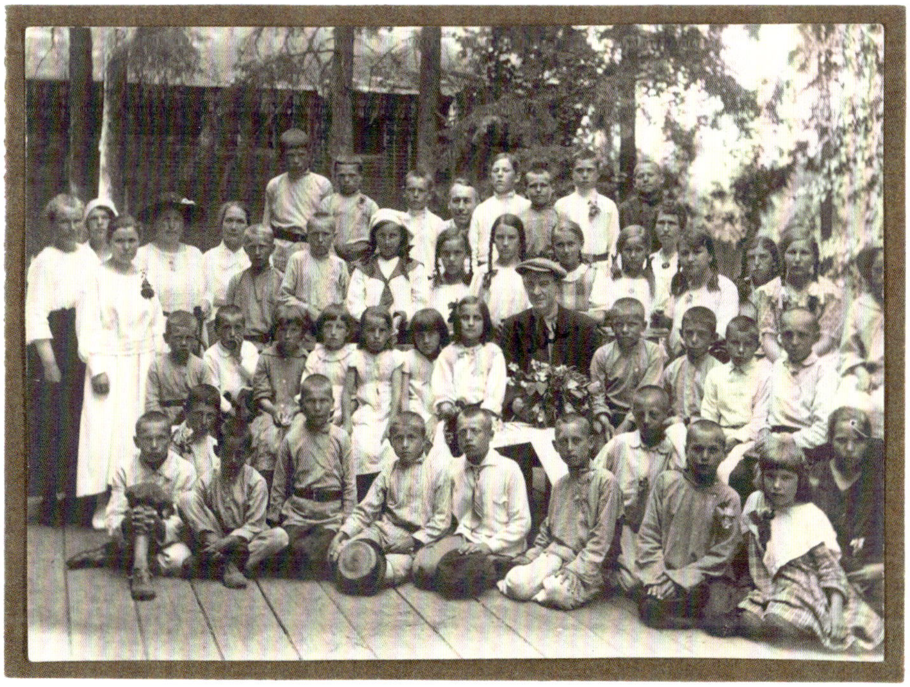

Colonel Walter Bell among children fed by the ARA, spring 1923.

Timeline of US Famine Relief to Soviet Russia, 1921–1923

1921

JUNE 26: Soviet newspaper *Pravda* (*Truth*) announces that famine threatens nearly 25 million Soviet citizens. The famine was triggered by a drought after years of economic disruption caused by war, revolution, and Communist agricultural policies.

JULY 13: Maxim Gorky's appeal "To All Honest People" for help in combating the famine is published in European and American newspapers.

JULY 23: Herbert Hoover responds to Gorky's appeal, stating his willingness to offer assistance through the American Relief Administration (ARA) under certain conditions, first and foremost American control over the distribution of food inside Soviet Russia.

AUGUST 10: Negotiations between representatives of the Soviet government and the ARA begin in Riga, Latvia.

AUGUST 20: Riga Agreement is signed between ARA representative Walter Lyman Brown and Deputy People's Commissar of Foreign Affairs Maxim Litvinov.

AUGUST 25: ARA advance party of seven departs Riga for Moscow, arriving August 27.

SEPTEMBER 1: First American relief ship, the *Phoenix*, arrives in Petrograd (today called St. Petersburg) carrying 700 tons of balanced food rations.

SEPTEMBER 2: Agreement signed in Washington between the ARA and the American Red Cross serves as the foundation for the ARA's medical relief program in Soviet Russia. The Red Cross undertakes to furnish supplies and funds at a combined value of $3 million, a total later increased to $3.8 million.

SEPTEMBER 6: First American kitchen in Soviet Russia opens in Petrograd.

OCTOBER 19: Food Remittance Agreement is signed in Moscow between the ARA and the Soviet government.

DECEMBER 22: US Congress appropriates $20 million for Russian relief, to be used mostly for the purchase of corn. This marks a dramatic expansion of the ARA mission to include the feeding of adults as well as children.

DECEMBER 30: Agreement between the ARA and the Soviet government for the purchase by the Kremlin of American wheat seed in the amount of $10 million. On February 1, 1922, the Ukrainian Soviet Socialist Republic makes a supplemental purchase of $2 million in seed.

1922

JANUARY 10: Agreement between the ARA and the Ukrainian Soviet Socialist Republic authorizing American food relief operations throughout Ukraine.

JANUARY 20: US Congress appropriates $4 million toward the purchase of surplus government medical supplies for distribution by the ARA in Soviet Russia.

FEBRUARY 2: The Laura Spelman Rockefeller Memorial pledges an appropriation of up to $500,000 to cover the expense of inspecting and packing the surplus Army supplies and transporting them from the medical supply depots to the Eastern Seaboard for shipment to Soviet Russia. The total donation amounted to $267,392.88.

FEBRUARY 6: The first corn ship, the *Winnebago*, carrying 6,000 tons of corn, arrives in the Black Sea port of Novorossiysk.

MARCH 7: First corn train arrives in Ufa, in the Ural Mountains.

MARCH 13: First corn train arrives in Samara, on the Volga.

APRIL 1: First corn train arrives in Simbirsk, on the Volga.

MAY 17: Death of Harold Blandy, from typhus, in Ufa.

JULY 30: Herbert Hoover and the officers of the ARA, at a conference in New York, decide to continue the ARA's Soviet Russia operations, on a reduced scale, until the harvest of 1923.

AUGUST 1: The ARA reaches the peak of its feeding activity, providing a daily meal to 10.5 million beneficiaries, the adults receiving daily rations of corn grits, the children being served their balanced daily meals.

OCTOBER 26: Clothing Remittance Agreement is signed in Moscow between the ARA and the Soviet government.

1923

JUNE 12: Colonel Beeuwkes departs Moscow for the United States.

JUNE 15: Liquidation Agreement is signed in Moscow between the ARA and the Soviet government.

JULY 17: Dr. John Toole, the last of the American medical staff, departs Moscow for the United States.

Selected Bibliography

Hoover Institution Archives

American Relief Administration Russian operational records
American Relief Administration European operational records
Poster Collection
Frank A. Golder papers
Charles L. Hall papers
Raymond McKnight Sloan papers
F. Dorsey Stephens papers
John E. Toole diary

Secondary Sources

Adamets, Sergueï. "Famine in Nineteenth- and Twentieth-Century Russia: Mortality by Age, Cause, and Gender." In *Famine Demography*, edited by Tim Dyson and Cormac Ó Gráda, 158–80. New York: Oxford University Press, 2002.

———. *Guerre civile et famine en Russie: Le pouvoir bolchevique et la population face à la catastrophe démographique 1917–1923*. Paris: Institut d'études slaves, 2003.

American Medical Association. *A Handbook of Useful Drugs*. Chicago: Press of the American Medical Association, 1914.

Argenbright, Robert. "Lethal Mobilities: Bodies and Lice on Soviet Railroads, 1918–1922." *Journal of Transport History* 29, no. 2 (September 2008): 259–76.

Bechah, Yassina, Christian Capo, Jean-Louis Mege, and Didier Raoult. "Epidemic Typhus." *The Lancet Infectious Diseases* 8, no. 7 (July 2008): 417–26.

Beeuwkes, Henry, MD. *American Medical and Sanitary Relief in the Russian Famine, 1921–1923*. American Relief Administration Bulletin series 2, no. 45 (April 1926).

Conroy, Mary Schaeffer, and Valentina Federovna Soskina. "Rescuers in Another Time." *Hoover Digest* no. 3 (Summer 2020): 177–91.

Davenport, Major Walter P. "General Health Conditions and Medical Relief Work in Armenia." *Military Surgeon* 48 (January–June 1921): 139–58.

Epidemiological Intelligence 4 (1922).

Epidemiological Intelligence 7 (1923).

Fisher, H. H. *America and the New Poland*. New York: MacMillan, 1928.

———. *The Famine in Soviet Russia, 1919–1923*. New York: MacMillan, 1927.

Foster, Gaines M. *The Demands of Humanity: Army Medical Disaster Relief.* Washington, DC: Center of Military History, United States Army, 1983.

———. "Typhus Disaster in the Wake of War: The American-Polish Relief Expedition, 1919–1920." *Bulletin of the History of Medicine* 55, no. 2 (Summer 1981): 221–32.

Foucar, Major F. H. "Resume of Experiences and Work Accomplished in Russia with the American Relief Administration, 1921–1923, part 1." *Military Surgeon* 54 (January–June 1924): 680–98.

———. “Resume of Experiences and Work Accomplished in Russia with the American Relief Administration, 1921–1923, part 2.” *Military Surgeon* 55 (July–December 1924): 20–38.

Frith, Dr. John, RFD. “Arsenic—the ‘Poison of Kings’ and the ‘Saviour of Syphilis.’ ” *Journal of Military and Veterans’ Health* 21, no. 4 (December 2013): 11–17.

Gantt, W. Horsley. *A Medical Review of Soviet Russia*. London: British Medical Association, 1928.

Golder, Frank Alfred, and Lincoln Hutchinson. *On the Trail of the Russian Famine*. Stanford, CA: Stanford University Press, 1927.

Hionidou, Violetta. “Why Do People Die in Famines? Evidence from Three Island Populations.” *Population Studies* 56, no. 1 (March 2002): 65–80.

Hutchinson, John F. *Politics and Public Health in Revolutionary Russia, 1890–1918*. Baltimore: Johns Hopkins University Press, 1990.

———. “Tsarist Russia and the Bacteriological Revolution.” *Journal of the History of Medicine and Allied Sciences* 40, no. 4 (October 1985): 420–39.

Irwin, Julia F. “The Great White Train: Typhus, Sanitation, and US International Development during the Russian Civil War.” *Endeavor* 36, no. 3 (September 2012): 89–96.

Johnson, Steven. *Extra Life: A Short History of Living Longer*. New York: Riverhead Books, 2021.

Patenaude, Bertrand M. *The Big Show in Bololand: The American Relief Expedition to Soviet Russia in the Famine of 1921*. Stanford, CA: Stanford University Press, 2002.

Patterson, K. David. “Typhus and Its Control in Russia, 1870–1940.” *Medical History* 37, no. 4 (October 1993): 361–81.

Soloman, Susan Gross, ed. *Health and Society in Revolutionary Russia*. Bloomington: Indiana University Press, 1990.

Surface, Frank M., and Raymond L. Bland. *American Food in the World War and Reconstruction Period: Operations of the Organizations under the Direction of Herbert Hoover, 1914 to 1924*. Stanford, CA: Stanford University Press, 1931.

Tarassevitch, L. A. “Epidemics in Russia since 1914: Report to the Health Committee of the League of Nations by Professor L. Tarassevitch, part 1.” *Epidemiological Intelligence* 2 (March 1922).

———. “Epidemics in Russia since 1914: Report to the Health Committee of the League of Nations by Professor L. Tarassevitch, part 2.” *Epidemiological Intelligence* 5 (October 1922).

Trott, Margaret Akers. “Soviet Medicine and Western Medical Charity, 1917–1927.” PhD diss., University of Virginia, 1996.

Wheatcroft, S. G. “Famine and Epidemic Crises in Russia, 1918–1922: The Case of Saratov.” *Annales de démographie historique* (1983): 329–52.

Wolbach, S. Burt, John L. Todd, and Francis W. Palfrey. *The Etiology and Pathology of Typhus*. Cambridge, MA: League of Red Cross Societies at the Harvard University Press, 1922.

Index

Page numbers followed by the letter f *indicate figures and illustrations.*

About the Authors

Bertrand M. Patenaude is a research fellow at the Hoover Institution and a faculty fellow at the Center for Innovation in Global Health at Stanford University School of Medicine. He is the author of *The Big Show in Bololand: The American Relief Expedition to Soviet Russia in the Famine of 1921* (Stanford University Press, 2002).

Joan Nabseth Stevenson, an independent scholar, is the author of *Deliverance from the Little Big Horn: Doctor Henry Porter and Custer's Seventh Cavalry* (University of Oklahoma Press, 2012), winner of the 2013 High Plains Book Award for Best Nonfiction. She received her PhD in Slavic Languages and Literatures from Stanford University.